Schizophrenia and Mood Disorders

Schizophrenia and Mood Disorders:

the new drug therapies in clinical practice

Edited by
Peter F. Buckley MD
Professor of Psychiatry
Case Western Reserve University, Cleveland, Ohio, USA

and

John L. Waddington PHD DSC
Professor of Neuroscience, Department of Clinical Pharmacology
Royal College of Surgeons in Ireland, Dublin, Ireland

With a Foreword by
Ross J. Baldessarini MD DSC

A member of the Hodder Headline Group
LONDON

Lilly

Sponsored by an educational grant by
Eli Lilly and Company Limited

This edition first published in Great Britain in 2000 by Butterworth Heinemann.

This impression published in 2003 by
Arnold, a member of the Hodder Headline Group,
338 Euston Road, London NW1 3BH

http://www.arnoldpublishers.com

Distributed in the USA by
Oxford University Press Inc.,
198 Madison Avenue, New York, NY10016
Oxford is a registered trademark of Oxford University Press

© 2001 Arnold

Whilst the advice and information in this book are believed to be true and
accurate at the date of going to press, neither the authors nor the publisher
can accept any legal responsibility or liability for any errors or omissions
that may be made. In particular (but without limiting the generality of the
preceding disclaimer) every effort has been made to check drug dosages;
however, it is still possible that errors have been missed. Furthermore,
dosage schedules are constantly being revised and new side-effects
recognized. For these reasons the reader is strongly urged to consult the
drug companies' printed instructions before administering any of the drugs
recommended in this book.

British Library Cataloguing in Publication Data
A catalogue record for this book is available from the British Library

Library of Congress Cataloging-in-Publication Data
A catalog record for this book is available from the Library of Congress

ISBN 0 7506 4096 0

2 3 4 5 6 7 8 9 10

Printed and bound in Great Britain by MPG Books Ltd, Bodmin, Cornwall

What do you think about this book? Or any other Arnold title?
Please send your comments to feedback.arnold@hodder.co.uk

Contents

Foreword

This new, multiauthored, international textbook on the pharmacological treatment of major mental illnesses, edited by Peter Buckley of Cleveland, Ohio, and John Waddington, of Dublin, Republic of Ireland, includes 25 chapters organized into sections on schizophrenia, major mood disorders, and special problems. Individual chapters on specific topics were prepared by experts representing academic centres in nine nations. These include *Australia* (Melbourne), *Austria* (Innsbruck, Vienna), *Canada* (Calgary, Toronto), *Denmark* (Arrhus), *Germany* (Berlin, Hamburg), *Irish Republic* (Dublin, Galway), *Netherlands* (Utrecht), *United Kingdom* (Belfast, Cambridge, Crowthorne, London, Newcastle), and *United States* (Ann Arbor, Atlanta, Baltimore, Bethesda, Boston, Cincinnati, Cleveland, Dallas, Hanover, Irvine, Jacksonville, Los Angeles, New York, Palo Alto, Pittsburgh, Portland, San Antonio).

The initial sections open with the preclinical pharmacology of each major class of psychotropic drugs used to treat psychotic and major affective disorders, respectively, and consider the relevance of pharmacology to clinical decision-making. The first section on psychotic disorders provides separate chapters on the clinical use of traditional international neuroleptics (benzamides, butyrophenones, phenothiazenes, thioxanthenes, and others) and on each of the established and emerging modern antipsychotics (including clozapine, risperidone, clanzapine, quetiapine, sertindole, ziprasidone, zotepine), with a concluding look into the future of antipsychotic drug development.

The second section on mood-altering treatments, similarly, summarizes use of older antidepressants (tricyclics, monoamine oxidase inhibitors), with separate chapters covering modern antidepressants (serotonin reuptake inhibitors, nefazodone, mirtazapine, venlafaxine), as well as on lithium and alternative or proposed mood stabilizers (antipsychotics, carbamezepine, valproate, gabapentin, lamotrigine), again with a look into the future development of mood-altering agents.

The third, special section covers important topics that are often insufficiently addressed in textbooks on psychopharmacology. These include drug interactions, management of pregnant women as well as paediatric and geriatric patients, comorbid substance-use disorders, violence, treatment-compliance, and pharmacoeconomics.

The chapters are well organized and edited for stylistic consistency. Each chapter includes a brief summary, specific topics divided by subheadings, and an adequate, alphabetically organized bibliography of full reference citations. Some preclinical chapters provide highly detailed reviews of emerging scientific understanding of the neuropharmacology of antipsychotic and mood-altering agents. Most clinical chapters are brief but authoritative and reliable, usually without providing detailed summaries of research data to back up conclusions and therapeutic advice offered. The level of detail is appropriate both as a textbook for general readers new to the field, and as a reference for clinicians and other professionals.

The disorders addressed in this book represent leading problems for contemporary world health since, together, the psychotic and severe mood disorders afflict at least 1/20 citizens of all countries at any time, and more than 1/10, if less severe forms of the disorders are included. These disorders, with their commonly associated comorbidities and high fatality rates, account for very high proportions of morbidity, disability, and premature mortality, as well as enormous social and economic costs worldwide. Indeed, their overall societal impact compares well with that of cancer, all forms of cardiovascular disease, and many infectious diseases. Ironically, the impact of these major mental disorders on international health and global economics stands in gross disproportion to the limited resources available for their study and treatment, in that way still comparing very unfavorably with other leading health problems

Arguably, more than any other single factor, modern drug treatments for psychotic disorders, mania, and severe depression have had the greatest impact on their improved clinical management and increasingly favorable long-term prospects for their victims. Too, the modern treatments have had an enormous stimulating and heuristic effect on academic psychiatry and psychiatric research. They have challenged traditional nosologies and had a major impact on both the DSM-IV and ICD-10 international diagnostic systems followed in this book. Moreover, most biological theories concerning the causes or pathophysiology of the disorders discussed in the book owe much to our understanding of the actions of drugs that have proved effective in their treatment and led to more, essentially similar agents.

Psychopharmacology has developed and expanded enormously in the half-century since the introduction of lithium into modern psychiatry in 1949, to become a truly international field with an increasingly refined, restless, rapidly expanding and changing basic and scientific knowledge-base. Although most of the material in this book has emerged from academic departments of psychiatry or pharmacology, it is important to point out that the bulk of modern drug discovery and both preclinical and very costly and formidable clinical development have become largely the province of the multinational pharmaceutical industry.

The content, authorship, and organization of this new volume reflect well the current state of psychopharmacology for the common major mental disorders. The scientific, clinical and regional complexity of this field calls for the kind of expert, international collaborative effort represented in this volume. The editors and authors have efficiently and readably compiled information derived from extraordinarily high levels of scientific and clinical knowledge and experience, to provide essential, useful and reliable information on specific topics pertinent to the informed treatment of psychiatrically ill persons with psychotic and major affective disorders.

Ross J. Baldessarini, M.D., D.Sc.
Professor of Psychiatry and Neuroscience
Harvard Medical School, Boston, Massachusetts
October 25, 1999

Preface

Technological advances in computing and telecommunications now provide an unprecedented volume of educational information, derived from all corners of the world. This global perspective is particularly advantageous for psychiatry given historical precedents for continent-specific variations in diagnosis and treatment. Differences in the diagnosis of mood disorders and schizophrenia between European and American psychiatrists in the US–UK project exemplified this fundamental difficulty. Subsequent work to devise DSM-IV and ICD-10 diagnostic systems testifies to greater congruence now between continents. This book draws upon this heightened appreciation of global information on diagnosis and treatment to examine current knowledge, 'best practices' and clinical pearls from each continent, as well as overall future directions in the psychopharmacology of the major mental illnesses of schizophrenia and mood disorders. Most chapters are coauthored by American and European/Australasian experts in an effort to assimilate the breadth of clinical wisdom on each topic. The editors are particularly grateful to the Stanley Foundation, who provide support to both of them and to fellow researchers into schizophrenia and mood disorders across the continents.

In recognition that most clinicians treat patients with either condition in their practice, this book has a combined focus on schizophrenia and mood disorders. The organization of the book reflects this perspective. The first section covers the clinical use and experience with a variety of antipsychotic medications for the treatment of schizophrenia, including those most recently available as well as those under development. The second section covers the clinical use and experience with the range of antidepressant medications and mood stabilizers, including those under regulatory consideration or in advanced clinical development. The third section covers broader topics of drug interactions, psychopharmacology during pregnancy, psychopharmacology of the young and the old, pharmacoeconomics, medication compliance, and the management of difficult-to-treat patients with substance abuse and with violence.

We are most grateful to the contributors, each of whom provided a scholarly synthesis of clinical information from America and Europe/Australasia.

Peter F. Buckley
John L. Waddington

Contributors

Dr Ruth Allen MBBS MRCPsych
Department of Psychiatry, Royal Free Hospital, London, UK

Dr Daniel Andrews MRCPsych BSc
Honorary Lecturer in Psychiatry, Division of Neuroscience and
Psychological Medicine, Imperial College School of Medicine, London, UK

Professor A. George Awad MB BCh PhD FRCP(C)
Professor Emeritus, University of Toronto; Chief of Psychiatry, Department
of Psychiatry, Humber River Regional Hospital, Toronto, Canada

Professor Thomas R.E. Barnes MD FRCPsych
Professor of Clinical Psychiatry, Department of Psychiatry, Imperial
College School of Medicine, London, UK

Professor Charles Bowden MD
Chairman, Department of Psychiatry, The University of Texas Health
Science Center at San Antonio, Texas, USA

Dr Robert W. Buchanan MD
Professor of Psychiatry, Maryland Psychiatric Research Center, Baltimore,
USA

Dr Peter F. Buckley MD
Professor and Vicechair, Department of Psychiatry, Case Western Reserve
University; Medical Director, Northcoast Behavioral Healthcare System,
Cleveland, Ohio, USA

Professor Joseph Calabrese MD
Professor of Psychiatry, Director, Mood Disorders Program, University
Hospitals, Department of Psychiatry, Case Western Reserve University,
Ohio, USA

Professor Daniel Casey MD
Psychiatry Service, Veterans Affairs Medical Center, Oregon, USA

Dr Robert Conley MD
Associate Professor of Psychiatry, Maryland Psychiatric Research Center,
Baltimore, USA

Dr John Cookson MD PhD
Consultant Psychiatrist, Psychiatric Department, The Royal London
Hospital, St Clements, London, UK

Dr Stephen Cooper MD FRCPsych
Senior Lecturer, Department of Mental Health, The Queen's University of
Belfast, N. Ireland

Dr Ruth Dickson MD FRCP(C)
Associate Professor, Department of Psychiatry, University of Calgary,
Canada

Professor Ted Dinan MD PhD
Department of Psychiatry, Royal College of Surgeons in Ireland, Dublin,
Ireland

Professor Nicol Ferrier MD
Professor of Psychiatry, School of Neuroscience and Psychiatry, University
of Newcastle, Newcastle-upon-Tyne, UK

Professor W. Wolfgang Fleischhacker MD
Professor and Head of the Department of Biological Psychiatry,
Department of Psychiatry, Innsbruck University Clinics, Innsbruck, Austria

Dr Sophia Frangou MD MSc MRCPsych
Senior Lecturer in Psychiatry, Institute of Psychiatry, London, UK

Dr William Glazer MD
Associate Clinical Professor of Psychiatry, Harvard Medical School,
Boston, MA, USA

Professor Siegfried Kasper MD
Professor and Chairman, Department of General Psychiatry, University of
Vienna, Vienna, Austria

Professor Cornelius Katona MD FRCPsych
Department of Psychiatry and Behavioural Sciences, Royal Free and UCL
Medical School and Essex and Herts Community NHS Trust, London, UK

Professor Paul Keck MD
Professor and Vice Chairman for Research, University of Cincinnati College
of Medicine, Cincinnati, USA

Dr Jeffrey Kelsey MD PhD
Department of Psychiatry, Emory University School of Medicine, Atlanta,
Georgia, USA

Professor David King MD FRCPsych FRCP(I) DPM
Professor of Clinical Psychopharmacology, Department of Therapeutics
and Pharmacology, Belfast, N. Ireland

Dr Sanjiv Kumra MD, FRCP(C)
Center for Addictions and Mental Health and the Hospital for Sick
Children, University of Toronto, Toronto, Canada

Professor Brian Leonard PhD DSc
Pharmacology Department, National University of Ireland, Galway,
Ireland

Professor Shôn Lewis MD
Professor of Adult Psychiatry, The University of Manchester, Manchester,
UK

Professor Rasmus W. Licht MD
Chief Psychiatrist and Director of the Mood Disorders Research Unit at the
Psychiatric Hospital in Aarhus, Risskov, Denmark; Associate Professor in
Clinical Pharmacology at The University of Aarhus, Denmark

Dr Sheila Marcus MD
Director, Adult Ambulatory Division, University of Michigan Health
Systems, Michigan, USA

Professor Stephen R. Marder MD
Professor and Vice Chair, Department of Psychiatry and Biobehavioral
Sciences, University of California, Los Angeles, USA

Professor Patrick McGorry MB BS MRCP(UK) FRANZCP PhD
Professor of Psychiatry, University of Melbourne, Victoria, Australia

Dr Peter McKenna MD
Consultant Psychiatrist, Fulbourn Hospital, Cambridge, UK

Professor Kim Mueser PhD
Professor of Psychiatry, Dartmouth Medical School, New Hampshire-
Dartmouth Psychiatric Research Center, New Hampshire, USA

Professor Bruno Müller-Oerlinghausen MD
Forschergruppe Klinische Psychopharmakologie, Psychiatrische Klinik und
Poliklinik der Freien Universitat Berlin, Berlin, Germany

Professor Dieter Naber MD
Professor of Psychiatry and Head of Department, Psychiatrische Klinik,
Hamburg, Germany

Professor Charles Nemeroff MD PhD
Professor and Chairman, Department of Psychiatry, Emory University
School of Medicine, Atlanta, Georgia, USA

Professor Willem A. Nolen MD
Professor of Psychiatry, University Medical Centre Utrecht and H.C.
Rümke Groep, Willem Arntsz Huis, Utrecht, The Netherlands

Dr Robert Post MD
Chief, NIMH Biological Pyschiatry Branch Bethesda, Maryland, USA

Professor Steven Potkin MD
Professor, Department of Psychiatry; Director, Clinical Psychiatric
Research and Robert R. Sprague Director, Brain Imaging Center,
University of California, Irvine, California, USA

Dr Barbora Richardson MBBChir MRCGP MRCPsych
Department of Psychiatry and Behavioural Sciences, Royal Free and UCL
Medical School, London, UK

Professor Elliott Richelson MD
Professor of Psychiatry and Pharmacology, Mayo Medical School,
Rochester, MN Consultant in Psychiatry and Pharmacology, Mayo Clinic
Jacksonville, Jacksonville, Florida, USA

Dr Gary Sachs MD
Department of Psychiatry, Massachusetts General Hospital, Boston, USA

Professor Alan Schatzberg MD
Stanford University School of Medicine, Department of Psychiatry &
Behavioral Sciences, California, USA

Professor S. Charles Schulz MD
Chair, Department of Psychiatry, University of Minnesota, Minneapolis,
USA

Dr Tim Stevens MBBCh MRCPsych
Department of Psychiatry and Behavioural Sciences, Royal Free and UCL
Medical School and Essex and Herts Community NHS Trust, London, UK

Dr Trisha Suppes MD PhD
University of Texas Southwestern Medical Center, Associate Professor,
Department of Psychiatry; Director, Bipolar Disorder Clinic and Research
Program; Bipolar Module Director, Texas Medication Algorithm Project
(TMAP), Texas, USA

Dr Rajiv Tandon MD
Professor of Psychiatry, Department of Psychiatry, University of Michigan,
Michigan, USA

Professor Pamela J. Taylor MB BS MRCP FRCPsych
Professor of Special Hospital Psychiatry, Institute of Psychiatry, London, and Broadmoor Hospital, UK

Professor Michael E. Thase MD
Professor of Psychiatry, University of Pittsburgh School of Medicine, Western Psychiatric Institute and Clinic, Pittsburgh, Pennsylvania, USA

Dr Madhukar Trivedi MD
Associate Professor of Psychiatry, University of Texas Southwestern Medical Center; Director, Depression and Anxiety Disorders Program, and Director, Depression Module Texas Medication Algorithm Project, Southwest Medical Center, Dallas, Texas, USA

Professor John Waddington PhD DSc
Professor of Neuroscience, Department of Clinical Pharmacology, Royal College of Surgeons in Ireland, Dublin, Ireland

Schizophrenia

Comparative pharmacology of classical and novel (second-generation) antipsychotics

John Waddington and Daniel Casey

Key points

- New agents each show favourable characteristics in conventional models predictive of efficacy and low EPS liability; some share with clozapine favourable characteristics in new models held to predict broader efficacy.
- Amisulpride: selective antagonist at $D_{2/3}$ receptors, studied mainly in conventional models.
- Clozapine: multiple receptor antagonist, with defining second-generation characteristics in new models consistent with novel mechanism(s) of action.
- Olanzapine: multiple receptor antagonist, with characteristics in new models similar to, but not identical with, clozapine.
- Quetiapine: multiple receptor antagonist, with characteristics in new models which in part overlap with clozapine.
- Risperidone: antagonist at $5\text{-}HT_2/D_2/\alpha_1$ receptors, with characteristics in new models which in part overlap with clozapine.
- Sertindole: antagonist at $5\text{-}HT_2/D_2/\alpha_1$ receptors, studied mainly in conventional models.
- Ziprasidone: antagonist at $5\text{-}HT_2/D_2/\alpha_1$ and agonist at $5\text{-}HT_{1A}$ receptors, with inhibition of NA/5-HT reuptake, studied mainly in conventional models.
- Zotepine: multiple receptor antagonist, with inhibition of NA reuptake, studied mainly in conventional models

---

Introduction

While psychiatry is obliged frequently to debate issues of nosology, the status of pharmacology as a biomedical science usually insulates it from such introspection. However, over the past several years there has emerged, and continues to emerge, not one or even two but rather a considerably broader family of novel antipsychotic agents which challenges both clinical practice and pharmacological concepts that derive from some four decades of experience with classical (typical) neuroleptics: what molecular, cellular and psychopharmacological mechanisms underpin their improved clinical profiles? To what extent do they appear to share a fundamental property, or do they possess a diverse range of individually advantageous actions (Kinon and Lieberman, 1996; Waddington *et al.*, 1997; Arnt and Skarsfeldt, 1998)?

To what extent is it justified to continue to apply the widely adopted appellation 'atypical' to so many novel compounds when they are actually 'typical' of this new (second-) generation of agents (Gerlach and Casey, 1994; Waddington and O'Callaghan, 1997; Waddington *et al.*, 1997)? The purpose of this chapter is to introduce the new drug therapies for schizophrenia and related psychotic illnesses, and to consider similarities and differences among their pharmacological profiles *vis-à-vis* classical agents, as substrates for their individual profiles of therapeutic and adverse effects to be considered in subsequent chapters.

The pharmacology of classical neuroleptics is rooted in brain dopamine (DA) receptor antagonism that is evident in a number of traditional rodent models held to predict differentially antipsychotic efficacy and extrapyramidal side effect (EPS) liability (Ellenbroek, 1993; Waddington and Quinn, 1999). Over recent years, these concepts have been extended to encompass (i) occupancy of a broader family of D_2-like (D_2, D_3, D_4) receptors and, more variably, with non-DAergic receptors including particularly serotonergic (5-HT), but also noradrenergic (α), muscarinic (M) and histaminergic (H) subtypes, together with other sites (Bymaster *et al.*, 1996; Schotte *et al.*, 1996; Seeman *et al.*, 1997), and (ii) effects in new rodent models, some of which may relate more directly to aspects of the disease process, to confer face and possibly construct validity for schizophrenia (Waddington *et al.*, 1997; Higgins, 1998). These issues are important because of increasing emphasis for second-generation antipsychotics on broader concepts both of efficacy beyond attenuation of psychotic psychopathology, and of side effects beyond reduction in propensity to induce EPS (Waddington and O'Callaghan, 1997; Waddington *et al.*, 1997). Here, the second-generation antipsychotics amisulpride, clozapine, olanzapine, quetiapine, risperidone, sertindole, ziprasidone and zotepine are contrasted with classical agents.

Second-generation antipsychotics

Each agent is considered first in terms of its overall *in vitro* receptor binding profile; these are presented only in descriptive outline here, with exhaustive tables of K_i values (affinity constants) available elsewhere (Bymaster *et al.*, 1996; Schotte *et al.*, 1996; Seeman *et al.*, 1997; Arnt and Skarsfeldt, 1998). Thereafter, these agents are contrasted further in terms of their *in vivo* actions, with particular emphasis on new rodent models. Finally, they are contrasted further in terms of their *in vivo* actions at receptor sites in human brain, as evaluated by positron emission tomography (PET) and single photon emission computed tomography (SPECT), and the functional consequences of such actions in non-human primates as they relate particularly and importantly to clinical EPS liability (see Table 1.1). It is important to emphasize that no animal models uniformly predict all three dimensions of antipsychotic efficacy, adverse effects and appropriate clinical dose. However, several models have sufficiently high correlations with clinical outcomes that they are valuable tools for investigating potential antipsychotic drugs.

Table 1.1 Comparative pharmacology of classical and novel (second-generation) antipsychotics

	Receptor profile	c-fos[a]			PCP[b]		PET (SPECT)[c]	
		Nac	Str	Fcx	PPI	SI	D_2 (%)	5-HT_2 (%)
Haloperidol	Preferential D_2-like antagonist	+ +	+ + +	−	−	−	70–90	0
Amisulpride	Selective $D_{2/3}$ antagonist	?	?	?	?	?	38–76	0
Clozapine	Multiple antagonist	+ +	−	+ +	+ +	+ +	20–68	84–100
Olanzapine	Multiple antagonist	+ +	+	+	+ +	+ +	43–89	90–100
Quetiapine	Multiple antagonist	+ +	−	+ +	+ +	−	22–68	48–70
Risperidone	5-HT_2/D_2/α_1 antagonist	+ +	+	−	+ +	−	59–89	78–100
Sertindole	5-HT_2/D_2/α_1 antagonist	?	?	?	?	+	(50–74)	(90 +)
Ziprasidone	5-HT_2/D_2/α_1 antagonist + 5-HT_{1A} agonist + NA/5-HT reuptake	?	?	?	?	?	77	95
Zotepine	Multiple antagonist + NA reuptake	?	?	?	?	?	(57–61)	?

[a]Induction of c-fos in nucleus accumbens (Nac), dorsolateral striatum (Str) and frontal cortex (Fcx): prominent, + + +; moderate, + +; mild, +; absent, −; unknown, ?
[b]Antagonism of phencyclidine (PCP) effects on prepulse inhibition (PPI) and social isolation (SI): findings indicated as above[a].
[c]Occupancy (%) of basal ganglia D_2-like receptors and of cortical 5-HT_2 receptors in living patients receiving conventional antipsychotic doses, as estimated by positron emission tomography (PET) (or single photon emission computed tomography (SPECT)).

Models of EPS liability in non-human primates have considerable utility in predicting doses of typical and second-generation antipsychotics that produce EPS in patients (Casey, 1995, 1996a). However, it is not yet possible to predict the efficacious antipsychotic dose range in man even from studies in non-human primates. Therefore, it is necessary to combine data from both preclinical studies in animals and clinical trials in patients to characterize best the dose–response curves for relative efficacy and adverse effects to estimate benefit-risk ratios across a group of drugs. EPS in non-human primates are valuable models because monkeys develop the same types of motor system side effects as patients, have the EPS evoked by the same type of drugs and respond similarly to anti-EPS medications, such as anticholinergics (Casey, 1995). It should be assumed that each of these second-generation agents entered extensive clinical development on the basis of a favourable antipsychotic efficacy vs EPS liability profile in those more conventional preclinical (rodent) models used to predict and characterize classical antipsychotics (Ellenbroek, 1993;

Kinon and Lieberman, 1996; Waddington et al., 1997; Arnt and Skarsfeldt, 1998).

Amisulpride

This substituted benzamide analogue of sulpiride (Coukell et al., 1996) is a selective antagonist of D_2-like ($D_2 = D_3 \gg D_4$) receptors with little affinity for D_1-like or non-DAergic receptors. It has been argued on the basis of preclinical studies using conventional models that (i) lower doses of amisulpride preferentially block presynaptic D_2-like autoreceptors to give a relative *enhancement* of DAergic function, which may confer clinical effectiveness against 'negative' ('deficit' or 'psychomotor poverty') symptoms, while (ii) higher doses reduce certain post-synaptic DA receptor-mediated functions to predict antipsychotic efficacy, but with little or no induction of catalepsy to predict low EPS liability (see Waddington et al., 1997). However, there is as yet little in the way of data using the new preclinical models noted above.

Clinical studies have indicated that lower doses of amisulpride (50–300 mg) reduce negative symptom scores relative to placebo without any effect on positive symptoms and with little or no induction of EPS. Recently, more extensive trials have confirmed 100 mg sulpiride to produce a sustained reduction in negative symptom scores without EPS, relative to placebo, though with a high drop-out rate due to recrudescence of psychosis; conversely, 400–800 mg amisulpride was at least as effective as 16–20 mg haloperidol in reducing total psychopathology and positive symptom scores, and was more effective in reducing negative symptom scores with fewer EPS. In patients with predominantly negative symptoms, low-dose amisulpride was more effective than placebo over a 6-month period, while over a 1-year period it showed little advantage over low-dose haloperidol in reducing these symptoms. In terms of adverse effects, amisulpride can induce some dose-related EPS, insomnia–agitation, dry mouth, prolactin elevation and other endocrine effects, and weight gain, but few cardiovascular events (Coukell et al., 1996; Loo et al., 1997; Speller et al., 1997; Waddington et al., 1997).

In patients with schizophrenia, PET studies indicate lower doses of amisulpride (50–100 mg) to occupy only 4–26% of basal ganglia D_2-like receptors, while higher doses (200–800 mg) occupy 38–76% thereof, in comparison to 70–90% occupancy for classical antipsychotics with a putative threshold of 75–80% for induction of EPS (see Waddington et al., 1997); it has been confirmed recently that such occupancy of D_2-like receptors by 200–1200 mg amisulpride occurs in the absence of cortical 5-HT$_2$ receptor occupancy (Trichard et al., 1998).

Studies in non-human primates are not yet available with amisulpride. However, one report of an investigation with sulpiride, a compound closely related to amisulpride, found that sulpiride had an EPS profile that suggested a low EPS liability in patients at doses that had antipsychotic efficacy (Casey, 1995). This is consistent with the low EPS profile seen with amisulpride in the clinic, but further tests in non-human primates are needed to assess more accurately the preclinical EPS relationships between these two substituted benzamides.

Clozapine

As the archetype second-generation antipsychotic, this highly non-selective dibenzodiazepine demonstrates an extensive range of pharmacological actions at multiple levels of neuronal function involving diverse neurotransmitter systems, which have attracted extensive review; within this complex profile, so different from that of amisulpride, may reside important, even fundamental clues to improved antipsychotic activity (Ashby and Wang, 1996; Waddington *et al.*, 1997). At an *in vitro* level, clozapine is at best a modest antagonist both of D_2-like ($D_4 > D_2 > D_3$) and of D_1-like receptors; it has considerably higher antagonist affinity for α ($\alpha_1 > \alpha_2$), H_1, M and 5-HT_2 receptors.

Among new neurochemical models, expression of the intermediate-early gene *c-fos* is induced by numerous physiological and pharmacological stimuli, including antipsychotic drugs, in a manner that might reveal neuroanatomical sites and functional pathways of drug action. As do classical antipsychotics, clozapine induces *c-fos* in the nucleus accumbens; however, relative to such agents, which particularly induce *c-fos* in the dorsolateral striatum as a correlate of EPS liability, clozapine induces *c-fos* preferentially in the prefrontal cortex, while substantially sparing the striatum (see Waddington *et al.*, 1997). Among new behavioural models, the ability of a low intensity prepulse to inhibit the startle response to a subsequent higher intensity stimulus (prepulse inhibition; PPI) is disrupted in schizophrenia and can be disrupted in rodents by DA receptor agonists such as apomorphine and by the psychotogen and 'negative' symptom inducer phencyclidine (PCP). While restoration of apomorphine-induced disruption of PPI by clozapine remains controversial (see Waddington *et al.*, 1997; Swerdlow *et al.*, 1998), clozapine but not classical antipsychotics restores PCP-induced disruption thereof; it also attenuates PCP-induced social isolation (Sams-Dodd, 1997). In patients with schizophrenia, PET studies indicate clozapine to occupy 20–68% of D_2-like and 36–59% of D_1-like receptors in the basal ganglia at conventional clinical doses while occupying 84–100% of cortical 5-HT_2 receptors (Nordstrom *et al.*, 1995; Kapur *et al.*, 1999). Using SPECT, the range of D_2-like receptor occupancies by clozapine appears wider (Pickar *et al.*, 1996; Kasper *et al.*, 1998); while the issue of whether clozapine might exert higher D_2-like occupancy in extra-striatal regions such as the temporal lobe and thalamus remains controversial, it consistently demonstrates high occupancy of cortical 5-HT_2 receptors (Travis *et al.*, 1998a).

Clozapine studies in non-human primates contribute further to the unique profile of this drug. Administered across a very wide dose range, clozapine did not produce EPS of dystonia, whereas the typical antipsychotics readily caused EPS and other second-generation agents produced EPS at a relatively much higher dose (see below) (Casey, 1995, 1996a). Thus, clozapine is the only antipsychotic agent that does not produce EPS in non-human primates. This is consistent with the exceptionally low EPS of clozapine in the clinic. Furthermore, these data suggest that while other second-generation agents may have a favourable antipsychotic efficacy-adverse effect ratio, clozapine remains unique amongst such agents (Casey, 1996a). This 'no-low' EPS profile is consistent with low (less than 70%) D_2-like striatal binding of clozapine (Nordstrom *et al.*, 1995; Kapur *et al.*, 1999).

Olanzapine

This thienobenzodiazepine analogue of clozapine (Fulton and Goa, 1997) is a broad, high affinity antagonist of $5\text{-}HT_2 = M > H_1 > D_2$-like $(D_2 = D_3 = D_4) > D_1$-like $= \alpha(\alpha_1 > \alpha_2)$ receptors. It shares the action of clozapine to induce *c-fos* in the prefrontal cortex as well as in the nucleus accumbens, but unlike clozapine it slightly elevates *c-fos* in the dorsolateral striatum. Behaviourally, olanzapine shares the action of clozapine to restore PCP-induced disruption of PPI and may reverse PCP-induced social isolation (see Sams-Dodd, 1997; Waddington *et al.*, 1997). In patients with schizophrenia, PET studies indicate olanzapine to occupy 43–89% of D_2-like receptors in the basal ganglia at conventional clinical doses, while occupying 90–100% of cortical $5\text{-}HT_2$ receptors (Nordstrom *et al.*, 1998; Kapur *et al.*, 1999). Using SPECT, the range of D_2-like receptor occupancies appears similarly wide, in the face of a high degree of cortical $5\text{-}HT_2$ receptor occupancy (Travis *et al.*, 1998b).

Olanzapine has a favourable EPS profile in non-human primates. It produces dose-related EPS in a threshold dose range that is 20- to 40-fold higher than the dose of haloperidol that causes EPS in monkeys (unpublished data). Since both olanzapine and haloperidol have antipsychotic efficacy in the clinic over a similar dose range, the data in non-human primates comparing olanzapine and haloperidol suggest that olanzapine will be relatively free of EPS, perhaps by a factor of 20 compared to haloperidol, in the recommended clinical dose range.

Quetiapine

This dibenzothiazepine analogue of clozapine (Gunasekara and Spencer, 1998) is a broad, lower affinity antagonist of $H_1 > 5\text{-}HT_2 = \alpha_{1/2} > D_2$-like $(D_2 = D_3 > D_4) > D_1$-like $= M$ receptors. It shares the action of clozapine to induce *c-fos* in the prefrontal cortex, as well as in the nucleus accumbens, but not in the dorsolateral striatum. Behaviourally, quetiapine shares the action of clozapine to restore PCP-induced disruption of PPI but does not appear to reverse PCP-induced social isolation (see Sams-Dodd, 1997; Waddington *et al.*, 1997). In patients with schizophrenia, PET studies indicate quetiapine to occupy 22–68% of D_2-like receptors in the basal ganglia at conventional clinical doses, while occupying 48–70% of cortical $5\text{-}HT_2$ receptors (Gefvert *et al.*, 1998). Using SPECT, D_2-like occupancy appears somewhat lower (Kufferle *et al.*, 1997).

Quetiapine has been studied in several different paradigms in non-human primates, all of which show a favourable EPS profile (Migler *et al.*, 1993; Casey, 1996b; Peacock and Gerlach, 1999). These different research designs identified different EPS-inducing threshold doses of quetiapine, but comparing them within each study design with other antipsychotics, quetiapine is about 10-fold less likely to cause EPS than an equiefficacious antipsychotic dose of haloperidol or chlorpromazine.

Risperidone

This benzisoxazole is a very high affinity antagonist of 5-HT$_2$ and a high affinity antagonist of D$_2$-like (D$_2$ > D$_3$ = D$_4$), $\alpha(\alpha_1 > \alpha_2)$ and H$_1$ receptors; a metabolite, 9-OH-risperidone, shares a generally similar profile and likely contributes to its overall pharmacological activity (Schotte et al., 1996). Like other antipsychotics, risperidone induces c-fos in the nucleus accumbens; however, unlike clozapine, it modestly induces c-fos in the dorsolateral striatum in the absence of induction in the prefrontal cortex. Behaviourally, risperidone shares the action of clozapine to restore PCP-induced disruption of PPI, but does not appear to reverse PCP-induced social isolation (see Sams-Dodd, 1997; Waddington et al., 1997). In patients with schizophrenia, PET studies indicate risperidone to occupy 59–89% of D$_2$-like receptors in the basal ganglia at conventional clinical doses, while occupying 78–100% of cortical 5-HT$_2$ receptors (Farde et al., 1995; Kapur et al., 1999). Using SPECT, D$_2$-like and 5-HT$_2$ occupancies appear very similar (Busatto et al., 1995; Kufferle et al., 1996; Knable et al., 1997; Travis et al., 1998a).

Data with risperidone and EPS in non-human primates are consistent with clinical findings. The threshold dose for causing EPS in monkeys is similar to the haloperidol threshold dose and translates to about 5 mg/day p.o. in man (Casey, 1996a). Clinical data indicate that risperidone has a favourable EPS profile below 6 mg/day p.o. but at and above this dose there are dose-related EPS (Marder and Meibach, 1994).

Sertindole

This indole derivative (Dunn and Fitton, 1996) is a high affinity antagonist of 5-HT$_2$ > α_1 > D$_2$-like (D$_2$ = D$_3$ = D$_4$) receptors which may be a pseudo-irreversible α_1 antagonist (Ipsen et al., 1997); though otherwise little studied in new models, it appears to exert some reversal of PCP-induced social isolation (Sams-Dodd, 1997). In patients with schizophrenia, PET studies with sertindole have been undertaken so far only at subclinical doses, at which little D$_2$-like receptor occupancy was apparent (Farde et al., 1997). Using SPECT, D$_2$-like occupancy at conventional clinical doses is from 50–74% and upwards, with a high occupancy of cortical 5-HT$_2$ receptors (Pilowsky et al., 1997; Kasper et al., 1998; Travis et al., 1998b).

Sertindole has a favourable adverse effect profile in non-human primates (Casey, 1996a). The doses required to produce EPS in monkeys when converted to human oral dose equivalents were approximately five- to 10-fold higher for inducing EPS than for antipsychotic efficacy. These non-human primate results are consistent with clinical experience over the past few years that show sertindole to have antipsychotic efficacy at doses that do not consistently cause EPS.

Ziprasidone

This indole derivative (Davis and Markham, 1997) is a high affinity antagonist of 5-HT$_2$ > D$_2$-like (D$_2$ = D$_3$ > D$_4$) > $\alpha(\alpha_1 > \alpha_2)$ > H$_1$ receptors, which also exhibits 5-HT$_{1A}$ agonism and inhibits the reuptake of NA and

5-HT; it has been little studied using the new models considered above. In normal volunteers, PET studies indicate ziprasidone to occupy of the order of 77% of D_2-like receptors in the basal ganglia at conventional clinical doses, while occupying of the order of 98% of cortical 5-HT$_2$ receptors (Bench *et al.*, 1996; Fishman *et al.*, 1996); studies using either PET or SPECT in patients with schizophrenia have yet to be reported. To date no data are available for ziprasidone in non-human primate models of EPS or psychosis.

Zotepine

This dibenzothiepine analogue of clozapine (Prakash and Lamb, 1998) is a high affinity antagonist of 5-HT$_2 = \alpha_1 = H_1 > D_2$-like ($D_2 = D_3 = D_4$) > D_1-like, which also inhibits the reuptake of NA; it has been little studied using the new models considered above. No studies on zotepine using PET have yet been reported. In patients with schizophrenia, SPECT studies indicate zotepine to occupy 57–61% of D_2-like receptors in the basal ganglia at conventional clinical doses (Barnas *et al.*, 1997); there are as yet no such studies of 5-HT$_2$ receptor occupancy. Again, no studies in non-human primates have been reported.

Overview and context

In general terms, these second-generation antipsychotics appear to fall into one of three categories: (i) selective D_2-like antagonists (amisulpride); (ii) 5-HT$_2$/D$_2$-like/α_1 antagonists ± 5-HT$_{1A}$ agonism ± inhibition of NA/5-HT reuptake (risperidone, sertindole, ziprasidone); (iii) antagonists of these and multiple other receptor systems ± inhibition of NA reuptake (clozapine, olanzapine, quetiapine, zotepine). With these new agents come realistic clinical expectations beyond antipsychotic efficacy and materially reduced motor side effects liability: contemporary aspirations extend to alleviation of 'negative' ('deficit'/'psychomotor poverty') symptoms, cognitive impairment, affective symptoms and violent behaviour, including previously refractory patients, and to reduction in subjective dysphoria, sedation, autonomic/cardiac effects, prolactin elevation, sexual dysfunction and weight gain (see Waddington and O'Callaghan, 1997). The therapeutic challenge is to gain a clearer picture of the extent to which these second-generation antipsychotics satisfy these expectations, and how they should be used to maximize the likelihood of achieving such expectations; these issues are the topic of subsequent chapters. Pharmacologically, the challenge is to relate increasing insight into their diverse cellular and psychological effects, as described above, to those clinical expectations that prove realizable over the course of day-to-day clinical care.

From an era focusing on the primacy of D_2 (now D_2-like) receptor blockade in antipsychotic efficacy and extent of EPS liability, subsequent proposals in relation to second-generation agents have included D_2/D_4 antagonism (Seeman *et al.*, 1997), 5-HT$_2$/D$_2$-like antagonism (Kapur, 1998), D_2-like upregulation/D_1-like downregulation (Lidow *et al.*, 1998), and 'loose' as opposed to 'tight' D_2 antagonism (Seeman and Tallerico,

1998); it should be noted that each proposal involves some role for DA receptor antagonism and that each second-generation agent exerts at least some degree of D_2-like antagonism. The clinical findings with the selective 5-HT$_2$ antagonist MDL 100,907 (Kehne *et al.*, 1996) would constitute the first evidence from a double-blind, placebo-controlled trials on the effectiveness of an agent having essentially *no* affinity for any known DA receptor subtype; such data would clarify the viability of a third-generation of antipsychotics having no direct action on DAergic function.

Acknowledgements

The authors' studies are supported by the Research Committee of the Royal College of Surgeons in Ireland and the Stanley Foundation for JLW, and the VA Medical Research Program, the VA Mental Illness Research, Education, and Clinical Center (MIRECC), VISN 20, and US National Institutes of Mental Health Grant MH 36657 for DEC.

References

Arnt, J. and Skarsfeldt, T. (1998). Do novel antipsychotics have similar pharmacological characteristics? A review of the evidence. *Neuropsychopharmacology*, **18**, 63–101.

Ashby, C.R. and Wang, R.Y. (1996). Pharmacological actions of the atypical antipsychotic drug clozapine: a review. *Synapse*, **24**, 349–394.

Barnas, C., Tauscher, J., Kufferle, B., *et al.* (1997). ^{123}I-IBZM SPECT imaging of dopamine-2 receptors in psychotic patients treated with zotepine. *Eur. Neuropsychopharmacol.*, **7** (Suppl. 2), S215.

Bench, C.J., Lammerstma, A.A., Grasby, P.M., *et al.* (1996). The time-course of binding to striatal dopamine D_2 receptors by the neuroleptic ziprasidone (CP-88, 059-01), determined by positron emission tomography. *Psychopharmacology*, **124**, 141–147.

Busatto, G.F., Pilowsky, L.S., Costa, D.C., *et al.* (1995). Dopamine D_2 receptor blockade in vivo with the novel antipsychotics risperidone and remoxipride – an ^{123}I-IBZM single photon emission tomography (SPET) study. *Psychopharmacology*, **117**, 55–61.

Bymaster, F.P., Calligaro, D.O., Falcone, J.F., *et al.* (1996). Radioreceptor binding profile of the atypical antipsychotic olanzapine. *Neuropsychopharmacology*, **14**, 87–96.

Casey, D.E. (1995). The nonhuman primate model: focus on dopamine D2 and serotonin mechanisms. In: *Schizophrenia: An Integrated View* (R. Fog, J. Gerlach and R. Hemmingsen, eds), Copenhagen, Munksgaard, pp. 287–297.

Casey, D.E. (1996a). Behavioral effects of sertindole, risperidone, clozapine and haloperidol in cebus monkeys. *Psychopharmacology*, **124**, 134–140.

Casey, D.E. (1996b). Extrapyramidal syndromes and new antipsychotic drugs: findings in patients and nonhuman primate models. *Br. J. Psychiatry*, **168** (Suppl. 29), 32–39.

Coukell, A.J., Spencer, C.M. and Benfield, P. (1996). Amisulpride: a review of its pharmacodynamic and pharmacokinetic properties and therapeutic efficacy in the management of schizophrenia. *CNS Drugs*, **6**, 237–256.

Davis, R. and Markham, A. (1997). Ziprasidone. *CNS Drugs*, **8**, 153–159.

Dunn, C.J. and Fitton, A. (1996). Sertindole. *CNS Drugs*, **5**, 224–230.

Ellenbroek, B.A. (1993). Treatment of schizophrenia: a clinical and preclinical evaluation of neuroleptic drugs. *Pharmacol. Ther.*, **57**, 1–78.

Farde, L., Nyberg, S., Oxenstierna, G., *et al.* (1995). PET studies on D_2 and 5-HT$_2$ receptor binding in risperidone-treated schizophrenia patients. *J. Clin. Psychopharmacol.*, **15** (Suppl. 1), 19S–23S.

Farde, L., Mack, R.J., Nyberg, S., *et al.* (1997). D_2 occupancy, extrapyramidal side effects and antipsychotic drug treatment: a pilot study with sertindole in healthy subjects. *Int. Clin. Psychopharmacol.*, **12** (Suppl. 1), S3–S7.

Fishman, A.J., Bonab, A.A., Babich, J.W., *et al.* (1996). Positron emission tomographic analysis of central 5-hydroxytryptamine$_2$ receptor occupancy in healthy volunteers treated with the novel antipsychotic agent, ziprasidone. *J. Pharmacol. Exp. Ther.*, **279**, 939–947.

Fulton, B. and Goa, K.L. (1997). Olanzapine: a review of its pharmacological properties and therapeutic efficacy in the management of schizophrenia and related psychoses. *Drugs*, **53**, 281–298.

Gefvert, O., Bergstrom, M., Langstrom, B., *et al.* (1998). Time course of central nervous dopamine-D_2 and 5-HT$_2$ receptor blockade and plasma drug concentrations after discontinuation of quetiapine (Seroquel) in patients with schizophrenia. *Psychopharmacology*, **135**, 119–126.

Gerlach, J. and Casey, D.E. (1994). Drug treatment of schizophrenia: myths and realities. *Curr. Opinion Psychiatry*, **7**, 65–70.

Gunasekara, N.S. and Spencer, C.M. (1998). Quetiapine: A review of its use in schizophrenia. *CNS Drugs*, **9**, 325–340.

Higgins, G.A. (1998). From rodents to recovery: development of animal models of schizophrenia. *CNS Drugs*, **9**, 59–68.

Ipsen, M., Zhang, Y., Dragsted, N., *et al.* (1997). The antipsychotic drug sertindole is a specific inhibitor of α_{1A}-adrenoceptors in rat mesenteric small arteries. *Eur. J. Pharmacol.*, **336**, 29–35.

Kapur, S. (1998). A new framework for investigating antipsychotic action in humans: lessons from PET imaging. *Mol. Psychiatry*, **3**, 135–140.

Kapur, S., Zipursky, R.B. and Remington, G. (1999). Clinical and theoretical implications of 5-HT$_2$ and D_2 receptor occupancy of clozapine, risperidone and olanzapine in schizophrenia. *Am. J. Psychiatry*, **156**, 286–293.

Kasper, S., Tauscher, J., Kufferle, B., *et al.* (1998). Sertindole and dopamine D_2 receptor occupancy in comparison to risperidone, clozapine and haloperidol – a ^{123}I-IBZM SPECT study. *Psychopharmacology*, **136**, 367–373.

Kehne, J.H., Baron, B.M., Carr, A.A., *et al.* (1996). Preclinical characterization of the potential of the putative atypical antipsychotic MDL 100,907 as a potent 5-HT$_{2A}$ antagonist with a favourable CNS safety profile. *J. Pharmacol. Exp. Ther.*, **277**, 968–981.

Kinon, B.J. and Lieberman, J.A. (1996). Mechanisms of action of atypical antipsychotic drugs: a critical analysis. *Psychopharmacology*, **124**, 2–34.

Knable, M.B., Heinz, A., Raedler, T., *et al.* (1997). Extrapyramidal side effects with risperidone and haloperidol at comparable D2 receptor occupancy levels. *Psychiat. Res.* (Neuroimaging Section), **75**, 91–101.

Kufferle, B., Brucke, T., Topitz-Schratzberger, A., *et al.* (1996). Striatal dopamine-2 receptor occupancy in psychotic patients treated with risperidone. *Psychiat. Res.* (Neuroimaging Section), **68**, 23–30.

Kufferle, B., Tauscher, J., Asenbaum, S., *et al.* (1997). IBZM SPECT imaging of striatal dopamine-2 receptors in psychotic patients treated with the novel antipsychotic substance quetiapine in comparison to clozapine and haloperidol. *Psychopharmacology*, **133**, 323–328.

Lidow, M.S., Williams, G.V. and Goldman-Rakic, P.S. (1998). The cerebral cortex: a case for a common site of action of antipsychotics. *Trends Pharmacol. Sci.*, **19**, 136–140.

Loo, H., Poirier-Littre, M.-F., Theron, M., *et al.* (1997). Amisulpride versus placebo in the medium-term treatment of the negative symptoms of schizophrenia. *Br. J. Psychiatry*, **170**, 18–22.

Marder, S.R. and Meibach, R.C. (1994). Risperidone in the treatment of schizophrenia. *Am. J. Psychiatry*, **151** (6), 825–835.

Migler, B.M., Warawa, E.J. and Malick, J.B. (1993). Seroquel: behavioral effects in conventional and novel tests for atypical antipsychotic drugs. *Psychopharmacology*, **112**, 299–307.

Nordstrom, A.L., Farde, L., Nyberg, S., *et al.* (1995). D_1, D_2, and 5-HT$_2$ receptor occupancy in relation to clozapine serum concentration: a PET study of schizophrenic patients. *Am. J. Psychiatry*, **152**, 1444–1449.

Nordstrom, A.L., Nyberg, S., Olsson, H., *et al.* (1998). Positron emission tomography finding of a high striatal D_2 receptor occupancy in olanzapine-treated patients. *Arch. Gen. Psychiatry*, **55**, 283–284.

Peacock, L. and Gerlach, J. (1999). New and old antipsychotics versus clozapine in a monkey model: adverse effects and antiamphetamine effects. *Psychopharmacology* **144** (3), 189–197.

Pickar, D., Su, T.P., Weinberger, D.R., *et al.* (1996). Individual variation in D_2 dopamine receptor occupancy in clozapine-treated patients. *Am. J. Psychiatry*, **153**, 1571–1578.

Pilowsky, L.S., O'Connell, P., Davies, N., *et al.* (1997). In vivo effects on striatal dopamine D_2 receptor binding by the novel atypical antipsychotic drug sertindole – a ^{123}I IBZM single photon emission tomography (SPET) study. *Psychopharmacology*, **130**, 152–158.

Prakash, A. and Lamb, H.M. (1998). Zotepine: A review of its pharmacodynamic and pharmacokinetic properties and therapeutic efficacy in the management of schizophrenia. *CNS Drugs*, **9**, 153–175.

Sams-Dodd, F. (1997). Effect of novel antipsychotic drugs on phencyclidine-induced stereotyped behaviour and social isolation in the rat social interaction test. *Behav. Pharmacol.*, **8**, 196–215.

Schotte, A., Janssen, P.F.M., Gommeren, W., *et al.* (1996). Risperidone compared with new and reference antipsychotic drugs: in vitro and in vivo receptor binding. *Psychopharmacology*, **124**, 57–73.

Seeman, P. and Tallerico, T. (1998). Antipsychotic drugs which elicit little or no Parkinsonism bind more loosely than dopamine to brain D_2 receptors, yet occupy high levels of these receptors. *Mol. Psychiatry*, **3**, 123–134.

Seeman, P., Corbett, R. and Van Tol, H.H.M. (1997). Atypical neuroleptics have low affinity for dopamine D_2 receptors or are selective for D_4 receptors. *Neuropsychopharmacology*, **16**, 93–110.

Speller, J.C., Barnes, T.R.E., Curson, D.A., *et al.* (1997). One-year, low-dose neuroleptic study of in-patients with chronic schizophrenia characterised by persistent negative symptoms: amisulpride v. haloperidol. *Br. J. Psychiatry*, **171**, 564–568.

Swerdlow, N.R., Varty, G.B. and Geyer, M.A. (1998). Discrepant findings of clozapine effects on prepulse inhibition of startle: Is it the route or the rat? *Neuropsychopharmacology*, **18**, 50–56.

Travis, M.J., Busatto, G.F., Pilowsky, L.S., *et al.* (1998a). 5-HT$_{2A}$ receptor blockade in patients with schizophrenia treated with risperidone or clozapine. *Br. J. Psychiatry*, **173**, 236–241.

Travis, M.J., Busatto, G.F., Pilowsky, L.S., *et al.* (1998b). Serotonin: 5-HT$_{2A}$ receptor occupancy in vivo and response to the new antipsychotics olanzapine and sertindole. *Br. J. Psychiatry*, **173**, 290–291.

Trichard, C., Paillere-Martinot, M.L., Attar-Levy, D., *et al.* (1998). Binding of antipsychotic drugs to cortical 5-HT$_{2A}$ receptors: a PET study of chlorpromazine, clozapine, and amisulpride in schizophrenic patients. *Am. J. Psychiatry*, **155**, 505–508.

Waddington, J.L. and O'Callaghan, E. (1997). What makes an antipsychotic 'atypical'? *CNS Drugs*, **7**, 341–346.

Waddington, J.L., Scully, P.J. and O'Callaghan, E. (1997). The new antipsychotics, and their potential for early intervention in schizophrenia. *Schizophr. Res.*, **28**, 207–222.

Waddington, J.L. and Quinn, J.F. (1999). From first- to second-generation antipsychotics. In: *Atypical Antipsychotics* (B.A. Ellenbroek and A.R. Cools, eds), Basel, Birkhauser (in press).

2

Traditional antipsychotic medications: contemporary clinical use

Charles Schulz and Patrick McGorry

Key points

- Typical antipsychotic medications have had a profound impact on the treatment of schizophrenia and until recently have been the mainstay of treatment.
- Prescribing practices have altered over time.
- Low doses of these drugs are now considered as efficacious as the higher doses which were previously recommended.
- With the advent of new medications, the side-effect profile of traditional antipsychotics, particularly the propensity for developing tardive dyskinesia, is the major drawback for the continued use of these drugs.
- Typical antipsychotics still have, by virtue of the availability of intramuscular forms, a pre-eminent role in the acute management of agitated psychosis and in the treatment of patients who are non-compliant with oral medications.

Legacy of the traditional antipsychotics

Given the current era of rapid drug development, some reflection on the development and influence of the traditional ('first generation', 'typical') antipsychotics is instructive. The first specific antipsychotic medication (chlorpromazine), discovered by Laborit in 1949 in his attempt to develop a pre-anaesthetic agent for his patients, was fortuitously found (by Delay and Denicker) to have not only calmative factors (for review, see Ellenbroek, 1993), but also to reduce the positive symptoms of hallucinations and delusions. These new medications, shown in clinical trials to be better than placebo and better than sedating drugs, were rapidly introduced in a widespread fashion. The reduction in mental hospital populations was attributed initially to the efficacy of the new medications, and they were correctly seen as much more effective than electroconvulsive therapy (ECT) or psychotherapy in enduring psychosis. However several years later, a more sober assessment was possible (Ellard, 1963). This paper pointed out the new medications had been oversold, that they were only partially effective, had numerous adverse effects and that the emptying of the state hospitals was primarily due to earlier treatment, community-based facilities, and more sympathetic public attitudes (Stoller, 1996).

Among the important effects of the introduction of the traditional antipsychotic medications were the impact on neuroscience research and the development of clinical trials methodology. The observation of the central nervous system dopamine changes following antipsychotic medication administration, led to decades of research to find the aetiology and/or pathophysiology of schizophrenia. The involvement of institutions in multi-centre clinical studies to investigate the safety and efficacy of these new medications was another important outgrowth which resulted in the development of professional organizations and standardized rating instruments. These benefits continue to serve the field well.

Clinical studies all clearly indicated that positive symptoms of schizophrenia were substantially reduced when patients took adequate trials of antipsychotic medications. The impact of the traditional medicines on negative symptoms was much less, although there is some literature to suggest that negative symptoms are reduced with traditional antipsychotic medication treatment. Further studies clearly indicated that the antipsychotic medications were required to sustain remission. Placebo-controlled studies demonstrated that without a doubt there was a very high relapse rate (about 80% per year) when placebo was substituted for maintenance antipsychotic medication treatment (Kane, 1996). The importance of maintenance treatment led to the development of longer acting compounds, which are administered to patients around the world. In the USA fluphenazine and haloperidol decanoate preparations are frequently prescribed, although they may be used mostly for patients with problems with compliance. Other parts of the world probably use a higher amount of long-acting medication as they consider it an integral part of treatment.

Evolving experience with these medications revealed that nearly one-third of patients experience minimal clinical benefit (Schulz and Buckley, 1995). Numerous studies attempted to improve the response rate through assessment of neuroleptic blood levels (Baldessarini et al., 1988) and by use of augmentation strategies with non-neuroleptic agents such as lithium, carbamazepine, alprazolam, and propranolol (Angrist and Schulz, 1990). The issue of the poorly responsive patient has also been credited with playing a large role in the development of the new compounds, as described in subsequent chapters. An unfortunate effect of the introduction of the antipsychotic medications has been the impact of splitting many psychiatric practitioners. Rather than viewing the antipsychotic medications as an important somatic treatment which could assist schizophrenic patients in their overall psychosocial treatment, the field of psychiatry splintered into those who were 'biological' and those who were 'psychodynamic'. At the same time, subsequent clinical trials over the last 10–15 years have consistently demonstrated the synergy between psychosocial treatments when used in conjunction with adequate trials of antipsychotic medications (Penn and Meuser, 1996; Schooler et al., 1997). Important psychological approaches include individual therapy (Hogarty et al., 1995), family therapies (Falloon et al., 1985), and more recently cognitive behavioural approaches (Kemp et al., 1997).

Side effects

Side effects of the traditional antipsychotic medications and their management are highlighted in Table 2.1. Tardive dyskinesia and tardive dystonia

Table 2.1 Management of neuromuscular side effects from traditional antipsychotic medications

Adverse effect	Management
Acute dystonia	i.m. benztropine or diphenhydramine; reduce dose or change medication
Parkinsonism	Reduce dose; add benztropine
Akathisia	Reduce dose; add beta blocker, or benzodiazepine in low dose
Tardive dyskinesia	If mild/early, add vitamin E; switch to atypical drug. If established, switch to clozapine
Neuroleptic malignant syndrome	Stop drug, hospitalize. Rule out other causes. Give dantrolene or bromocriptine. Ensure supportive care and adequate hydration

are seen in 4–5% of patients during the first year of treatment and unfortunately 4–5% more each year for the first 5 years of treatment when the rate levels off (Kane, 1995). This observed clinical effect is supported by animal laboratory results demonstrating the dystonia to parkinsonism to tardive dyskinesia progression and their relationship to dopamine receptor functioning. Patients over the age of 65 have a marked increase in rates of tardive dyskinesia – rates of 50% over 2 years have been reported (Woerner *et al.*, 1998). On the other hand, a high prevalence of EPS (especially dystonia) has been documented in younger patients (adolescents and young adults) compared to older patients. These observed phenomena of the relationship of age to neurological side effects is important for clinical use of traditional agents. While there is some evidence that vitamin E may reduce abnormal involuntary movements of recent onset, most psychiatrists would favour switching from a traditional to an atypical antipsychotic medication if tardive dyskinesia emerges.

Akathisia, considered to be one of the leading causes of non-compliance with traditional antipsychotic medications, has not been clearly related to the dopamine receptor pathophysiology thought to underlie the above movement disorders. Moreover, the treatment for akathisia – propranolol or other beta-blockers – does not appear to act by an influence of the dopamine system. Non-neurological side effects of traditional antipsychotic medications include hypotension, liver enzyme abnormalities, galactorrhoea, eye changes, and sedation (for review see Sajatovic and Schulz, 1997). Many psychiatrists feel that the major basis to choose an antipsychotic medication is to match the antipsychotics side effects to the patient's needs. However, no data indicate that an agitated patient requires a sedating antipsychotic medication.

Effective doses of antipsychotics

Doses of antipsychotic medications vary around the world. In the mid-1980s, American psychiatrists prescribed antipsychotic medications at an approximate 1500 mg-chlorpromazine equivalence, while clinicians in other countries frequently used far less medication – even as low as 300–500 mg chlorpromazine equivalence. Faced with a growing concern of tardive dyskinesia and the lack of superior efficacy with high dose therapy, clinicians have struggled to find the lowest effective dose of the medication. Neuroleptic blood levels have been of some, but limited help. Using the emergence of extrapyramidal side effects in patients as an indirect measure of dopamine blockade – the 'neuroleptic threshold' (McEvoy *et al.*, 1991) – was also proposed. More recent positron emission tomography (PET) studies support the use of low doses of these drugs (53–74% dopamine receptor blockade at 2 mg of haloperidol (Kapur, 1998)) with no additional clinical improvement (Wolkin, 1990) and greater EPS when 70% or greater saturation of D_2 receptors occurs (Nyberg, 1998). Clinical studies of treatment response in first episode (Lieberman *et al.*, 1989) and more chronic patients (Kane, 1996) also demonstrate the efficacy of lower doses. A more recent comparative study of three doses of haloperidol with three doses of sertindole showed equiefficacy for a low 4 mg dose of haloperidol (Zimbroff *et al.*, 1997). On the other hand, discontinuation and targeted treatment studies confirm the higher risk of relapse for the majority of patients who discontinue medication altogether.

Appropriate use of antipsychotics

Findings from a recent review of care in the USA reveal that use of these drugs is still far from optimum (Lehman *et al.*, 1998). Only 29% of outpatients were receiving antipsychotic maintenance therapy within the recommended dose range (300–600 chlorpromazine equivalents). Only 24% of those patients who were candidates for depot antipsychotics were receiving an intramuscular medication. In a recently conducted audit of actual prescribing habits in the real world outpatient practice of Australian public sector psychiatry (routine psychiatrists and trainees, i.e. everyday practitioners, not 'experts'), the mean maintenance dose of neuroleptic in chlorpromazine equivalents was 390 mg (Parker *et al.*, 1999). Monotherapy was employed in about 90% of cases. Depot medications were used in about 45%, with a mean dose in chlorpromazine equivalents of 345 mg per day. In another Australian survey of practising psychiatrists (Lambert, 1999) which explored their responses to standard clinical scenarios in a similar way to the survey of American experts (Expert Consensus, 1996), psychiatrists tended to use lower doses than was the prevailing view over a decade ago when the Quality Assurance Project (QAP, 1984) advised that a standard dose for acute treatment was 400 mg chlorpromazine per day or 20 mg trifluoperazine. However, dosages were considered still too high (4–6 mg risperidone; 5–10 mg haloperidol) and inpatient prescribing showed that the time intervals between increases in dosage in the face of non-response were too short. Where depot medication was recommended for maintenance therapy, the doses were a little more appropriate (50–100 mg haloperiodol deconoate per month, 12.5–25 mg fluphenazine decanoate per fortnight).

An area of substantial international differences is the rate of use of injectable or long-acting medication. As noticed previously, practice in the USA is to reserve long-acting injectable medications for patients who are non-compliant with oral treatment (Glazer and Kane, 1992). In actuality, this may be a poor use of injectable medications, as patients still need to attend for their appointments to receive an injection. European psychiatrists more frequently rely on long-acting oral or injectable medication as a routine in their clinics. However, depot medications may still not be optimally used. For example, little effort has been made to use depot medications only after psychoeducation, cognitive behavioural therapy and other attempts to help the patient to accept the idea of maintenance therapy have been properly tried and shown to have no effect.

It is also important to note that since the new antipsychotic medications all cost substantially more than generic preparations of the traditional antipsychotic medications, there are parts of the world where the use of the new antipsychotic medications is simply not practical.

What are the current reasons for using traditional antipsychotic medications?

The availability of atypical antipsychotic medications with fewer neurological side effects and markedly reduced rates of tardive dyskinesia focus attention on the continued role for the traditional antipsychotic medications. At this time, the major reason to use traditional antipsychotic medications appears to be availability of short- or long-acting injectable preparations. The fast-acting intramuscular preparations of traditional antipsychotic medications such as haloperidol, fluphenazine and thiothixene make their use still important in the management of the severely disturbed schizophrenic patient (Buckley, 1999). The long-acting preparations of traditional antipsychotic medications – fluphenazine and haloperidol decanoate – are helpful to some patients who may be forgetful about their medications (Carpenter *et al.*, 1999) and are sometimes used in a forensic setting to ensure compliance between probation appointments (Buckley *et al.*, in press).

Some psychiatrists have indicated that the combination of a traditional antipsychotic medication can sometimes be helpful for individual patients. Theoretically, there may be some persistently ill schizophrenic patients who may need a small amount of added traditional antipsychotic medication for best results. It must be remembered that clinical trials to demonstrate efficacy and safety of an augmented strategy are complicated and require control of time and added drug. Although this practice is utilized, there are no empiric data to support this use at present.

As alluded to above, the cost of the new medications may be prohibitive for some countries or some states around the world. Even though pharmacoeconomic considerations suggest that the more expensive atypical antipsychotic medications could reduce overall cost (Glazer and Dickson, see Chapter 25), some countries may still not be able to afford the new drugs.

Finally, some patients feel well stabilized on traditional antipsychotic medications and/or may request them after having tried new medications. In these cases, in our opinion, the patient's wishes must be respected.

With the continued development of newer drugs of more varied pharmacological profiles, it is likely that the use of traditional antipsychotics will continue to be refined and probably become more specific over time.

References

Angrist, B. and Schulz, S.C. (eds) (1990). *The neuroleptic nonresponsive patient: Characterization and Treatment*, Washington, DC, American Psychiatric Association.

Baldessarini, R.J., Cohen, B.M. and Teicher, M.H. (1988). Significance of neuroleptic dose and plasma level in pharmacological treatment of psychoses. *Arch. Gen. Psychiatry*, **45**, 79–91.

Buckley, P.F. (1999). The role of typical and atypical antipsychotics in the management of agitation and aggression. *J. Clin. Psychiatry*, **60**, 52–60.

Buckley, P.F., Noffsinger, S., Knoll, J. (in press). Treatment of the psychiatric patient who is violent. In: *Psychopharmacology and Serious Mental Illness* (R.W. Buchanan, R.B. Conley, eds.) Gordon and Breach: Newark, USA.

Carpenter, W.T., Buchanan, R.W., Kirkpatrick, B., *et al.* (1999). Comparative effectiveness of fluphenazine decanoate injections every 2 weeks versus every 6 weeks. *Am. J. Psychiatry*, **156**, 412–418.

Ellard, J. (1963). Psychotropic drugs in general practice. *Med. J. Aust.*, **2**, 773–777.

Ellenbroek, B.A. (1993). Treatment of schizophrenia: a clinical and preclinical evaluation of neuroleptic drugs. *Pharmacol. Ther.*, **57**, 1–78.

Falloon, I.R.H., Boyd, J.L., McGill, C.W *et al.*, (1985). Family management in the prevention of schizophrenia. *Arch. Gen. Psychiatry.*, **42**, 887–896.

Glazer, W.M. and Kane, J.M. (1992). Depot neuroleptic therapy: an underutilized treatment option. *J. Clin. Psychiatry*, **53**, 426–433.

Hogarty, G.E., Kornblith, S.J., Greenwald, D., *et al.* (1995). Personal therapy: a disorder-relevant psychotherapy for schizophrenia. *Schizophr. Bull.*, **21**, 379–393.

Kane, J.M. (1995). Tardive dyskinesia. In: *Psychopharmacology the Fourth Generation of Progress* (F. Bloom and D. Kupfer, eds) Raven Press, New York.

Kane, J.M. (1996). Schizophrenia. *N. Engl. J. Med.*, **334**, 34–41.

Kapur, S. (1998). A new framework for investigating antipsychotic action in humans: lessons from PET imaging. *Mol. Psychiatry.*, **3**, 135–140.

Kemp, R., Chua, S., McKenna, P., *et al.* (1997). Reasoning and delusions. *Br. J. Psychiatry*, **170**, 398–405.

Lehman, J.A., Steinwachs, D.M. and Co-Investigators of the PORT Project (1998). Initial results from the schizophrenia Patient Outcomes Research Team (PORT) Client Survey. *Schizophr. Bull.*, **24**, 11–20.

Lieberman, J.A., Jody, D., Geisler, S., *et al.* (1989). Treatment outcome of first-episode schizophrenia. *Psychopharmacol. Bull.*, **25**, 92–96.

McEvoy, J.P., Hogarty, G. and Steingard, S. (1991). Optimal dose of neuroleptic in acute schizophrenia. A controlled study of the neuroleptic threshold and higher haloperidol dose. *Arch. Gen. Psychiatry*, **48**, 739–745.

Nyberg, S. (1998). Relationships among extrapyramidal symptoms, antipsychotic drug doses and neuroreceptor occupancy. *Int. J. Psych. Clin. Pract.*, **2** (Supp 2), S33–S39.

Parker, G., Lambert, T., McGrathy, J., *et al.* (1999). Neuroleptic management of schizophrenia: a survey and commentary on Australia psychiatric practice. In: *Australia results of Audit of psychotropic prescribing in community psychiatric clinics* (T.J.R. Lambert, ed.) NorthWestern Healthcare Network.

Penn, D.L. and Meuser, K.T. (1996). Research update of the psychosocial treatment of schizophrenia. *Am. J. Psychiatry*, **153**, 607–617.

Quality Assurance Project (1984). Treatment outlines for the treatment of schizophrenia. *Aust. NZ J. Psychiatry*, **18**, 19–38.

Sajatovic, M. and Schulz, S.C. (1997). In: *Comprehensive Textbook of Psychiatry* (D.L. Dunner, ed.) 2nd edn.

Schooler, N.R., Keith, S.J., Severe, J.B., *et al.* (1997). Relapse and rehospitalization during maintenance treatment of schizophrenia. *Arch. Gen. Psychiatry*, **54**, 453–458.

Schulz, S.C. and Buckley, P.F. (1995). Treatment-resistant schizophrenia. In: *Schizophrenia* (S.R. Hirsch and D.W. Weinberger, eds), Cambridge, Blackwell Science, pp. 469–484.

Stoller, A. (1996). The first tranquilizer decade. *Aust. J. Pharmacy*, **47**, 2–6.

Woerner, M.G., Alvir, J.M.J., Saltz, B.L., *et al.* (1998). Prospective study of tardive dyskinesia in the elderly: rates and risk factors. *Am. J. Psychiatry*, **155**, 1521–1528.

Wolkin, A. (1990). Positron emission tomography, and the study of neuroleptic response. In: *The neuroleptic nonresponsive patient: characterization and treatment* (B. Angrist and S.C. Schulz, eds), Washington, DC, American Psychiatric Association, pp. 35–49.

Zimboff, D.L., Kane, J.M., Tamminga, C.A., *et al.* (1997). Controlled, dose-response study of sertindole and haloperidol in the treatment of schizophrenia. *Am. J. Psychiatry*, **154**, 773–781.

3

Clozapine: clinical use and experience*

Robert Buchanan and Peter McKenna

Key points

- Clozapine is the only drug that has been specifically approved for the treatment of positive symptoms in treatment-resistant patients.
- The effect of clozapine on negative symptoms is limited to secondary negative symptoms.
- Clozapine is effective for affective and hostility symptoms.
- Clozapine has a mixed effect on cognitive processes, with improvement seen in some and worsening observed in others.
- Clozapine treatment is associated with enhanced social and occupational functioning.
- Clozapine is a rare cause of tardive dyskinesia and may actually be an effective treatment for these symptoms.

The introduction of clozapine has revolutionized our conceptualization of the treatment of schizophrenia, both at the level of pharmacological mechanism and at the level of the evaluation of treatment outcome. Although the mechanism of action of clozapine is still a matter of hypothetical conjecture, its atypical pharmacological profile, in particular its relatively enhanced antagonistic activity at the dopamine D_1 and D_4 receptors and the serotonin 5-HT_{2A} receptor, combined with its superior efficacy for positive symptoms and low incidence of extrapyramidal symptoms (EPS), has stimulated the development of a whole new generation of antipsychotic agents. Each of these new agents was designed to try to capture clozapine's unique efficacy profile, while avoiding its side effects, especially agranulocytosis, which have limited the therapeutic impact of this agent.

Prior to the introduction of clozapine, there were very few clinical trials that included outcomes other than positive symptoms and measures of global function. After the introduction of clozapine, there has been a marked expansion in the scope of outcomes that are evaluated in the context of clinical trials (Meltzer, 1992). This expansion was due, in part, to the hope that clozapine's unique pharmacological profile and positive symptom superior efficacy would translate to efficacy for negative symptoms, affective symptoms, quality of life, social and occupational functioning, and cognitive impairments. There is now quite a large body of clinical research covering the effects of clozapine in all these areas.

*Supported in part by grant number MH45074 from the National Institute of Mental Health.

In this chapter, we review the efficacy of clozapine for a broad range of outcomes, and describe its appropriate clinical use, including acute and maintenance dosage and the management of side effects. The first section evaluates the efficacy profile of clozapine, based on the available research findings, while the second presents a more informal account of nearly 10 years' clinical experience with clozapine in the USA and the UK.

The efficacy profile of clozapine

Clozapine is a dibenzodiazepine derivative that was first manufactured in 1959. The efficacy of clozapine has been examined for positive, negative, and affective symptoms, quality of life, and social and occupational functioning, and cognitive impairment (Table 3.1).

Positive symptoms

Nine double-blind clinical trials have demonstrated that clozapine is at least as effective as conventional antipsychotics for the treatment of the acutely psychotic patient with schizophrenia (McKenna and Bailey, 1993; Buchanan, 1995). There have also been eight long-term follow-up studies, which suggest that clozapine is effective as a maintenance treatment for positive symptoms (Buchanan, 1995). These latter studies have tended to be open-labelled or retrospective in design, but the uniformity of the results and subsequent clinical experience support clozapine's efficacy as a maintenance agent.

The results of some of the early clinical trials on clozapine raised the possibility that it may have superior efficacy for positive symptoms that have failed to respond to conventional antipsychotics (McKenna and Bailey, 1993). In a landmark multicentre study, Kane and colleagues demonstrated beyond reasonable doubt that clozapine was more effective

Table 3.1 Clozapine treatment and outcome dimensions

	Efficacy
Positive symptoms	
Acute	+ + +
Treatment-resistant	+ +
Negative symptoms	
Primary	−
Secondary	+ / + +
Other symptoms	
Hostility/violence	+ +
Affective symptoms	+ +
Social/occupational functioning	+ / + +
Cognitive impairments	+ /−
Tardive dyskinesia	+ +

+ :   mild improvement
+ + :   modest improvement
+ + + :   marked improvement
− :   no effect

than chlorpromazine for positive symptoms in treatment-resistant inpatients (Kane *et al.*, 1988). In a subsequent study, clozapine was shown to be more effective for positive symptoms in partially responsive outpatients with schizophrenia (Breier *et al.*, 1994; Buchanan *et al.*, 1998). These results have been confirmed in multiple other double-blind and open-labelled studies (e.g. Pickar *et al.*, 1992; Kuoppasalmi *et al.*, 1993; Lieberman *et al.*, 1994; Lindenmayer *et al.*, 1994). To date, clozapine remains the only drug that has been specifically approved by the FDA for use in treatment-resistant patients.

Negative symptoms

The multicentre study by Kane *et al.* (1988) also raised the possibility that clozapine may be effective for negative symptoms. These symptoms, which include blunted affect, alogia, avolition, anhedonia, and decreased social drive, are responsible for much of the social and occupational impairment found in patients with schizophrenia (Buchanan and Gold, 1996). The development of an effective treatment for these symptoms would represent a major therapeutic advance.

The evaluation of the effectiveness of a drug for negative symptoms is complicated by the fact that these symptoms may be either primary to the illness or secondary to other factors, including positive and depressive symptoms, and antipsychotic side effects (e.g. EPS, sedation) (Carpenter *et al.*, 1985). The majority of studies subsequent to the Kane *et al.* multicentre study have either found the effect of clozapine on negative symptoms to be associated with its antipsychotic effectiveness or reduction in EPS (Tandon *et al.*, 1993; Lieberman *et al.*, 1994; Miller *et al.*, 1994). Moreover, two studies have prospectively examined the efficacy of clozapine for primary, enduring negative or deficit symptoms (Breier *et al.*, 1994; Conley *et al.*, 1994; Buchanan *et al.*, 1998). In neither of these studies was an effect on deficit symptoms observed. Taken together, these studies suggest that the effect of clozapine is limited to secondary negative symptoms, and may be especially helpful for those patients characterized by high levels of EPS.

Other symptoms

Clozapine has been shown to be effective for the reduction of hostility and violence. These results have been observed in both double-blind and open-labelled studies (Kane *et al.*, 1988; Mallya *et al.*, 1992; Wilson, 1992; Volavka *et al.*, 1993; Buchanan *et al.*, 1998). Of particular interest are the observations that suggest that clozapine may be useful in reducing the use and duration of seclusion and restraint (Mallya *et al.*, 1992) and episodes of violence (Wilson, 1992), and in increasing privilege level (Wilson, 1992) in chronically hospitalized inpatients. These results suggest that clozapine may be particularly effective for violent patients.

Clozapine has also been shown to alleviate depressed mood and other symptoms of depression (Kane *et al.*, 1988; Meltzer and Okayli, 1995). Clozapine may also be effective in reducing the number and severity of suicide attempts (Meltzer and Okayli, 1995). However, it is unclear to what extent the reduction in suicidality is a direct effect of clozapine treatment or an indirect effect related to increased clinical monitoring and level of psychosocial programme participation.

Quality of life/social and occupational functioning

There have been several studies that have examined whether clozapine has any impact on the quality of life and social and occupational functioning of patients with schizophrenia. In two open-labelled studies, clozapine treatment was associated with significant improvement in quality of life (Meltzer et al., 1990; Galletly et al., 1997). A third study found a non-significant improvement in quality of life, which was mainly observed in patients without primary, enduring negative or deficit symptoms (Buchanan et al., 1998). This latter study also included an assessment of the impact of clozapine on social and occupational functioning. In contrast to the findings on quality of life, clozapine treatment was observed to produce a significant improvement in these functional dimensions (Buchanan et al., 1998). In patients whose quality of life improves with clozapine treatment, the improvement appears to be associated with enhanced memory function (Buchanan et al., 1994). However, the results of an ongoing meta-analysis have so far failed to reveal significant differences between clozapine and conventional antipsychotics on a broad range of outcomes, including drug acceptability, ability to work or even suitability for discharge at end of the study period (Essali et al., 1997). Future studies are required to clarify the meaning of these conflicting results.

Cognitive impairment

Patients with schizophrenia are characterized by a broad range of cognitive impairments, including abstract problem solving, working memory, and visual and auditory perception, attention, learning, and memory impairments (see Goldberg and Gold, 1995). Conventional antipsychotics have restricted beneficial or deleterious effects on cognitive function. The unique pharmacological profile of clozapine has led to an interest in examining whether it has any effect on these functions.

The results of open-labelled and double-blind studies that employed comprehensive assessment batteries are summarized in Table 3.2 (Goldberg et al., 1993; Hagger et al., 1993; Buchanan et al., 1994; Grace et al., 1996; Hoff et al., 1996; Galletly et al., 1997). These studies suggest that clozapine has a mixed effect on cognitive impairments. Verbal memory, visual attention, and verbal fluency have been almost universally observed to improve. In contrast, patient performance on measures of visual memory and executive functions has tended to worsen with clozapine treatment. These effects, regardless of direction, have been modest, despite often marked improvement on symptom measures (Goldberg et al., 1993).

Tardive dyskinesia

Clozapine's lack of acute extrapyramidal side effects (i.e. acute dystonia, akathisia and parkinsonism) was noted in the earliest clinical trials of the drug (see Casey, 1989). There is now a consensus that the drug causes no

Table 3.2 Clozapine treatment and cognitive function

Study	Sample size	Verbal memory	Visual memory	Visual attention	Visuospatial measures	Executive functions	Verbal fluency
Goldberg et al. (1993)	9–14	↓	=	=	=	=	NA
Hagger et al. (1993)	25–36	↑	NA	↑	NA	↑	↑
Buchanan et al. (1994)	33–38	=	=	↑	↑	↓	↑
Hoff et al. (1996)	20	↑	↓	=	NA	↓	↑
Grace et al. (1996)	22	↑	↑	↑	NA	NA	↑
Galletly et al. (1997)	19	↑	NA	↑	NA	NA	↑

↑: improves performance
↓: worsens performance
=: no effect
NA: not assessed

more parkinsonism than placebo; acute dystonic reactions are rare; and akathisia is considerably less common than with conventional antipsychotic treatment. Over the years, clozapine's apparent lack of propensity to cause tardive dyskinesia has also attracted comment. Reviewing the literature prior to the world-wide re-introduction of the drug in 1989–90, Casey (1989) found that there were no convincing case reports of tardive dyskinesia on treatment with clozapine. Juul-Povlsen et al. (1985) also found that none of 85 patients treated with clozapine alone for up to 12 years had tardive dyskinesia documented in their case notes, compared to 4% of 131 patients treated with clozapine plus other drugs. There continues to be a paucity of case reports of clozapine causing tardive dyskinesia: one reported 'tardive oculogyric crises' (recurrent acute dystonias responsive to anticholinergic treatment) after 18 months' treatment with clozapine (Davé, 1994a); and another by the same author reported two cases of typical tardive dyskinesia appearing after months or years of treatment with clozapine (Davé, 1994b) – one of these could, however, have represented withdrawal dyskinesia due to previous treatment. As part of their ongoing incidence study of tardive dyskinesia, Kane and co-workers have followed up 28 patients whose treatment was changed to clozapine for 6.2 ± 4.2 years (Kane et al., 1993). Two (7.2%) developed mild tardive dyskinesia; however, both of these patients were rated as having questionable dyskinesia at entry to the study.

Clozapine may also be a treatment for tardive dyskinesia. Several case reports have documented improvement of established tardive dyskinesia on treatment with clozapine (Casey, 1989; Wittenberg et al., 1996; see also Levkovitch et al., 1995; Adityanjee and Estrera, 1996) or a combination of clozapine and clonazepam (Blake et al., 1991; Shapleske et al., 1996). There have also been a number of controlled studies (see Wittenberg et al., 1996); these have had variable findings, but taken together point to full remission or considerable improvement in dyskinesia in up to one-third of patients treated with the drug.

Clinical experience with clozapine

The authors have treated over 200 patients with clozapine. The following represents their accumulated experience of use of the drug. Some general observations are followed by specific issues, which follow the headings of the first part of the chapter.

In general, it is well known that clozapine has to be started at low dosages – typically 25 mg per day – and built up slowly. In the USA, increments of up to 25 mg daily or every other day have been advocated, but in the UK a typical regimen would be increments of 25 mg weekly. It is less well known that 'tapering' of previous antipsychotic medication has proved unnecessary in the authors' experience – surprisingly, problems are rarely, if ever, encountered even when large doses of conventional neuroleptics are stopped abruptly and replaced with an initially tiny and non-therapeutic dose of clozapine.

Clinical experience, as well as several studies (Meltzer, 1992; Lieberman et al., 1994) indicates that the response to clozapine can be slow, and some patients require up to 6 months of treatment to show improvement. This delay in response is usually related to the time it takes to titrate patients to what will be their therapeutic dosage. Upon reaching their eventual therapeutic dose, time to response is usually less than 2 months (Conley et al., 1994). There is less clarity about when to stop increasing the dose of clozapine. A rule of thumb is that if there has been little clinical improvement when a dose of 600 mg per day has been reached, there is little prospect of improvement with further dose increases. This is particularly true if plasma clozapine levels are above 350 ng/ml (Perry et al., 1991). There is less clarity still about whether clozapine can be reduced to a lower maintenance dose after a stable improvement has been achieved.

As noted above there is preliminary evidence to suggest that clozapine reduces the frequency of relapse in patients who respond to it. This is certainly borne out by clinical experience – patients who do well on clozapine generally remain well – but there is no doubt that relapse may occur despite good medication compliance. The management of relapse may require increasing the dose of clozapine and adding adjunctive medications to the treatment regimen. In our experience, such an approach has led to recovery back to the previous level of improvement each time.

Clozapine can be combined with lithium or anticonvulsants, other than carbamazepine, without difficulty. Combination treatment with carbamazepine is contraindicated on the grounds that both drugs can cause agranulocytosis. With respect to concomitant use of other antipsychotics, clozapine monotherapy is recommended as a general rule; this is received wisdom from Scandinavian psychiatry where the drug has had the longest clinical use. Recently, combination treatment with clozapine and sulpiride has been advocated as a measure to enhance clinical response (Shiloh et al., 1997). There appear to be minimal complications with this approach. Inevitably, there are patients who clinicians find themselves treating with clozapine plus a conventional antipsychotic for other reasons. The authors have run into few problems with concomitant use of a variety of other conventional antipsychotics, including haloperidol, chlorpromazine and trifluoperazine but, as mentioned above, monotherapy is recommended as a general rule.

Positive symptoms

In a review of the effects of clozapine on a sample of 66 treatment-refractory patients with schizophrenia, Lieberman *et al.* (1994) concluded that a favourable response was associated with short duration of illness and a paranoid, as opposed to other, presentation. Clinical experience to some extent echoes these findings: clozapine tends to be most effective in patients with a presentation of persistent positive symptoms, rather than those who have developed the typical picture of chronic schizophrenia with prominent negative symptoms.

According to Meltzer (1992) the response to clozapine is dramatic in about 10% of cases. This experience is also borne out by the present authors, both of whom can easily identify corresponding numbers of patients who have shown complete or nearly complete remission of symptoms. Such patients invariably show the features associated with favourable response by Lieberman *et al.* (1994) outlined above; they tend to have florid, persistent, treatment-resistant positive symptoms, but underneath their personality and social function is relatively preserved. The case history of one of the author's patients, a young woman who had had protracted episodes of illness over 12 years and had been continuously floridly ill for nearly 2 years prior to treatment with clozapine, has been described in detail (McKay *et al.*, 1996).

Negative symptoms

As noted above, it is uncertain whether clozapine has any effect on negative symptoms. Initial positive findings in the study by Kane *et al.* (1988) have given way to pessimism in the face of findings that any such apparent effects reflect improvement in 'secondary' negative symptoms due to EPS, depression, etc. In spite of this, clinical impression suggests that the effect on secondary negative symptoms may be important for some patients. They may seem more alert and interested. Nursing staff often report an increase in motivation which allows rehabilitation to become a meaningful option. Sometimes, when there has been no discernible improvement from a clinical point of view, the patients' relatives will insist that there has been a notable increase in his or her warmth and communication.

Other symptoms

One of the first clues that clozapine was atypical came from early clinical studies, where the drug acquired a reputation for being particularly useful in behaviourally disturbed patients. As noted above, several recent controlled studies have confirmed that treatment is associated with significant reductions in violence and need for seclusion. Clinical experience suggests that clozapine may sometimes reduce hostility, threats and violence in the absence of any other evidence of improvement.

In line with research findings, depression, which is part of schizophrenia or a 'mainly schizophrenic' schizoaffective presentation, appears to improve along with other symptoms on treatment with clozapine. The results are more controversial for patients with 'mainly affective' schizoaffective presentations and occasional patients with affective disorder (in the UK clozapine can be used on a named patient basis for treatment-resistant affective disorder). Despite reports of effectiveness in patients with affective disorders (Kimmel et al., 1994; Ranjan and Meltzer, 1996), the authors have only had limited success with these patients.

Quality of life/social and occupational functioning

It is difficult to add meaningfully to the conflicting research findings on clozapine's effects on quality of life. It can, however, be pointed out that this does not always accord with clinical experience, and this applies particularly in the small percentage of cases where the response is dramatic. It might be that the enhancement in social and occupational functioning that occurs in such patients tends to be swamped by the far larger proportion with less clinical improvement who show no change.

Cognitive impairment

In line with the research evidence suggesting that clozapine and other atypical antipsychotics bring about only modest gains in cognitive function, no obvious gains in cognitive function tend to be seen in clozapine-treated schizophrenic patients. This appears to hold true even when there the clinical improvement is marked: Laws and McKenna (1997) reported on two patients who became essentially symptom-free after clozapine treatment. On testing they both exhibited surprising degrees of impairment in memory and/or frontal function.

It is worth noting that clozapine has anticholinergic properties and has been found to worsen memory function in some studies (see Goldberg and Weinberger, 1994). This may have clinical implications: patients or their caregivers occasionally report forgetfulness as a side effect of treatment. In one such case there was improvement when the dose was lowered (Carter et al., 1994).

Tardive dyskinesia

When a schizophrenic patient is found to be developing tardive dyskinesia, the clinician faces the dilemma of either continuing treatment, or withdrawing this with the near certainty of relapse. Until recently, this dilemma was resolved by continuing treatment in most if not all patients, and taking the chance that the movements will not prove to be socially disabling or follow a progressively worsening course. Clozapine has transformed this gloomy algorithm. As described above it does not cause tardive dyskinesia (or does so only rarely), and so patients showing initial signs can be changed to this drug with the reasonable expectation that it will not progress and may even remit.

As described above, clozapine is also useful in the treatment of established tardive dyskinesia. Clinical experience on a small number of cases of severe tardive dyskinesia or tardive dystonia suggests that it is sometimes strikingly effective, and is usually greatly superior to the other therapeutic measures such as tetrabenazine. Nevertheless, it has to be emphasized that it is by no means always effective.

References

Adityanjee, and Estrera, A. (1996). Successful treatment of tardive dyskinesia with clozapine. *Biol. Psychiatry*, **39**, 1064–1065.

Blake, L.M., Marks, R.C., Nierman, P., *et al.* (1991). Clozapine and clonazepam in tardive dyskinesia. *J. Clin. Psychopharmacol.*, **11**, 268–269.

Breier, A., Buchanan, R. W., Kirkpatrick, B., *et al.* (1994). Effects of clozapine on positive and negative symptoms in outpatients with schizophrenia. *Am. J. Psychiatry*, **151**, 20–26.

Buchanan, R. W. (1995). Clozapine: efficacy and safety. *Schizophr. Bull.*, **21**, 579–591.

Buchanan, R. W. and Gold, J.M. (1996). Negative symptoms: diagnosis, treatment and prognosis. *Int. Clin. Psychopharmacol.*, **11**, 3–11.

Buchanan, R. W., Holstein, C. and Breier, A. (1994). The comparative efficacy and long-term effect of clozapine treatment on neuropsychological test performance. *Biol. Psychiatry*, **36**, 717–725.

Buchanan, R. W., Breier, A., Kirkpatrick, B., *et al.* (1998). Positive and negative symptom response to clozapine in schizophrenic patients with and without the deficit syndrome. *Am. J. Psychiatry*, **155**, 751–760.

Carpenter, W.T., Heinrichs, D.W. and Alphs, L.D. (1985). Treatment of negative symptoms. *Schizophr. Bull.*, **11**, 440–452.

Carter, J., Thrasher, S. and Thornicroft, G. (1994). Cognitive impairment and clozapine. *Br. J. Psychiatry*, **164**, 132–133.

Casey, D. E. (1989). Clozapine: neuroleptic-induced EPS and tardive dyskinesia. *Psychopharmacology*, **99** (suppl.), S47–S53.

Conley, R., Gounaris, C. and Tamminga, C. A. (1994). Clozapine response varies in deficit versus non-deficit schizophrenic subjects. *Biol. Psychiatry*, **35**, 746–747.

Davé, M. (1994a). Tardive oculogyric crises with clozapine. *J. Clin. Psychiatry*, **55**, 264–265.

Davé, M. (1994b). Clozapine-related tardive dyskinesia. *Biol. Psychiatry*, **35**, 886–887.

Essali, M.A., Rezk, E., Wahlbeck, K., *et al.* (1997). Clozapine vs atypical neuroleptic medication for schizophrenia. In: *Schizophrenia Module of the Cochrane Database of Systematic Reviews* (updated 04 Mar 1997) (C. E. Adams, J. de Jesus Mari and P. White, eds). Available in the Cochrane Library (database on disk and CDROM). The Cochrane Collaboration; Issue 2. Oxford: Update Software.

Galletly, C. A., Clark, C. R., McFarlane, A. C., *et al.* (1997). Relationships between changes in symptom ratings, neuropsychological test performance and quality of life in schizophrenic patients treated with clozapine. *Psychiatry Res.*, **72**, 161–166.

Goldberg, T.E. and Gold, J.M (1995). Neurocognitive deficits in schizophrenia. In: *Schizophrenia* (S.R. Hirsch and D.R. Weinberger, eds.). Blackwell: Oxford, 146–162.

Goldberg, T.E. and Weinberger, D.R. (1994). The effects of clozapine on neurocognition: an overview. *J. Clin. Psychiatry*, **55** (suppl. B), 88–90.

Goldberg, T. E., Greenberg, D. R., Griffin, S. J., *et al.* (1993). The effect of clozapine on cognition and psychiatric symptoms in patients with schizophrenia. *Br. J. Psychiatry*, **162**, 43–48.

Grace, J., Bellus, S. B., Raulin, M. L., *et al.* (1996). Long-term impact of clozapine and psychosocial treatment on psychiatric symptoms and cognitive functioning. *Psychiatric Services*, **47**, 41–45.

Hagger, C., Buckley, P., Kenny, J. T., *et al.* (1993). Improvement in cognitive functions and psychiatric symptoms in treatment-refractory schizophrenic patients receiving clozapine. *Biol. Psychiatry*, **34**, 702–712.

Hoff, A. L., Faustman, W. O., Wieneke, M., *et al.* (1996). The effects of clozapine on symptom reduction, neurocognitive function, and clinical management in treatment-refractory state hospital schizophrenic inpatients. *Neuropsychopharmacology*, **15**, 361–369.

Juul-Povlsen, U., Noring, U., Fog, R., *et al.* (1985). Tolerability and therapeutic effect of clozapine. A retrospective investigation of 216 patients treated with clozapine for up to 12 years. *Acta Psychiatr. Scand.*, **71**, 176–185.

Kane, J., Honigfeld, G., Singer, J., Meltzer, H. and the Clozaril Collaborative Study Group (1988). Clozapine for the treatment-resistant schizophrenia: a double-blind comparison with chlorpromazine. *Arch. Gen. Psychiatry*, **45**, 789–796.

Kane, J.M., Woerner, M.G., Pollack, S., *et al.* (1993). Does clozapine cause tardive dyskinesia? *J. Clin. Psychiatry*, **54**, 327–330.

Kimmel, S.E., Calabrese, J.R., Woyshville, M.J., *et al.* (1994). Clozapine in treatment refractory mood disorders. *J. Clin. Psychiatry*, **55** (suppl. B), 91–93.

Kuoppasalmi, K., Rimon, R., Neukkarinen, H., *et al.* (1993). The use of clozapine in treatment-refractory schizophrenia. *Schizophr. Res.*, **10**, 29–32.

Laws, K. and McKenna, P.J. (1997). Psychotic symptoms and cognitive deficits: what relationship? *Neurocase*, **3**, 41–50.

Levkovitch, Y., Kronenberg, J., Kayser, N., *et al.* (1995). Clozapine for tardive dyskinesia in adolescents. *Brain and Development*, **17**, 213–215.

Lieberman, J. A., Safferman, A. Z., Pollack, S., *et al.* (1994). Clinical effects of clozapine in chronic schizophrenia: response to treatment and predictors of outcome. *Am. J. Psychiatry*, **151**, 1744–1752.

Lindenmayer, J-P., Grochowski, S. and Mabugat, L. (1994). Clozapine effects on positive and negative symptoms: a six-month trial in treatment-refractory schizophrenics. *J. Clin. Psychopharmacol.*, **14**, 201–204.

Mallya, A. R., Roos, P. D. and Roebuck-Colgan, K. (1992). Restraint, seclusion, and clozapine. *J. Clin. Psychiatry*, **53**, 395–397.

McKay, A. P., McKenna, P. J. and Laws, K. (1996). Severe schizophrenia: what is it like? In: *Methods in Madness: Case Studies in Cognitive Neuropsychiatry* (P. Halligan and J. Marshall, eds). Hove: Erlbaum, 95–122.

McKenna, P.J. and Bailey, P.E. (1993). The strange story of clozapine. *Br. J. Psychiatry*, **162**, 32–37.

Meltzer, H. Y. (1992). Dimensions of outcome with clozapine. *Br. J. Psychiatry*, **160**, 46–53.

Meltzer, H. Y. and Okayli, G. (1995). Reduction of suicidality during clozapine treatment of neuroleptic-resistant schizophrenia: impact on risk-benefit assessment. *Am. J. Psychiatry*, **152**, 183–190.

Meltzer, H. Y., Bernett, S., Bastani, B., *et al.* (1990). Effects of six months of clozapine treatment on the quality of life of chronic schizophrenic patients. *Hosp. Comm. Psychiatry*, **41**, 892–897.

Miller, D. D., Perry, P. J., Cadoret, R. J., *et al.* (1994). Clozapine's effect on negative symptoms in treatment-refractory schizophrenics. *Compr. Psychiatry*, **35**, 8–15.

Perry, P.J., Miller, D.D., Arndt, S.V., *et al.* (1991). Clozapine and norclozapine plasma concentrations and clinical response of treatment-refractory schizophrenic patients. *Am. J. Psychiatry*, **148**, 231–235.

Pickar, D., Owen, R. R., Litman, R. E., *et al.* (1992). Clinical and biologic response to clozapine in patients with schizophrenia: crossover comparison with fluphenazine. *Arch. Gen. Psychiatry*, **49**, 345–353.

Ranjan, R. and Meltzer, H.Y. (1996). Acute and long-term effectiveness of clozapine in treatment-resistant psychotic depression. *Biol. Psychiatry*, **40**, 253–258.

Shapleske, J., McKay, A. P. and McKenna, P. J. (1996). Successful treatment of tardive dystonia with clozapine and clonazepam. *Br. J. Psychiatry*, **168**, 516–518.

Shiloh, R., Zemishlany, Z., Aizenberg, D., *et al.* (1997). Sulpiride augmentation in people with schizophrenia partially responsive to clozapine. *Br. J. Psychiatry*, **171**, 569–573.

Tandon, R., Goldman, R., DeQuardo, J. R., *et al.* (1993). Positive and negative symptoms covary during clozapine treatment in schizophrenia. *J. Psychiatr. Res.*, **27**, 341–347.

Volavka, J., Zito, J. M., Vitrai, J., *et al.* (1993). Clozapine effects on hostility and aggression in schizophrenia. *J. Clin. Psychopharmacol.*, **13**, 287–289.

Wilson, W. H. (1992). Clinical review of clozapine treatment in a state hospital. *Hosp. Comm. Psychiatry*, **343**, 700–703.

Wittenberg, N., Stein, D., Barak, Y., *et al.* (1996). Clozapine and tardive dyskinesia: analysis of clinical trials. *Pathophysiology*, **3**, 241–245.

4

Risperidone and olanzapine: clinical use and experience

W. Wolfgang Fleischhacker and Stephen Marder

Key points

- Risperidone and olanzapine are each widely used both in USA and Europe for treating psychosis.
- Risperidone dosages have decreased to below the original recommended dose since its introduction, while the opposite has occurred with olanzapine.
- Risperidone has a dose-related EPS profile and causes prolactin elevation. Olanzapine has a less pronounced EPS profile and does not elevate prolactin. However, it is more sedating and causes more weight gain than typical and other atypical antipsychotics (except clozapine).
- Currently, the efficacy of risperidone and olanzapine in treatment-refractory schizophrenia is not well established.

Introduction

The introduction of risperidone and olanzapine in the early 1990s resulted in a substantial improvement in the pharmacotherapy of schizophrenia and other psychotic disorders. Both of these agents are effective antipsychotics and both result in substantially less extrapyramidal side effects (EPS) than older antipsychotic agents. Moreover, there is substantial evidence that these characteristics are related to the activity of these agents at both 5-HT_{2A} and D_2 receptors. In contrast to clozapine, risperidone and olanzapine have a mild side-effect profile and neither requires blood monitoring. For these reasons, both agents have been widely accepted by clinicians and patients and are commonly prescribed as 'first-line' agents. Recent research, focusing mainly on the clinical profiles of the two drugs, is outlined in the following chapter.

Overview of risperidone

Risperidone is a structurally and pharmacologically novel antipsychotic introduced in 1994. As a benzisoxazole derivative, it is structurally different from most of the other novel antipsychotics, including clozapine. Risperidone blocks serotonin, dopamine and noradrenaline receptors with a stronger anti-5-HT_2 than anti-D_2 activity (Leysen *et al.*, 1988). The half-life of the drug is reported to be between 2.8 and 16 hours. The main metabolite, 9-hydroxy-risperidone, has a half-life of 20–22 hours (Heykants *et al.*, 1994). As 9-hydroxy-risperidone is pharmacologically active to a similar extent as its parent compound, both agents together constitute the biologically active moiety (Heykants *et al.*, 1994). The main metabolism route of risperidone is via the hepatic cytochrome P450-2D6 system. 9-Hydroxy-risperidone is mainly eliminated through the kidneys (Mannens *et al.*, 1993). Older patients have been reported to have a reduced plasma clearance by about 30% (Snoeck *et al.*, 1995) which would suggest use of lower doses in the elderly.

In clinical trials 1–16 mg risperidone daily have been evaluated. Current recommendations state to use 1–8 mg risperidone per day.

Efficacy of risperidone for acute schizophrenia

Two large multicentre trials including over 1700 patients were the pivotal studies for the registration of risperidone (Marder and Meibach, 1994; Peuskens and the Risperidone Study Group, 1995). Both trials, one placebo-controlled and using 20 mg haloperidol as the reference antipsychotic (Marder and Meibach, 1994), the other employing a 10 mg haloperidol reference group (Peuskens and the Risperidone Study Group, 1995), and risperidone doses of 1–16 mg daily, reported antipsychotic efficacy that was significantly better than placebo and similar to haloperidol at most dosages. This was true both if Positive and Negative Symptom Scale (PANSS, Kay *et al.*, 1987) total scores were compared between groups, and if a 20% improvement criterion on the PANSS was employed. A number of other controlled double-blind clinical trials have been reported comparing risperidone to placebo or various other antipsychotics including haloperidol (Borison *et al.*, 1992; Claus *et al.*, 1992; Chouinard *et al.*, 1993), perphenazine (Høyberg *et al.*, 1993), zuclopenthixol (Huttunen *et al.*, 1995), olanzapine (Tran *et al.*, 1997) and clozapine (Heinrich *et al.*, 1994). In a recent meta-analysis, Bech *et al.* (1998) have reported that the antipsychotic effect size favours risperidone over various comparators (haloperidol, zuclopenthixol and perphenazine). Two studies were carried out with patients suffering from first episode schizophreniform or schizophrenic disorder (Kopala *et al.*, 1997; Emsley and the Risperidone Working Group, 1999). Both studies have found considerably higher response rates than those reported in the trials with more chronically ill patient groups. This amounted to 63% of risperidone treated patients improving more than 50% on the PANSS in the report by Emsley and the Risperidone Working Group (1999). In both studies patients on lower doses of risperidone (2–4 mg/day, Kopala *et al.*, 1997; less than 6 mg/day, Emsley and the Risperidone Working Group, 1999) fared better than patients on higher doses, suggesting that patients with first episode schizophrenia may require lower doses of risperidone. The same appears to hold true for older patients. In an open trial in schizophrenic or schizoaffective patients with a mean age of 71 years, a mean of 2.4 mg risperidone daily led to a more than 20% PANSS total reduction in 50% of the patients (Madhusoodanan *et al.*, 1999). PANSS reductions were higher in patients treated with less than 3 mg/day than in patients treated with 3–6 mg/day. Risperidone has also been shown to be efficacious against negative symptoms of schizophrenia in acutely ill patients who suffered from both positive and negative symptoms concomitantly (Marder and Meibach, 1994; Peuskens and the Risperidone Study Group, 1995). This is considered to be at least partially independent of an improvement in extrapyramidal motor symptoms (Möller et al., 1995).

When evaluated in terms of its efficacy against cognitive dysfunction in schizophrenia, risperidone was shown to improve verbal memory to a significantly higher degree than haloperidol (Green et al., 1997).

Risperidone has also been used successfully in psychotic children and adolescents (Mandoki, 1995; Simeon et al., 1995; Sternlicht and Wells, 1995) according to case reports.

Risperidone was also compared with a combination of haloperidol and amitriptyline in a 6-week study in patients with coexisting psychotic and depressive symptoms suffering from either schizoaffective disorder, depressive type, major depression with psychotic features or non-residual schizophrenia with major depressive symptoms. While patients suffering from depression with psychotic features did better when receiving the haloperidol–amitriptyline combination, both types of treatment were equally helpful for patients with the other two diagnoses. In the overall sample, the combination was significantly better than risperidone monotherapy. The authors state that this is mostly due to the advantages of the combination in the treatment of depressive patients with psychotic features (Müller-Siecheneder et al., 1998).

Maintenance therapy with risperidone

Only limited published data are available concerning the long-term efficacy of risperidone. Preliminary evidence from an open 1-year continuation study suggests that risperidone maintained its antipsychotic effect beyond the 8-week double-blind study period (Lindström et al., 1995).

When choosing a worsening in the PANSS total score of more than 20% as the relevant event, 67.7% of all patients treated with risperidone in the above mentioned study by Tran et al. (1997) maintained response over 28 weeks. This was significantly less than the 87.9% maintaining response on olanzapine.

In a retrospective pharmacoeconomic evaluation Chouinard et al. (1993) calculated a better cost utility ratio for risperidone than haloperidol.

Side effects of risperidone

The most striking advantage of the novel antipsychotics as a group is their significantly reduced propensity to induce extrapyramidal motor side effects (EPS) (Fleischhacker and Hummer, 1997; Fleischhacker, 1999). This is also a characteristic of risperidone, which is evident in most of the above mentioned trials comparing the drug to a traditional antipsychotic. When comparing risperidone to olanzapine, it was found, at a rather high mean dose of 7.2 mg/day, to induce more EPS than 17.2 mg olanzapine daily (Tran et al., 1997). Two clozapine comparison studies (Heinrich et al., 1994; Bondolfi et al., 1998) found no differences in terms of EPS risk between risperidone and clozapine. These latter findings could not be substantiated by a point prevalence study in which patients on a stable regimen of either clozapine, risperidone or traditional antipsychotics were evaluated for EPS risk (Miller *et al.*, 1998). In this study, risperidone was found to have a higher EPS risk than clozapine and a lower risk compared to conventional antipsychotics.

In a combined analysis of 12 double-blind studies including a total of 2074 risperidone-treated patients assessed by the Extrapyramidal Symptom Rating Scale (ESRS, Chouinard *et al.*, 1980) EPS severity was found to be significantly greater in patients receiving haloperidol or other traditional antipsychotics than in those receiving 4–8 mg/day of risperidone. Risperidone patients also required significantly less antiparkinsonian medication (Lemmens *et al.*, 1999).

Summarizing the available evidence, it can be concluded that doses amounting to less than 8 mg risperidone daily lead to a significantly lower risk of acute EPS than treatment with classical antipsychotic drugs. Risperidone appears to be different from the other novel antipsychotics in so far as there is a well defined dose/EPS-risk relationship with risperidone, which so far has not been reliably demonstrated for any other of the new drugs.

Unfortunately, few published data on risperidone-induced tardive dyskinesia are available. Lemmens *et al.* (1999), reporting an incidence rate of 0.1%, concede themselves that these numbers may underestimate true indicence rates as they are based on spontaneous reporting rather than rating scale based findings.

Despite the fact that novel antipsychotics carry significant advantages over classical drugs in terms of EPS risk, it must not be forgotten that non-EPS associated adverse events are also of clinical relevance. With risperidone treatment, these include weight gain, orthostatic hypotension and increased prolactin levels. Weight gain has been consistently found in clinical trials. Orthostatic hypotension is most likely due to risperidone's alpha-antagonism. Patients are at highest risk during the early stages of treatment; therefore the manufacturer has recommended a dose titration schedule over the first days of treatment, starting at 1 or 2 mg daily with 1–2 mg dose increments on the following treatment days.

In an analysis of four randomized double-blind clinical trials of risperidone, prolactin levels following risperidone treatment were significantly higher than those measured in patients treated with haloperidol 10 mg/day (Kleinberg *et al.*, 1999). Again, there appears to be a dose dependency for this effect. In an attempt to correlate prolactin increase with potentially prolactin-related sexual adverse effects, no correlations between plasma prolactin and these side effects could be detected in females. In male patients, on the other hand, who showed a higher incidence of sexual dysfunctions, there was a significant correlation between prolactin levels and decreased libido in the overall sample. In female patients, amenorrhoea was the most commonly reported sexual adverse event; in male patients erectile and ejaculatory dysfunctions were most commonly found, albeit at a similar rate to haloperidol.

Risperidone in treatment-refractory patients

Bondolfi *et al.* (1998) studied schizophrenic patients who were either resistant or intolerant to treatment with classical antipsychotics. They compared the efficacy of 6.4 mg of risperidone daily to a mean of 291 mg/day of clozapine and found that over 65% of patients in both groups showed 20% or more improvement on the PANSS in an 8-week study of 86 inpatients.

Overview of olanzapine

Olanzapine is an antipsychotic agent which was introduced in the USA and Europe in 1996. It can be classified as a serotonin-dopamine antagonist since it has substantial affinity for both 5-HT_{2a} and D_2. However, olanzapine is also a complex agent with activity at 5-HT_{2c}, 5HT_3, 5HT_6, α_1, D_1, D_4, M_1 and H_1 receptors. Studies using positron emission tomography indicate that at its effective dose range of 5–20 mg/day it occupies approximately 43–80% of D_2 and near saturation of 5-HT_{2A} receptors (Kapur *et al.*, 1998; Nordstrom *et al.*, 1998). This suggests that its antipsychotic efficacy is associated with greater dopamine receptor activity than clozapine, an agent that has a similar receptor profile. Despite this profile, olanzapine is associated with minimal extrapyramidal side effect (EPS) in its effective antipsychotic dose range.

Orally administered olanzapine has a half-life about 31 hours which indicates that patients can be treated with a single daily dose. Since it has relatively weak affinity for hepatic P450 cytochromes, it is unlikely to be associated with significant drug–drug interactions.

Efficacy of olanzapine for acute schizophrenia

The largest study of olanzapine was an international trial in which patients received 5–20 mg of either haloperidol or olanzapine (Tollefson *et al.*, 1997). Clinicians titrated olanzapine patients to a mean dose of 13.2 mg daily and haloperidol patients were titrated to 11.8 mg. Since this study included 1996 patients, it provides useful information regarding the relative efficacy of the two agents. Olanzapine was significantly more effective than haloperidol in improving total scores on the Brief Psychiatric Rating Scale (BPRS). In addition, negative symptoms on the PANSS demonstrated greater improvement on olanzapine. Depressive symptoms as measured by the Montgomery-Asberg Depression Rating Scale (MADRS) also demonstrated significantly greater improvement with olanzapine. There was no significant difference in positive symptoms.

Olanzapine's effectiveness was also evaluated in a double-blind comparison of three dose ranges of olanzapine (2.5–7.5, 7.5–12.5, 12.5–17.5 mg/day), haloperidol (10–20 mg/day) or placebo in 335 patients with schizophrenia (Beasley *et al.*, 1996). The middle and highest doses of olanzapine and haloperidol (that is, 7.5–17.5 mg/day) were more effective than placebo on total BPRS as well as positive symptoms. Both the low dose and high dose ranges of olanzapine (but not the middle range or haloperidol) were more effective than placebo on the Scale for the Assessment of Negative Symptoms (SANS). This study indicates that the higher dose range of 12.5–17.5 mg/day is probably the most appropriate for treating acute psychosis in schizophrenia. This is also consistent with the experiences of clinicians who have prescribed olanzapine since its introduction. In the USA, the average dose of olanzapine for acute schizophrenia is in the range of 15–20 mg daily.

Side effects of olanzapine

One of the most striking advantages of olanzapine is its side-effect profile. Since antipsychotics in the pre-clozapine era were nearly always associated with discomforting side effects at their most effective doses, one of the difficult dilemmas for clinicians was how to convince patients to continue taking medications that made them feel miserable. This discomfort resulted from the activity of drugs at a number of receptor sites, but was usually related to extrapyramidal effects resulting from D_2 blockade.

An overview of a drug's side-effect profile can be gained from comparing the agent to placebo. In the study by Beasley and co-workers (Beasley *et al.*, 1996), the most common side effects of olanzapine were somnolence (39% versus 16% on placebo), dizziness (17% versus 3% on placebo) and constipation (15% versus 0% on placebo). Only 5.8% of the patients who received the higher dose range (12.5–17.5 mg daily) were discontinued because of adverse effects (compared to 10.3% on placebo). This indicates that olanzapine is very well tolerated in acute treatment.

The large study ($n = 1996$) comparing 5–20 mg of olanzapine and haloperidol provides an opportunity to compare olanzapine with a conventional antipsychotic (Tollefson *et al.*, 1997). Patients who received haloperidol were more likely to experience extrapyramidal side effects, psychomotor activation, vomiting, and weight loss whereas those who received olanzapine were more likely to experience dry mouth, weight gain, and increased appetite (Beasley *et al.*, 1997). Those who received haloperidol were more likely to have their medication discontinued for adverse effects (7.3%) than those who received olanzapine (4.5%).

Measures of EPS support olanzapine's low liability. In the above mentioned double-blind studies (Beasley *et al.*, 1996; Tollefson *et al.*, 1997) rates of EPS as measured by the Simpson-Angus Scale were substantially and significantly higher on haloperidol. In the study by Beasley *et al.*, EPS ratings were no greater on olanzapine than on placebo. Another method of comparing EPS on two agents is to compare the use of anticholinergic medications for EPS. The proportion of patients receiving anticholinergics on olanzapine and placebo was similar. In addition, rates of akathisia as measured by the Barnes Akathisia Scale were similar on olanzapine and placebo. These findings, as well as clinical experience, indicate that olanzapine is associated with very little EPS in doses up to 17.5 mg. There are no data available regarding EPS at doses of 20 mg or more daily.

As mentioned earlier, olanzapine is associated with a risk for weight gain. In acute studies weight gain was in the range of 2–3 kg (Beasley *et al.*, 1997). When the results of several studies were combined, 40.5% of olanzapine patients gained 7% or more of their weight compared to 12.4% of patients who received haloperidol. These data are consistent with the observations of clinicians who have confirmed that weight gain is one of the most common adverse effects associated with olanzapine treatment.

Olanzapine appears to be less likely to elevate prolactin above normal levels when compared with conventional dopamine receptor antagonists. Although it is associated with transient prolactin elevation, patients treated with olanzapine had levels that returned to the normal range (Beasley *et al.*, 1997). This is an important advantage of olanzapine since women on conventional agents tend to develop irregular menstrual periods or galactorrhoea.

Starting patients on olanzapine

Olanzapine can be prescribed at an initial dose of 5 mg in the elderly or patients who have a history of being sensitive to medications. Others can be treated with a starting dose of 10 mg. Most patients with schizophrenia will respond to doses in the range of 10–20 mg daily but some will require 25 mg. Case reports suggest that some patients respond to higher doses. Elderly patients should be treated with 2.5–7.5 mg/day. As mentioned earlier, olanzapine can be administered in a single daily dose.

Maintenance therapy with olanzapine

The effectiveness of olanzapine in preventing relapse was evaluated in double-blind extensions of acute studies (Dellva *et al.*, 1997). The first study included individuals who were treated with one of three dose ranges of olanzapine (2.5–7.5, 7.5–12.5, or 12.5–17.5 mg/day) or placebo. The subjects were those individuals who were defined as responders during the acute phase. Among the patients who entered the 46-week extension, 71.4% of olanzapine patients and 30.1% of placebo patients maintained their response ($P = 0.002$). Olanzapine was also compared with haloperidol in an analysis that pooled trials that compared olanzapine ($n = 627$) and haloperidol ($n = 180$). Survival rates were 80.3% on olanzapine and 72.0% on haloperidol ($P = 0.03$). Taken together, these studies provide strong support that olanzapine is effective for preventing relapse in schizophrenia.

There is also evidence that olanzapine can lead to improvements in quality of life. In a study using the Quality of Life Scale (QLS) (Heinrichs *et al.*, 1984), the authors found that total QLS was significantly improved on the medium ($P = 0.01$) and higher ($P = 0.04$) doses of olanzapine compared to placebo (Hamilton *et al.*, 1998).

Olanzapine in treatment-refractory patients

Twenty-five per cent or more of patients with schizophrenia demonstrate minimal or no improvement when they receive an antipsychotic. As a result, these treatment-resistant patients represent one of the most common problems in the management of schizophrenia. In a study using severely-ill hospitalized patients, Conley and co-workers (1998) compared 25 mg/day of olanzapine with 1200 mg of chlorpromazine (combined with benztropine). The two agents showed similar effectiveness with both treatment groups having relatively low rates of response. However, olanzapine was better tolerated. A more recent paper (Breier and Hamilton, 1999) found that olanzapine was more effective than haloperidol in treatment-refractory patients. In addition to demonstrating greater improvement in both positive and negative symptoms, olanzapine-treated patients also experienced milder side effects.

Conclusion

In summary, both olanzapine and risperidone are important additions to the therapeutic armamentarium for the treatment of patients suffering from schizophrenia and related disorders. Especially for olanzapine, but also to a certain extent for risperidone, most of the published evidence stems from phases II and III of clinical development. This may lead to problems as current changes in risperidone and olanzapine dosing show. While the dosing recommendations for risperidone are being lowered following post-marketing research, olanzapine, which has been shown to be effective at 10 mg daily in phase III, is being used at considerably higher doses in clinical practice.

As both drugs appear to be safer alternatives to traditional neuroleptics, most hope is based in their use in the long-term management of patients. Given better EPS profiles and a potential advantage in terms of enhancing cognitive functions they should also help to enhance the results of psycho-rehabilitative measures, whereby the outcome of schizophrenia may be improved.

References

Beasley, C.M. Jr, Tollefson, G., Tran, P., et al. (1996). Olanzapine versus placebo and haloperidol: acute phase results of the North American double-blind olanzapine trial. Neuropsychopharmacology, 14, 111–123.

Beasley, C.M. Jr, Tollefson, G. and Tran, P. (1997). Safety of olanzapine. J. Clin. Psychiatry, 58 (suppl. 10), 13–17.

Bech, P., Peuskens, J., Marder, S.R., et al. (1998). Meta-analytic study of the benefits and risks of treating chronic schizophrenia with risperidone or conventional neuroleptics. Europ. Psychiatry, 13, 310–314.

Borison, R.L., Pathiraja, A.P., Diamond, B.I., et al. (1992). Risperidone: clinical safety and efficacy in schizophrenia. Psychopharmacol. Bull., 28, 213–218.

Breier, A. and Hamilton, S.H. (1999). Comparative efficacy of olanzapine and haloperidol for patients with treatment-resistant schizophrenia. Biol. Psychiatry 45 (4), 403–411.

Chouinard, G., Ross-Chouinard, A., Annable, L., et al. (1980). Extrapyramidal Symptoms Rating Scale. Can. J. Neurol. Sci., 7, 233.

Chouinard, G., Jones, B., Remington, G., et al. (1993). A Canadian mulicenter placebo-controlled study of fixed doses of risperidone and haloperidol in the treatment of chronic schizophrenic patients. J. Clin. Psychopharmacol., 13, 25–40.

Claus, A., Bollen, J., De Cuyper, H., et al. (1992). Risperidone versus haloperidol in the treatment of chronic schizophrenic inpatients: a multicentre double-blind comparative study. Acta Psychiatr. Scand., 85, 295–305.

Conley, R.R., Tamminga, C.A., Bartko, J.J., et al. (1998) Olanzapine compared with chlorpromazine in treatment resistant schizophrenia. Am. J. Psychiatry, 155, 914–921.

Dellva, M.A., Tran, P., Tollefson, G.D., *et al.* (1997). Standard olanzapine versus placebo and ineffective-dose olanzapine in the maintenance treatment of schizophrenia. *Psychiatr. Serv.*, **48**, 1571–1577.

Emsley, R.A. and the Risperidone Working Group (1999). Risperidone in the treatment of first-episode psychotic patients: a double-blind multicenter study. *Schizophr. Bull.* (in press).

Fleischhacker, W.W. (1999). The pharmacology of schizophrenia. *Curr. Opinion Psychiatry*, **12**, 53–59.

Fleischhacker, W.W. and Hummer, M. (1997). Drug treatment of schizophrenia in the 1990s. *Drugs*, **53**, 915–929.

Green, M., Marshall, B., Wirshing, W., *et al.* (1997). Does risperidone improve verbal working memory in treatment-resistant schizophrenia? *Am. J. Psychiatry*, **154**, 799–804.

Hamilton, S.H., Revicki, D.A., Genduso, L.A., *et al.* (1998). Olanzapine versus placebo and haloperidol: quality of life and efficacy results of the North American double-blind trial. *Neuropsychopharmacology*, **18**, 41–49.

Heinrich, K., Klieser, E., Lehmann, E., *et al.* (1994). Risperidone versus clozapine in the treatment of schizophrenic patients with acute symptoms: a double-blind, randomized trial. *Prog. Neuropsychopharmacol. Biol. Psychiatry*, **18**, 129–137.

Heinrichs, D.W., Hanlon, T.E. and Carpenter, W.T. (1984). The quality of life scale: An instrument for rating the schizophrenic deficit syndrome. *Schizophr. Bull.*, **10**, 388–398.

Heykants, J., Huang, M.L., Mannens, G., *et al.* (1994). The pharmacokinetics of risperidone in humans: a summary. *J. Clin. Psychiatry*, **55**, 13–17.

Høyberg, O.J., Fensbo, C., Remvig, J., *et al.* (1993). Risperidone versus perphenazine in the treatment of chronic schizophrenic patients with acute exacerbation. *Acta Psychiatr. Scand.*, **88**, 395–402.

Huttunen, M.O., Pieponne, T., Rantanen, H., *et al.* (1995). Risperidone versus zuclopenthixol in the treatment of acute schizophrenic episodes: a double-blind parallel-group trial. *Acta Psychiatr. Scand.*, **91**, 271–277.

Kapur, S., Zipursky, R.B., Remington, G., *et al.* (1998). $5HT_2$ and D_2 receptor occupancy of olanzapine in schizophrenia: A PET investigation. *Am. J. Psychiatry*, **155**, 921–928.

Kay, S.R., Fiszbein, A. and Opler, L.A. (1987). The Positive and Negative Syndrome Scale (PANSS) for schizophrenia. *Schizophr. Bull.*, **13**, 261–276.

Kleinberg, D.L., Davis, J.M., De Coster, R., *et al.* (1999). Prolactin levels and adverse events in patients treated with risperidone. *J. Clin. Psychopharmacol.*, **19** (1), 57–61.

Kopala, L.C., Good, K.P. and Honer, W.G. (1997). Extrapyramidal signs and clinical symptoms in first-episode schizophrenia: response to low-dose risperidone. *J. Clin. Psychopharmacol.*, **17**, 308–313.

Lemmens, P., Brecher, M. and Van Baelen, B. (1999). A combined analysis of double-blind studies with risperidone versus placebo and other antipsychotic agents: Factors associated with extrapyramidal symptoms. *Acta Psychiatr. Scand.* **99** (3), 160–170.

Leysen, J.E., Gommeren, W., Eens, A., *et al.* (1988). The biochemical profile of risperidone, a new antipsychotic. *J. Pharmacol. Exp. Ther.*, **247**, 661–670.

Lindström, E., Eriksson, B., Hellgren, A., *et al.* (1995). Efficacy and safety of risperidone in the long-term treatment of patients with schizophrenia. *Clin. Ther.*, **17**, 402–412.

Madhusoodanan, S., Brecher, M., Brenner, R., *et al.* (1999). Risperidone in the treatment of elderly patients with psychotic disorders. *Am. J. Geriatr. Psychiatry*, **7**, 132–138.

Mandoki, M.W. (1995). Risperidone treatment of children and adolescents: increased risk of extrapyramidal side effects? *J. Child Adolesc. Psychopharmacol.*, **5**, 49–67.

Mannens, G., Huang, M.L., Meuldermans, W., *et al.* (1993). Absorption, metabolism, and excretion of risperidone in humans. *Drug Metab. Dis.*, **21**, 1134–1141.

Marder, S.R. and Meibach, R.C. (1994). Risperidone in the treatment of schizophrenia. *Am. J. Psychiatry*, **151**, 825–835.

Miller, C.H., Mohr, F., Umbricht, D., *et al.* (1998). The prevalence of acute extrapyramidal signs and symptoms in patients treated with clozapine, risperidone, and conventional antipsychotics. *J. Clin. Psychiatry*, **59**, 69–75.

Möller, H.J., Müller, H., Borison, R.L., *et al.* (1995). A path-analytical approach to differentiate between direct and indirect drug effects on negative symptoms in schizophrenic patients: a re-evaluation of the North American risperidone study. *Eur. Arch. Psychiatry Clin. Neurosci.*, **245**, 45–49.

Müller-Siecheneder, F., Müller, M.J., Hillert, A., *et al.* (1998). Risperidone versus haloperidol and amitriptyline in the treatment of patients with a combined psychotic and depressive syndrome. *J. Clin. Psychopharmacol.*, **18**, 111–119.

Nordstrom, A.L., Nyberg, S., Olsson, H., *et al.* (1998). Positron emission tomography finding of a high striatal D2 receptor occupancy in olanzapine-treated patients. *Arch. Gen. Psychiatry*, **55**, 283–284.

Peuskens, J. and the Risperidone Study Group (1995). Risperidone in the treatment of patients with chronic schizophrenia: a multi-national, multi-centre, double-blind, parallel-group study versus haloperidol. *Br. J. Psychiatry*, **166**, 712–726.

Simeon, J.G., Carrey, N.J., Wiggins, D.M., *et al.* (1995). Risperidone effects in treatment-resistant adolescents: preliminary case reports. *J. Child Adolesc. Psychopharmacol.*, **5**, 69–79.

Snoeck, E., Van Peer, A., Sack, M., *et al.* (1995). Influence of age, renal and liver impairment on the pharmacokinetics of risperidone in man. *Psychopharmacology*, **122**, 223–229.

Sternlicht, H.C. and Wells, S.R. (1995). Risperidone in childhood schizophrenia. *J. Am. Acad. Child Adolesc. Psychiatry*, **34**, 5.

Tollefson, G.D., Beasley, C.M. Jr, Tran, P.V., *et al.* (1997). Olanzapine versus haloperidol in the treatment of schizophrenia and schizoaffective and schizophreniform disorders: results of an international collaborative trial. *Am. J. Psychiatry*, **154**, 457–465.

Tran, F.V., Hamilton, S.H., Kuntz, A.J., *et al.* (1997). Double-blind comparison of olanzapine versus risperidone in the treatment of schizophrenia and other psychotic disorders. *J. Clin. Psychopharmacol.*, **17**, 408–417.

5

Quetiapine and sertindole: clinical use and experience

Peter Buckley and Dieter Naber

Key points

- Quetiapine is available in both Europe and the USA. Current prescribing practices for quetiapine are to use doses of 300–750 mg daily for most patients. Sertindole, not available in the USA and currently of restricted use in Europe, is prescribed at doses of 12–24 mg daily.
- Both quetiapine and sertindole have favourable (placebo-like) EPS profiles with no evidence of dose-related EPS in clinical studies.
- Unlike typical antipsychotics, both of these drugs are free of sustained hyperprolactinaemia.
- Sertindole is associated with retrograde ejaculation in approximately 5% of male patients.
- Quetiapine is less likely than other antipsychotics to cause sexual dysfunction.
- Both drugs are effective for treating positive and negative symptoms of schizophrenia, with sertindole showing superiority over typical antipsychotics in the amelioration of negative symptoms.

Clinical pharmacology

Quetiapine is a dibenzothiazepine compound which has affinity for multiple CNS receptors, most particularly serotonin receptor subtypes 5-HT_{2A} and 5-HT_6 (Meats, 1997). In contrast to the low potency typical antipsychotics and the newer agents clozapine and olanzapine, quetiapine has very low affinity for muscarinic receptors and consequently its propensity for anticholinergic side effects is negligible. It is also noteworthy that quetiapine's mild D_2 receptor blockade is associated with an absence of sustained hyperprolactinaemia in clinical practice. This is likely to account for the relative absence of sexual side effects during quetiapine therapy.

Quetiapine has a short half-life of approximately 7 hours. As a consequence, a twice daily (bid) dosing schedule is recommended. The drug is metabolized by the P450 hepatic cytochrome system, specifically the CYP3A4 pathway. While haloperidol, risperidone or lithium do not affect quetiapine's metabolism, coadministration of thioridazine, carbamazepine, or phenytoin may lower quetiapine levels (Weiden, 1997). There is no evidence yet that determining plasma levels of quetiapine or its metabolites is of benefit in predicting treatment response. Although quetiapine has several metabolites, its therapeutic effect is confined to the primary drug.

Sertindole is a phenylindol derivative with high affinity for serotonin-5-HT_2: dopamine D_2 and α_1-adrenergic receptors. It has a low affinity for α_2-adrenergic, histamine H_1 and σ-receptors; its affinity for 5-HT_{1A}, cholinergic or β-adrenergic receptors is negligible (Sanchez et al., 1991; Hyttel et al., 1992). In vivo, sertindole has demonstrated approximately 100-fold selectivity in the inhibition of activity of ventral segmental area over substantia nigra pars compacta dopaminergic neurons (Skarsfeldt and Perregaard, 1990). These data indicate that sertindole might have an antipsychotic effect with limited if any motor side effects.

Its steady-state clearance is 10–12 hours and the half-life is 73 hours; time to peak plasma level is approximately 10 hours. The drug is well absorbed with oral administration and highly protein-bound. The two major metabolites, dehydrosertindole and norsertindole, account for approximately 60% and 40% of the parent compound at steady-state. However, neither metabolite participates significantly in the drug's clinical effects (Hyttel et al., 1992).

Efficacy in clinical practice

Quetiapine was made available in the USA in 1997 and in Europe during 1998. Accordingly, there is limited experience over time with the use of this drug in clinical practice. Moreover, available data from clinical studies are predominantly from short-term, placebo-controlled trials of quetiapine compared with either haloperidol or chlorpromazine (Arvantis et al., 1997; Meats, 1997; Small et al., 1997). These studies consistently confirm quetiapine's efficacy as an antipsychotic. It has been shown to be superior to placebo across positive and negative symptoms and in global functioning. In a 6-week placebo controlled comparison study of low dose quetiapine (less than 250 mg daily; mean dose 209 mg) versus high dose quetiapine (up to 750 mg daily; mean dose 360 mg), the high dose outperformed the lower dose of quetiapine (Small et al., 1997). In a placebo-controlled comparative, 6-week study of quetiapine (5 doses: 75 mg up to 750 mg daily) versus haloperidol (12 mg daily), quetiapine at doses of above 150 mg daily was superior to placebo and equiefficacious to haloperidol (Arvantis et al., 1997). Results of a quetiapine–chlorpromazine trial also showed equiefficacy (Meats, 1997). In contrast to results from clinical trials on other new antipsychotics, these studies have not shown any clinical superiority (on the measures above) for quetiapine over the comparator drugs. On current evidence, quetiapine appears equiefficacious to typical antipsychotics. In

Table 5.1 A schematic representation of the comparative efficacy of antipsychotic medications

Drug	Positive symptoms	Negative symptoms	Cognitive deficits	Quality of life	Suicidality	Aggression
Haloperidol	+	0	0	−	+	+
Quetiapine	+	+/−	?	+	?	+/−
Sertindole	+	+	?	+	?	?

this regard, it is surprising in view of its excellent EPS profile that this drug did not show superiority over the atypicals in global measures of negative symptoms which are often confounded (and conflated) by high EPS scores. There are, as yet, no data on quetiapine's efficacy in first-episode psychosis. This is an important subgroup given the good tolerability of this drug. No data are available on quetiapine's efficacy in treatment-refractory schizophrenia. Information is emerging on the use of quetiapine in elderly patients (Arvantis and Rak, 1997). In an open-labelled study of 151 patients (mean age 76.8 years) with psychosis, substantial symptomatic improvement was observed in over half of the patients. The mean daily dose of quetiapine was 100 mg. Rates of emergent EPS were comparable to placebo. The most frequently noted adverse effects were somnolence (30%), dizziness (13%) and orthostatic hypotension (12%).

Sertindole has been available in European countries since 1997/1998 but at the time of writing its use is restricted due to regulatory concern about cardiac adverse effects (see below). The antipsychotic efficacy of orally administered sertindole has been evaluated in several controlled clinical trials. They all demonstrated that sertindole is effective against both the positive and negative symptoms of schizophrenia and is associated with a similar level of EPS to that seen under placebo (van Kammen et al., 1996; Zimbroff et al., 1997; Daniel et al., 1998). The study of particular interest is the double-blind, placebo-controlled study comparing three doses of sertindole (12, 20, and 24 mg/day) and haloperidol (4, 8, and 16 mg/day) in the treatment of psychotic symptoms in 497 hospitalized patients suffering from schizophrenia (Zimbroff et al., 1997). Both drugs were comparably effective in the treatment of psychosis, and all dose levels were significantly better than placebo. For the treatment of negative symptoms, only sertindole, 20 mg/day, was significantly more effective than placebo. Another large scale multicentre study, conducted in Europe, compared four doses of sertindole (8, 16, 20 and 24 mg/day) with 10 mg haloperidol in 595 schizophrenic patients (Hale et al., 1996). Sertindole at 16, 20 or 24 mg and haloperidol at 10 mg each produced significantly greater improvement on the Positive and Negative Symptom Scale (PANSS) total score than sertindole at 8 mg. On the PANSS negative symptoms subscale, the 16 mg sertindole dose induced a significant improvement compared with a 10 mg haloperidol dose. The only long-term study assessed time to treatment failure with 24 mg/day sertindole or 10 mg/day haloperidol in 282 clinically stable neuroleptic-responsive outpatients with schizophrenia (Daniel et al., 1998). Time to treatment failure was 'numerically superior', but not statistically significantly different, in sertindole-treated patients. These patients remained free of hospitalization for exacerbation of schizophrenia and remained medically compliant significantly longer than the haloperidol patients. Data on special populations such as first episode, elderly or treatment resistant patients are not available yet.

Prescribing practices

Quetiapine has a wide dose range, from 100 mg to 750 mg daily. Effective doses for patients with schizophrenia fall within the 300–750 mg range, with most clinicians in the USA aiming for a target dose of 300–400 mg daily during the initial trial period (Weiden, 1997). Because of orthostasis and sedation, lower doses of 50–200 mg daily are more appropriate for elderly patients. Consistent with our growing experience with other novel antipsychotics, it is best to start quetiapine by overlapping with the other medication, ideally over a few weeks' duration in a cross-tapering of dose. Abrupt discontinuation of drug followed by the gradual titration of quetiapine exposes the patient to the possibility of neuroleptic withdrawal symptoms (especially given quetiapine's lack of anticholinergic effects) and the risk of worsening of psychosis (Weiden *et al.*, 1997). This regimen is well tolerated. A starting dose of 25 mg bid of quetiapine is appropriate. In general, a prolonged period of overlap is a better way to begin quetiapine. On the other hand, it is important to discontinue the other medication so that inadvertent and protracted polypharmacy is avoided. With regard to pre-screening tests, a baseline ocular examination (preferably a slit-lamp ophthalmoscopic assessment) should be performed in all patients who are at high risk for developing cataracts (e.g. coexisting diabetes mellitus) or those who have pre-existing eye disease. This should be repeated at regular intervals (as yet undetermined; see below) during quetiapine therapy. For all other patients, it is reasonable to perform the eye examination shortly after commencing quetiapine and when it is clear that the patient will require maintenance therapy (there is no evidence of quetiapine-induced ocular changes from short-term therapy; see below).

The effective dosage of sertindole is between 12 and 20 mg/day. Sixteen to 20 mg seems to be the best dosage in the treatment of acutely psychotic patients; for maintenance treatment a dosage of 12 mg is probably sufficient for most patients. Due to the marked initial effect on α_1-adrenergic receptors with a resulting risk of orthostasis, a starting dose of 4 mg and titration rate with 4 mg dose increases every 3 days is recommended. If the patient is treated with a typical or with another atypical neuroleptic and a change to sertindole is considered because of EPS, sedation, weight gain or other side effects of the currently used neuroleptic, it is highly recommended to start sertindole by overlapping with the previous medication over 1–2 weeks. Anti-parkinsonian drugs should be continued for 2–3 weeks.

Adverse effects

In comparison with other novel antipsychotics, quetiapine is not associated with significant EPS, cardiac, haematological, or seizure complications. Additionally, the absence of hyperprolactinaemia may account for its low incidence of sexual side effects (less than 1%). However, in tandem with the newer drugs, this agent has higher sedation (approximately 15% of patients), orthostatic hypotension (7%) and weight gain (average weight gain of 1.7–2.3 kg) than the typical antipsychotics. Because of the results of ocular studies conducted in dogs, there has been concern about a risk of developing cataracts during quetiapine therapy. These results have not been confirmed in either subsequent animal studies or in experience during an open-labelled maintenance trial of quetiapine. Nevertheless, eye examina-

Table 5.2 A schematic representation of the comparative side-effect profile of antipsychotic medications

Drug	Extrapyramidal effects	Tardive dyskinesia	Sedation	Weight gain	ECG abnormalities	Ejaculatory dysfunction
Haloperidol	+	+	+	−	+	−
Quetiapine	−	?	+ +	+	+	−
Sertindole	−	?	+	−	+ +	+

tions are recommended for patients considered for long-term quetiapine therapy (see above).

All double-blind controlled studies found that, regarding EPS, sertindole is indistinguishable from placebo. Sertindole was generally well tolerated. The study by Zimbroff *et al.* (1997) revealed that 5.6% of sertindole patients discontinued because of adverse effects, while 9.1% discontinued haloperidol and 1.4% discontinued placebo. Nasal congestion and, in men, reduced ejaculatory volume occurred more frequently under sertindole. Similar to other novel antipsychotics, sertindole also increases body weight. However, weight gain seems to be not as high as with most other atypical neuroleptics (Buckley, 2000). With regard to cardiovascular safety, sertindole was associated with a significant prolongation of the QT and QTc intervals of 2–5% from baseline; mean QT and QTc intervals remained below the upper limit of normal for both men (440 ms) and women (480 ms). Analysis of 10 600 ECGs revealed that 1.7% of short-term treated patients and 2.3% of long-term treated patients had at least once a clinically relevant QTc prolongation of more than 500 ms (Lunkbeck A/S; sertindole product monograph). QT interval prolongations are also observed under other neuroleptic drugs, and it is not obvious yet whether clinically relevant cardiac side effects are more frequent under sertindole than under other drugs. This issue is currently under regulatory review.

Clinical niche

Quetiapine and sertindole both have a clinical indication for the treatment of psychosis and, accordingly, could be used as a first-line agent and in all stages of the illness. Their favourable adverse effects profile, particularly the negligible EPS, may be of note in this first-episode patients and could help to enhance compliance from the onset of therapy. These same clinical characteristics are also advantageous in the elderly patient subgroup wherein complexity of use and side effects are major determinants of choice of medication. Presently, their role and efficacy as maintenance therapy for schizophrenia is unclear because of the absence of longitudinal data. Likewise, there are no data on efficacy in treatment-refractory schizophrenia or on efficacy relative to clozapine for severe schizophrenia. Similarly, both drugs have not yet been compared with risperidone, olanzapine, or other agents with respect to efficacy and outcome over the phases of the illness.

There is an indication, from a subanalysis of clinical trials data, that quetiapine may be effective in treating agitation and hostility in schizophrenic patients. Accordingly, quetiapine is at present best distinguished clinically by its favourable EPS profile and its use may in time turn out to be most advantageous in patient subgroups who are most EPS susceptible (e.g. elderly, Parkinson's related psychosis, acute schizophreniform psychosis) (Parsa and Bastani, 1998). Results of ongoing studies with quetiapine as well as similar studies for the other new drugs will ultimately determine quetiapine's place within the pharmacological armamentarium for psychosis.

Sertindole is an effective antipsychotic, with a particularly favorable EPS profile, whose clinical niche remains to be determined. It does not sedate and it does not induce major weight gain. Regarding quality of life, a significant improvement under sertindole, but no change under haloperidol, has been found (Naber and Lambert, 1998).

References

Arvantis, L.A. and Rak, I.W. (1997). Efficacy, safety and tolerability of seroquel (quetiapine) in elderly subjects with psychotic disorders. Poster presented at the International Congress on Schizophrenia Research, April 12–14.

Arvantis, L.A., Miller, B.G. and the Seroquel Trial-13 Study Group (1997). Multiple fixed doses of 'seroquel' (quetiapine) in patients with acute exacerbation of schizophrenia: a comparison with haloperidol and placebo. *Biol. Psychiatry*, **42**, 233–246.

Buckley, P.F. (2000). Endocrine and metabolic effects of typical and atypical antipsychotics: contemporary clinical experience. In: *Adverse Effects of Antipsychotic Medications*. (J.M. Kane, ed.) Life Science: London.

Daniel, D.G., Wozniak, P., Mack, R.J., *et al.* (1998). Long-term efficacy and safety comparison of sertindole and haloperidol in the treatment of schizophrenia. *Psychopharmacol. Bull.*, **34**, 61–69.

Hale A., Van der Burght, M., Wehnert, A., *et al.* (1996). A European dose-range study comparing the efficacy, tolerability and safety of four doses of sertindole and one dose of haloperidol in schizophrenic patients (abstract). In: 35th American College of Neuropsychopharmacology Annual Meeting, San Juan, Puerto Rico, December 1996. Nashville (TN): American College of Neuropsychopharmacology. p. 252.

Hyttel J., Nielsen, J.B. and Nowak, G. (1992). The acute effect of sertindole on brain 5-HT$_2$, D$_2$ and alpha 1 receptors (ex vivo radioreceptor binding studies). *J. Neural Transmission (General Section)*, **89**, 61–69.

Meats, P. (1997). Quetiapine (seroquel); an effective and well-tolerated atypical antipsychotic. *Int. J. Psychiatry Clin. Practice*, **1**, 231–239.

Naber, D. and Lambert, M. (1998). Sertindole decreases hospitalization and improves the quality of life of schizophrenic patients. *Int. J. Psychiatry Clin. Practice*, **2** (Suppl. 2), 573–577.

Parsa, M.A. and Bastani, B. (1998). Quetiapine in the treatment of psychosis in patients with Parkinson's disease. *J. Neuropsychiatry Clin. Neurosci.*, **10**, 216–219.

Sanchez, C., Arnt, J., Dragsted, N., *et al.* (1991). Neurochemical and in vivo pharmacological profile of sertindole, a limbic-selective neuroleptic compound. *Drug Dev. Res.*, **22**, 239–250.

Skarsfeldt, T. (1992). Electrophysiological profile of the new atypical neuroleptic, sertindole, on midbrain dopamine neurons in rats: acute and repeated treatment. *Synapse*, **10**, 25–33.

Skarsfeldt, T. and Perregaard, J. (1990). Sertindole, a new neuroleptic with extreme selectivity on A10 versus A9 dopamine neurons in the rat. *Eur. J. Pharmacol.*, **182**, 613–614.

Small, J., Hirsch, S., Arvantis, L., *et al.* (1997). Quetiapine in patients with schizophrenia: a high and low-dose double blind comparison with placebo. *Arch. Gen. Psychiatry*, **54**, 549–557.

Weiden, P.J. (1997). Quetiapine ('seroquel'): A new 'atypical' antipsychotic. *J. Practical Psychiatry Behav. Hlth.*, **3**, 368–374.

Weiden, P.J., Aquila, R., Standard, J., *et al.* (1997). Switching antipsychotic medications. *J. Clin. Psychiatry*, **58**, 63–72.

van Kammen, D.P., Targum, S.D. and Sebree, T.B. (1996). A randomized, controlled, dose-ranging trial of sertindole in parents with schizophrenia. *Psychopharmacology*, **124**, 168–175.

Zimbroff, D.L., Ane, J.M., Tamminga, C.A., *et al.* (1997). Controlled, dose-response study of sertindole and haloperidol in the treatment of schizophrenia. *Am. J. Psychiatry*, **154**, 782–791.

6

Ziprasidone and zotepine: clinical use and experience

Steven Potkin and Stephen Cooper

Key points

Ziprasidone
- Efficacy in treating acutely ill patients with schizophrenia or schizoaffective disorder.
- Accumulating evidence of efficacy for depressive and negative symptoms associated with schizophrenia.
- Evidence of efficacy for relapse prevention and reducing negative symptoms in treatment of stable outpatients.
- No increase in prolactin.
- Well tolerated; low incidence of extrapyramidal side effects.
- Sedation may be observed when treatment is initiated but usually does not persist.
- Patients treated long-term with ziprasidone do not usually gain weight.
- Rapid acting i.m. formulation actively being developed.

Zotepine
- Clinical antipsychotic profile similar to other atypicals.
- Trials suggest benefits for depression, negative symptoms and cognition, but these are not yet adequately studied.
- Well tolerated; low incidence of extrapyramidal side effects.
- Sedation occurs, which may benefit some patients and be a problem for others.
- Increased seizure frequency above 300 mg daily.
- Increases plasma prolactin.

Ziprasidone

Compound development:

Ziprasidone is a dibenzothzolylpiperazine that is chemically unrelated to other antipsychotic compounds currently available or described in this text. The clinical development programme for oral ziprasidone in the treatment of psychotic disorders involved over 4000 subjects, 2878 of whom were exposed to ziprasidone, providing an unusual amount of clinical data. The separate development programme for the rapid-acting intramuscular formulation for the short-term management of agitated psychotic patients involved 671 patients. Its pharmacological properties are summarized in Chapter 1.

Human studies

Pharmacokinetics

Administration with food, especially fat, increases the absorption of ziprasidone by 69 to 97% (Lebel *et al.*, 1993; Miceli *et al.*, 1994), although there are no effects on absorption when ziprasidone is taken with aluminum and magnesium hydroxide antacids or with cimetidine. Ziprasidone is highly protein bound, i.e. >99%. With multiple dosing, the T_{max} occurs at 6–8 hours post dose with dose-proportionality over 20–80 mg bid with corresponding C_{max} of 66 and 202 ng/ml. The terminal half-life is 5–10 hours suggesting suitability for twice-daily dosing. In specifically designed pharmacokinetic studies, no clinically significant effects of age, gender, moderate hepatic or renal impairment were observed. Thus, no requirement for dose adjustment is expected in the elderly or those with moderate hepatic and renal impairment. Ziprasidone is extensively metabolized into inactive metabolites. Ziprasidone does not appreciably inhibit cytochrome 450 isoforms: 1A2, 2C9, 2C19, and 2D6. Ziprasidone is metabolized by CYP3A4 but *in vitro* inhibition is only observed at concentrations many-fold greater than clinically relevant concentrations. Neither ketoconazole (a potent CYP3A4 inhibitor) nor carbamazepine (a potent inducer of CYP3A4) produces clinically relevant effects on ziprasidone exposure in volunteers (change in area under curve ≤36%), suggesting that ziprasidone is metabolized by an alternative pathway (Laurent and Miceli, 1999; Laurent and Wilner, 1999). Its lack of metabolism by 1A2 suggests that smoking, a 1A2 inducer, should not alter pharmacokinetics.

Initial clinical trials

In a 4-week double-blind clinical trial in schizophrenic and schizoaffective subjects with an acute exacerbation of their illness ($n = 90$) treated with 4, 10, 40, or 160 mg/day ziprasidone or 15 mg/day haloperidol, the 160 mg dose of ziprasidone was better than 4 mg/day and had equal efficacy to haloperidol treatment in reducing positive symptoms. Concomitant benztropine use, however, was 15% with 160 mg ziprasidone compared with 53% for haloperidol. Further, post-ziprasidone dose plasma prolactin concentrations did not differ from pretreatment levels, although small transient post-dose increases in prolactin were observed in the 160 mg/day group, unlike the expected dramatic increases observed with haloperidol (Goff *et al.*, 1998).

A placebo-controlled 4-week trial in 139 acutely ill patients evaluated 40 and 120 mg/day of ziprasidone. The 40 mg dose could not be differentiated from placebo, indicating that 40 mg is too low for acutely exacerbated patients. A dose of 120 mg/day was consistently more effective than placebo (Keck *et al.*, 1998). Overall, Phase II clinical trials in 375 patients demonstrate that ziprasidone is well tolerated with a lower overall incidence of movement disorders than is seen with traditional antipsychotic agents (Gunn and Harrigan, 1995).

Principal clinical trials

In a large 6-week double-blind clinical trial ($n = 302$) in acutely exacerbated schizophrenic and schizoaffective disorder patients treated with 80 and 160 mg of ziprasidone, both doses were more effective than placebo, including improving total Positive and Negative Symptom Scale (PANSS) and negative subscale scores. Depressive symptoms, measured by the Montgomery-Asberg depression rating scale (MADRS), were significantly improved with ziprasidone 160 mg/day in the subset of patients who had clinically relevant levels of depression at baseline (MADRS $\geq$ 14). A low incidence of EPS and sexual dysfunction was also observed. (Daniel et al., 1999).

A 1-year, randomized, double-blind European study compared 40, 80 and 160 mg ziprasidone with placebo in stable patients in the prevention of acute exacerbation (a surrogate of relapse) of schizophrenia and in the long-term treatment of negative symptoms. The probability of experiencing an acute exacerbation was approximately half that of the placebo group (70.8%) in ziprasidone-treated patients (Arato et al., 1997). A significant reduction in core negative symptoms was also observed with ziprasidone with gradual ongoing improvement being observed throughout the 1-year study. The reduction in negative symptoms with ziprasidone corresponded to a significant improvement in global function, as measured by the Global Assessment of Functioning. Tolerability of ziprasidone was excellent with low use of anticholinergics and beta-blockers, no group differences in EPS ratings, and no pattern of laboratory abnormalities including prolactin. There were lower discontinuations for adverse events in the ziprasidone groups than with placebo, confirming its excellent tolerability in long-term treatment.

In a small subset of patients who had cognition assessments in an open-label randomized trial, there was a suggestion that ziprasidone-treated patients experienced greater improvement than risperidone-treated patients (Hagger et al., 1997). Double-blind comparison trials, however, are required before the relative efficacy in the neurocognitive and negative symptom domains can be determined.

Adverse effects

Based on ziprasidone's strong serotonergic effects one would predict a relatively high incidence of headache and gastrointestinal symptoms, such as nausea and dyspepsia. Surprisingly, these symptoms were mild or moderate in severity and rarely led to discontinuation. Comparing ziprasidone treated patients ($n = 702$) with placebo ($n = 273$) studied in short-term clinical trials of acutely ill patients, headache occurred 22% in both groups. Dyspepsia and nausea occurred slightly more frequently in the ziprasidone group (8% and 10%, respectively) compared with placebo (7% each), resulting in three discontinuations compared to one for placebo. Generally, side effects decreased with length of treatment. Sexual side effects commonly associated with serotonergic medications, prolactin elevation and alpha 1 blockade were also rare with ziprasidone: abnormal ejaculation and impotence (0% and 0.3%) for ziprasidone, (0.4% each) for placebo.

Weight gain is observed with several of the new antipsychotic compounds but less so with ziprasidone. As reviewed by Tandon *et al.* (1997), 9.8% of ziprasidone-treated patients gained more than 7% body weight in the 6–8-week studies compared to 4% for placebo. However, the ziprasidone weight gain appears to be far less than observed with other comparably studied compounds when compared to placebo, e.g. risperidone (18 v 9%), olanzapine (29 v 3%), and quetiapine (25 v 4%) (Allison *et al.*, 1998). Relative low H_1 affinity and serotonin reuptake properties may explain the lack of significant weight gain with ziprasidone. While this assertion requires confirmation in comparative long-term trials, relatively long-term clinical experience with ziprasidone supports the short-term study results. In a randomized, double-blind 1-year study, median weight decreased slightly (≤ 3 kg) with ziprasidone 40, 80 and 160 mg/day and with placebo (Arato *et al.*, 1998).

Dizziness occurs less frequently than predicted based on the moderate alpha 1 binding, 8% versus 6%. Somnolence was more frequent in the ziprasidone-treated patients than with placebo (14% vs 7%, respectively) but responsible for discontinuation in only two patients and was noted to attenuate over the course of short-term studies.

In 4- and 6-week studies, extrapyramidal syndrome (EPS) and akathisia were more frequent with ziprasidone (5% and 8%, respectively) than placebo (1% and 7%), but were relatively rare. Simpson-Angus EPS rating and Barnes Akathesia rating score changes were similar with ziprasidone and placebo with small mean reductions observed in both groups. Similarly, the percentages of patients with any increase in these scores with ziprasidone (23.2% and 15.3%, respectively) was similar to placebo (20.1% and 15.4%, respectively). Benztropine use at any time was 22.4% for ziprasidone-treated patients and 18.3% for placebo. Similarly, beta-blocker use was 7.1% for ziprasidone and 6.2% for placebo. These data suggest a favourable clinical EPS profile for ziprasidone, as predicted from its 5-HT_2 to D_2 affinity ratio. Additionally, no dose-related pattern of laboratory abnormalities has been observed with ziprasidone, including blood dyscrasias.

Much recent attention has focused on the effects of the newer atypical antipsychotic compounds on cardiac conduction, namely the QTc interval. Sertindole's new drug application (NDA) was reported to have been withdrawn because of QTc prolongation, which may set the stage for torsades de pointes and sudden death. However, the effect of sertindole appears to contrast with that of other novel antipsychotics, including ziprasidone. In short-term fixed-dose clinical studies of sertindole the mean increase in QTc was 21 ms and an interval of ≥ 500 ms was observed in 7–8% of patients (FDA, 1998). The average increase in QTc with ziprasidone is only 2.86 ms and no cases of torsades de pointes have been reported. Mean QTc increases have also been observed with other atypicals such as risperidone, quetiapine and olanzapine as well as more conventional neuroleptics, especially thioridazine. The Summary Basis for Approval (SBA) document (FDA, May 11, 1993) reported that 4.3% of risperidone-treated patients with baseline QTc values of less than 450 ms had QTc measures of ≥ 450 ms during treatment. For olanzapine the average QTc increase is 2.82 ms (SBA, 1996) and for quetiapine less than 10 ms (SBA, 1997). Unfortunately, it is not possible to make an appropriate comparison across studies. No results from any well-designed comparative ECG studies are yet available to clarify the relative QTc effects of these compounds and to elucidate the degree of potential cardiac risk.

Clinical uses

The usual starting dose is 40 mg bid, which is usually well-tolerated in patients with schizophrenia and schizoaffective disorder. This dosage can be increased to 60 or 80 mg bid over a 2-day period. In the first several days of treatment, patients occasionally experience some initial activation similar to that seen in the initial treatment days with selective serotonin reuptake inhibitors (SSRIs). Patients describe this as an 'inner restlessness' that can be distinguished from akathisia. This activation can be accompanied by insomnia and is easily treated by short-term use of benzodiazepines or increasing the dose of ziprasidone.

Sedation can be observed, usually at 80 mg bid. This may be useful for treating acute psychotic exacerbations. Adequate antipsychotic treatment can often be achieved with 40 mg bid, especially during maintenance treatment.

Patients with alternative diagnoses such as bipolar disorder and other psychotic disorders have not been well studied and dosage adjustments need to be determined, as is the case with other antipsychotic medications. Adolescents and children with Tourette's syndrome were satisfactorily treated with 40 mg/day (Sallee et al., 1997). Its efficacy in treatment-refractory schizophrenic patients and in affective disorder has not been determined.

Nausea, vomiting, dyspepsia and headache, symptoms commonly observed with serotonergic medications, are relatively rare but occur occasionally. Orthostatic hypotension is rare, despite affinity for alpha receptors. Sexual dysfunction and weight gain are infrequently encountered, and weight loss is more characteristic.

Intramuscular ziprasidone

A rapid-acting, intramuscular (i.m.) formulation of ziprasidone for the short-term management of the agitated psychotic patient has been investigated. In randomized, double-blind, 24-hour clinical trials ziprasidone i.m. 10 mg and 20 mg rapidly and significantly reduced the symptoms of acute agitation associated with psychosis for at least 4 hours. The effect was dose-related: neither dose was associated with dystonia, extrapyramidal syndrome or excessive sedation. Studies comparing ziprasidone i.m. with haloperidol i.m. indicated important tolerability advantages for ziprasidone, particularly in assessments of extrapyramidal symptoms. Ziprasidone i.m. is at least as effective as haloperidol i.m. in reducing symptoms and efficacy is maintained in the transition from i.m. to oral treatment. Patients treated with ziprasidone i.m. are rapidly calmed but not excessively sedated and remain rousable and lucid. The availability of a short-acting i.m. and an oral formulation will allow clinicians to keep patients on the same medication through the different stages of the illness.

Summary

Ziprasidone is an effective antipsychotic with good tolerability and low EPS. Its unique receptor profile offers the potential of enhanced efficacy for depression associated with schizophrenia and schizoaffective disorder, although comparative trials are required to confirm this potential advantage. The lack of weight gain offers another benefit, especially given the weight increases typically observed with other antipsychotics.

Zotepine

Compound development

Zotepine is a dibenzothiepine derivative from a phenothiazine type structure. It is a tricyclic compound with a seven membered central ring and is thus structurally similar to clozapine.

The compound was initially synthesized in Japan in 1970 and has been marketed there since 1982. It has subsequently been granted a product licence in Germany (1990), Austria (1996) and the UK (1998). The development of this compound has been unusual as almost two million patients had been treated with it before a more standard series of clinical trials was performed for the purpose of submission to European and US regulatory authorities. Many of the early clinical studies reported with zotepine would not be regarded as adequate tests of efficacy. However, well controlled clinical trials carried out during the last 10 years provide convincing evidence of its antipsychotic efficacy in schizophrenia. In addition, its extensive use means that any serious, but rare, adverse effects (such as agranulocytosis) should by now have become evident through post-marketing surveillance. None have been reported. Its pharmacological properties are summarized in Chapter 1.

Human studies

Human volunteers tolerate antipsychotic drugs poorly. Low doses of zotepine, however, were well tolerated in volunteer studies with sedation being the main effect, probably reflecting antihistamine and antiadrenergic effects. The sedation is reflected in increased slow wave activity seen on EEG in volunteers given zotepine (Saletu et al., 1987). There was a slight, but not significant, effect on blood pressure in volunteers compared to placebo, while clozapine at roughly equivalent doses induced a statistically significant decrease. These findings reflect some of the adverse effects reported by patients in clinical trials which will be discussed later.

Single dosing studies in human volunteers indicate an increase in plasma prolactin that parallels the peak plasma concentration of zotepine (Tanaka et al., 1998). Chronic dosing studies in patients with schizophrenia suggest persistent elevation of plasma prolactin to levels approximately two to three times normal which is similar to what is found with standard antipsychotic drugs and many of the atypicals (Bardeleben et al., 1987).

Pharmacokinetics

Studies of pharmacokinetics in patients and human volunteers have produced similar findings. Maximum plasma concentration following a single dose is achieved in 2–4 hours. This may be slightly delayed by food, though this does not affect the extent of absorption. The elimination half-life is in the region of 14 hours with figures from 13 to 21 hours found in different studies. There is extensive first pass metabolism to inactive metabolites as well as the active metabolite norzotepine. Both zotepine and norzotepine are 97% bound to plasma proteins.

Zotepine is principally metabolized via the CYP1A2 and CYP3A4 hepatic isoenzymes with no involvement of CYP2D6. Hepatic and renal impairment can both result in some elevation of plasma concentrations. Single dose studies also suggest that plasma levels are elevated in the elderly.

Initial clinical trials

The first clinical trials of zotepine were conducted in Japan and were comparisons with standard neuroleptics. Some were open studies and, in many, interpretation of the results was complicated by use of concomitant medication. Overall, however, these suggested comparable clinical efficacy for doses of zotepine between 75 mg and 450 mg with the comparator neuroleptic drugs. Five further trials, conducted in Austria and Germany, also indicated equivalent efficacy for daily doses of zotepine between 50 mg and 600 mg against an active comparator, with a trend in favour of zotepine (e.g. Fleischhacker et al., 1989). These were double-blind studies employing random allocation to treatment group and standard symptom rating scales. The principal comparator employed was haloperidol at doses between 2 mg and 30 mg daily. A further study compared zotepine and clozapine in 50 patients and found a similar degree of improvement in symptoms with both (Meyer-Lindenberg et al., 1997). Additionally in this study, assessments of a wide variety of cognitive functions suggested more consistent improvements with zotepine.

Principal clinical trials

Three major clinical trials have been conducted to examine efficacy for acute episodes of schizophrenia. These all recruited patients with an acute first episode or an acute exacerbation of long-standing schizophrenia and used DSM III-R criteria for patient selection. One of these in the USA compared zotepine at daily doses of either 75 mg, 150 mg or 300 mg with placebo in 289 patients and demonstrated statistically significant improvement from baseline for all doses of zotepine compared to placebo but no dose response effect. A comparison of zotepine (150 mg or 300 mg) versus chlorpromazine (300 mg or 600 mg) and placebo demonstrated greater efficacy for zotepine against both (Cooper et al., 1996). Comparison of zotepine (150 mg to 300 mg daily) versus haloperidol (6 mg to 20 mg) demonstrated equivalent efficacy (Petit et al., 1996). In the last two of these there was an improvement of around 25% in the total brief psychiatric rating scale (BPRS) scores. Of note was a concomitant improvement in mood ratings of around 30% and in negative symptom ratings of around 25%.

Longer-term efficacy has been confirmed by a 26-week study comparing zotepine (150 mg or 300 mg) versus placebo in patients with a history of relapse on their previous treatment. Only four out of 60 patients on zotepine had a recurrence versus 21 out of 58 on placebo (Cooper *et al.*, 1998).

Adverse effects

The degree of EPS, as assessed by standard rating scales, is no greater than for placebo and less than with haloperidol in the clinical trial data. Using data from controlled trials, the relative risk for all EPS compared to placebo is 1.30 (not statistically significant) and compared to haloperidol is 0.32 ($P < 0.001$).

Adverse effects reported significantly more frequently with zotepine than placebo are listed in Table 6.1. Other adverse events are similar to those reported with other antipsychotic drugs but occur less frequently. At doses below 300 mg per day the incidence of seizures is no greater than for other antipsychotic drugs. However, above this dose there appears to be a dose related increase in risk.

Clinical use

Dosing is usually commenced at 25 mg three times daily (tid) and increased to 50 mg tid if tolerated. Most patients appear to require doses between 150 mg and 300 mg daily. In practice, sedation appears to be the principal adverse effect that may result in stopping zotepine. It may have a place in the management of patients with depressive symptoms but, as yet, there is inadequate evidence to make a strong case for this or for particular benefits in relation to negative symptoms. The lack of extensive use in the UK, where a product licence has only recently been granted, makes it difficult to comment in more detail on practical issues.

Table 6.1 Adverse events reported significantly more frequently with zotepine than placebo in clinical trials

Adverse event	Relative risk compared with placebo
Dry mouth	17.1
Weight increase	14.8
Dizziness	6.9
Somnolence	5.6
Tachycardia	3.3
Asthenia	2.9

References

Allison, D.B., Mentore, J.L., Heo, M., *et al.* (1998). Weight gain associated with conventional and newer antipsychotics: a meta-analysis. *Eur. Neuropsychopharmacol.*, **8** (Suppl. 2), S216.

Arato, M., O'Connor, R., Meltzer, H. and Bradbury, J. (1997). Ziprasidone: efficacy in the prevention of relapse and in the long-term treatment of negative symptoms of chronic schizophrenia. *Eur. Neuropsychopharmacol.*, **7** (Suppl. 2), S214.

Arato, M., O'Connor, R., Bradbury, J.E., *et al.* (1998). Ziprasidone in the long-term treatment of negative symptoms and prevention of exacerbation of schizophrenia. *Eur. Psychiatry*, **13**, 303s.

Bardeleben, U. von, Benkert, F. and Holsboer, F. (1987). Clinical and neuroendocrine effects of zotepine – a new neuroleptic drug. *Pharmacopsychiatry*, **20**, 28–34.

Cooper, S.J., Raniwalla, J. and Welch, C. (1996). Zotepine in acute exacerbation of schizophrenia: a comparison versus chlorpromazine and placebo. *Eur. Neuropsychopharmacol.*, **6** (suppl. 3), 148.

Cooper, S.J., Butler, A., Tweed, J.A., *et al.* (1998). Zotepine is effective in preventing recurrence in patients with chronic schizophrenia. *Eur. Neuropsychopharmacol.*, **8** (Suppl. 2), S232.

Daniel, D.G., Zimbroff, D.L., Potkin, S.G., Reeves, K., *et al.* and the Ziprasidone Study Group (1999). Ziprasidone 40 mg bid and 80 mg bid in the acute exacerbation of schizophrenia and schizoaffective disorder: Results of a 6-week placebo-controlled trial (in press).

FDA (1993). Risperdal (risperidone) Summary Basis of Approval, FDA, May 11, 1993.

FDA (1998). Serdolect (sertindole) FDA Advisory Committee Report, 1998.

Fleischhacker, W., Barnas, C., Stuppack, C.H., *et al.* (1989). Zotepine versus haloperidol in paranoid schizophrenia: a double-blind trial. *Psychopharmacol. Bull.*, **25**, 97–100.

Goff, D.C., Posever, T., Herz, L. *et al.* (1998). An exploratory haloperidol-controlled dose-finding study of ziprasidone in hospitalized patients with schizophrenia or schizoaffective disorder, *J. Clin. Psychopharmacol.*, **18**, 296–304.

Gunn, K.P. and Harrigan, E.P. (1995). The safety and tolerability of ziprasidone in phase II clinical trials. *Int. Acad. Biomed. Drug Res.*, **10**, 73.

Hagger, C., Mitchell, D., Wise, A.L., *et al.* (1997). Effects of oral ziprasidone and risperidone on cognitive functioning in patients with schizophrenia or schizoaffective disorder: preliminary data. *Eur. Neuropsychopharmacol.*, **7** (Suppl. 2), S219.

Keck, Jr. P., Buffenstein, A., Ferguson, J., *et al.* (1998). The Ziprasidone Study Group. *Psychopharmacology*, **140** (2), 173–184.

Laurent, A. and Miceli, J.J. (1999). The effects of ketoconazole on ziprasidone pharmacokinetics: a placebo-controlled crossover study in healthy volunteers. *Br. J. Clin. Pharmacol.*, (Suppl.), (in press).

Laurent, A. and Wilner, K.D. (1999). The effect of carbamazepine on the steady-state pharmacokinetics of ziprasidone in healthy volunteers. *Br. J. Clin. Pharmacol.*, (Suppl.), (in press).

Lebel, M., Prouix, M., Allard, S., *et al.* (1993). Influence of a high fat breakfast on the absorption and the pharmacodynamics of CP-88; 059; a new antipsychotic. *Clin. Invest. Med.*, **16** (Abstract No. 117), B18.

Miceli, J.J., Hunt, T., Cole, M.J., *et al.* (1994). The pharmacokinetics (PK) of CP-88 059 (CP) in healthy male volunteers following oral (PO) and intravenous (IV) administration. *Clin. Pharmacol. Therapeutics*, **55**, 142.

Meyer-Lindenberg, A., Gruppe, H., Bauer, U., *et al.* (1997). Improvement in cognitive function in schizophrenic patients receiving clozapine or zotepine: results from a double-blind study. *Pharmacopsychiatry*, **30**, 35–42.

Petit, M., Raniwalla, J., Lutteneger, E., *et al.* (1996). A comparison of an atypical and typical antipsychotic, zotepine versus haloperidol in patients with acute exacerbation of schizophrenia. *Psychopharmacol. Bull.*, **32**, 81–87.

Saletu, B., Grunberger, J., Linzmayer, L., *et al.* (1987). Comparative placebo-controlled pharmacodynamic studies with zotepine and clozapine utilizing pharmaco-EEG and psychometry. *Pharmacopsychiatry*, **20**, 12–27.

Sallee, F., Kurlan, R., Goetz, C., *et al.* (1997). The tolerability and efficacy of ziprasidone in the treatment of children and adolescents with Tourette's syndrome. Presented at the 36th ACNP.

SBA (1996). Zyprexa (olanzapine) Summary Basis of Approval, NDA-20-592, 1996.

SBA (1997). Seroquel (quetiapine) Summary Basis of Approval, NDA-20-639, 1997.

Tanaka, O., Kondo, T., Otani, K., *et al.* (1998). Single oral dose kinetics of zotepine and its relationship to prolactin response and side effects. *Therap. Drug Monitoring*, **20**, 117–119.

Tandon, R., Harrigan, E. and Zorn, S.H. (1997). Ziprasidone: a novel antipsychotic with unique pharmacology and therapeutic potential. *J. Serotonin Res.*, **4**, 159–177.

7

Future directions in novel antipsychotics

Robert Conley

Key points

- Because of their pharmacology, current atypical antipsychotics may have broader indication and efficacy in patients with affective disorders and substance abuse.
- The development of acute and long-acting intramuscular forms of atypical antipsychotics is a major focus of current research.
- Continued drug development includes new directions such as selective 5-HT_{2A} receptor antagonists, sigma receptor antagonism, and drugs which inhibit degradation of membrane fatty acids.

We have begun what may be a paradigm shift in the pharmacological treatment of psychoses. Novel antipsychotics are replacing the mainstays of treatment for almost 40 years, namely traditional antipsychotic drugs. Why is this happening and what does it mean? Traditional antipsychotics were truly breakthrough medications. They provided effective therapy for a common affliction, psychosis, which had been almost impossible to treat in the past. However, the limitations of these drugs were rapidly recognized. They did not completely treat the syndrome of schizophrenia, having little benefit in the domains of cognitive dysfunction and negative symptoms. Conventional antipsychotics also cause severe side effects, particularly involving disregulation of voluntary motor function. Parkinsonian symptoms, akathisia and tardive dyskinesia are common in people who take these medications.

The search for antipsychotic drugs

The searches for more effective and safe antipsychotic medications first led to a better understanding of their mechanism of action, which was not known when they were first used. It was found that the clinical dose potency of these agents was directly correlated with their ability to bind to, and inhibit, post-synaptic D_2 dopamine receptors (Carlsson, 1972). This led to the 'dopamine theory' of psychosis which has been tremendously useful in understanding and modelling this disorder. However, this paradigm was seriously challenged by the demonstration of antipsychotic efficacy of two drugs which were weak dopamine antagonists, clozapine (Simpson and Varga, 1974; Gerlach *et al.*, 1974) and remoxipride (McCreadie *et al.*, 1988). These drugs are not only effective antipsychotics, but have few, if any parkinsonian side effects. Clozapine is also more effective than conventional antipsychotics in people who do not respond to these medications (Kane *et al.*, 1988). This may also be true of remoxipride (Conley *et al.*, 1994). These findings together suggest that these drugs may be acting at a different site of action than conventional drugs, or are interacting with this site in a very different way. Clozapine is limited in its clinical use, however, primarily because of the side effect of agranulocytosis, and remoxipride was withdrawn from human use because of the side effect of aplastic anaemia.

The new drugs risperidone, olanzapine and quetiapine are all effective antipsychotics that resulted from a re-invigorated drug discovery process that began with the work on clozapine and remoxipride. These drugs, while all D_2 antagonists, appear to have optimal clinical effects at much lower levels of D_2 receptor occupancy than conventional antipsychotics (Nyberg *et al.*, 1999; Remington and Kapur, 1999). Their mechanism of action is still uncertain. They may interact with D_2 receptors in ways that are more like endogenous dopamine (Seeman and Tallerico, 1999) or may interact with multiple receptors simultaneously (Meltzer, 1995) as their primary mode of action.

What does this mean clinically? First, newer medications are not 'haloperidol without side effects'. Their clinical actions in schizophrenia are likely to be different from conventional antipsychotics. On the positive side, novel antipsychotics, particularly when combined with psychosocial treatment, hold the promise of improving outcome and reducing the economic burden on society. Evidence exists that new antipsychotics not only reduce positive and negative symptoms and cause fewer side effects than conventional neuroleptics, but also lessen cognitive impairment, lead to a better quality of life, and have antidepressant effects (Meltzer, 1999). Rehospitalization rates are much lower with these medications than with conventional antipsychotics (Conley *et al.*, 1999). Because of their improved tolerability, these drugs hold more promise in patients with affective disorders, substance abusers, the young and elderly patients. Thus, one important future direction will be the careful study of the use of antipsychotic medications in disorders beyond the schizophrenia spectrum.

A second important future direction involves addressing the limitations of the current compounds. We still are not certain of the most effective dose of most of these medications. They have side effects of note, particularly the propensity to cause more weight gain than conventional antipsychotics (Beasley *et al.*, 1997; Kelly *et al.*, 1998). The most important deficiency these drugs have is that they are often not as effective in acutely aggressive patients as typical drugs and should be used concomitantly with a benzodiazepine in acutely agitated patients (Buckley, 1999). Dosing, weight gain and efficacy in acute agitation should therefore be of particular concern in the evaluation of any new antipsychotic. Another real limitation of the new drugs is a practical one: they are available in relatively few dosage forms, compared to traditional medications. Depot formulations of antipsychotic medications are often seen to be useful and are currently not available for the newer medications. Depot formulations of risperidone and olanzapine are currently under study. Oral solutions and/or rapidly adsorbed oral preparations of these new drugs are also needed. Oral solution risperidone is now available. The other new drugs have rapid adsorption formulations under study.

Finally, what is new? Since the field of antipsychotic research has now expanded beyond traditional D_2 antagonists, many exciting new compounds are in the pipeline. Ziprasidone is in a final review process and may be approved in the future. Its receptor binding profile is similar to that of risperidone (Seeger *et al.*, 1995). However, it is being studied in acute parenteral dosage forms and oral formulations, and thus may have increased flexibility of use if released. Amisulpride, a chemical cousin of remoxipride, has some similarities to that drug. It appears to have a selectivity for limbic, compared to striatal dopamine receptors, which should reduce its likelihood of causing parkinsonian side effects or secondary negative symptoms. It also has very different effects on dopamine type nerve conduction. At high doses, conduction is reduced, but at low doses it is enhanced. This low dose effect may be beneficial for people with primary negative symptoms. There is preliminary evidence that this is the case (Rein and Turjanski, 1997).

Drugs in development

There are several other drugs in development that also share some similarities to currently released agents. Iloperidone is another agent with a receptor binding profile that is similar to risperidone (Sainati *et al.*, 1995) and is currently in Phase III testing. Finally, ORG-5222 has been shown to also have a risperidone-like binding profile (Andree *et al.*, 1997), but there are few clinical data available for this drug yet.

A number of new compounds with novel biochemical approaches are under early review. One of particular interest is MLD-100907, under development by Aventis. This drug is a selective antagonist of the 5-HT$_{2a}$ receptor. If it is effective as an antipsychotic, it would further demonstrate that direct blockade of D_2 neurons is not required for antipsychotic efficacy. The Otsuka drug company has aripiprazole under development. This drug is a presynaptic agonist and post-synaptic antagonist of dopamine receptors (Lawler *et al.*, 1999). Thus it should inhibit the release of dopamine, and oppose its action. This could lead to anatomical selectivity different from any currently used compound.

Antagonism of central sigma receptors has long been considered a possible antipsychotic mechanism. It was one of the biochemical properties of remoxipride, besides that drug's weak D_2 antagonism. Many antipsychotics have sigma activity, but potency at this receptor does not appear to correlate directly with antipsychotic effects. There is now a potent, selective inhibitor of this receptor (SR-31742) that is being studied in humans by Sanofi which should provide evidence that will directly answer this question of the clinical effect of sigma blockade. Other areas of continuing interest are the modification of glutamate and also of nicotinic receptor function. There is a great deal of interesting preclinical data about both areas, but no clinical trials of candidate drugs have begun yet.

There are areas of interest that extend beyond receptor blockade. One particularly interesting area is that of fatty acid metabolism. It is now known that people with schizophrenia appear to have abnormal fatty acid profiles in their cell membranes (Doris *et al.*, 1998) and an overall deficiency of omega-3 fatty acids in their neuronal cell membranes (Warner *et al.*, 1999). Clozapine therapy causes increases in the concentrations of fatty acids in red blood cell membranes. If this is true, schizophrenia could be due to a potentially reversible brain lipid disorder. There is at least one drug, SC-111 from Scotia, that inhibits the breakdown of fatty acids in cell membranes that may be of use if this is true.

As we consider these exciting new possible medications, we need to keep in mind the continuing marked limitations of current drug therapy for psychosis. Most people with schizophrenia today still experience marked limitations in life functioning secondary to their illness. It is very likely that new, effective therapies for psychotic illnesses may be relatively ineffective against acute agitation, much as antibiotics treat infections well but are not good antipyretics. We must be aware that new, effective therapies for this complex problem are unlikely to be simple in their clinical use. As the field works to identify more accurately people who are vulnerable to psychosis, and to understand brain regions associated with this illness, we should work to integrate more effectively current treatment options with active psychosocial and rehabilitative programming to attempt to provide beneficial treatment for the people we see today.

References

Andree, B., Halldin, C., Vrijmoed-de Vries, M., et al. (1997). Central 5-HT2A and D2 dopamine receptor occupancy after sublingual administration of ORG 5222 in healthy men. *Psychopharmacology (Berl)*, **131**, 339–345.

Beasley, C.M. Jr, Tollefson, G.D. and Tran, P.V. (1997). Safety of olanzapine. *J. Clin. Psychiatry*, **58** (Suppl. 10), 13–17.

Buckley, P.F. (1999). The role of typical and atypical antipsychotic medications in the management of agitation and aggression. *J. Clin. Psychiatry*, **60** (Suppl. 10), 52–60.

Carlsson, A. (1972). Biochemical and pharmacological aspects of Parkinsonism. *Acta Neurol. Scand. Suppl.*, **51**, 11–42.

Conley, R.R., Tamminga, C.A. and Nguyen, J.A. (1994). Clinical action of remoxipride. *Arch. Gen. Psychiatry*, **51**, 1001.

Conley, R.R., Love, R.C., Kelly, D.L., et al. (1999). Rehospitalizations rates of patients recently discharged on to a regimen of risperidone or clozapine. *Am. J. Psychiatry*, **156**, 863–868.

Doris, A.B., Wahle, K., MacDonald, A., et al. (1998). Red cell membrane fatty acids, cytosolic phospholipase-A2 and schizophrenia. *Schizophr. Res.*, **25**, 185–196.

Gerlach, J., Koppelhus, P., Helweg, E., et al. (1974). Clozapine and haloperidol in a single-blind cross-over trial: therapeutic and biochemical aspects in the treatment of schizophrenia. *Acta Psychiatr. Scand.*, **50**, 410–424.

Kane, J., Honigfeld, G., Singer, J., et al. and the Clozaril Collaborative Study Group (1988). Clozapine for the treatment-resistant schizophrenic. *Arch. Gen. Psychiatry*, **45**, 789–797.

Kelly, D.L., Conley, R.R., Love, R.C., et al. (1998). Weight gain in adolescents treated with risperidone and conventional antipsychotics over six months. *J. Child Adolescent Psychopharmacol.*, **8**, 151–159.

Lawler, C.P., Prioleau, C., Lewis, M.M., et al. (1999). Interactions of the novel antipsychotic aripiprazole (OPC-14597) with dopamine and serotonin receptor subtypes. *Neuropsychopharmacology*, **20**, 612–627.

McCreadie, R.G., Todd, N., Livingston, M., et al. (1988). A double blind comparative study of remoxipride and thioridazine in the acute phase of schizophrenia. *Acta Psychiatr. Scand.*, **78**, 49–56.

Meltzer, H.Y. (1995). The role of serotonin in schizophrenia and the place of serotonin-dopamine antagonist antipsychotics. *J. Clin. Psychopharmacol.*, **15** (Suppl. 1), 2S–3S.

Meltzer, H.Y. (1999). Outcome in schizophrenia: beyond symptom reduction. *J. Clin. Psychiatry*, **60** (Suppl. 3), 3–7.

Nyberg, S., Erikson, B., Oxenstierna, G., *et al.* (1999). Suggested minimal effective dose of resiperidone based on PET-measured D_2 and $5HT_{2a}$ receptor occupancy in schizophrenic patients. *Am. J. Psychiatry*, **156**, 869–875.

Rein, W. and Turjanski, S. (1997). Clinical update on amisulpride in deficit schizophrenia. *Int. Clin. Psychopharmacol.*, **12** (Suppl. 2), S19–S27.

Remington, G. and Kapur, S. (1999). D2 and 5-HT2 receptor effects of antipsychotics: bridging basic and clinical findings using PET. *J. Clin. Psychiatry*, **60** (Suppl. 10), 15–19.

Sainati, S.M., Hubbard, J.W., Chi, E., *et al.* (1996). Safety, tolerability, and effect of food on the pharmacokinetics of iloperidone (HP 873), a potential atypical antipsychotic. *J. Clin. Pharmacol.*, **35**, 713–720, published erratum appears in *J. Clin. Pharmacol.*, 1996, **36**, 92.

Seeger, T.F., Seymour, P.A., Schmidt, A.W., *et al.* (1995). Ziprasidone (CP-88,059): a new antipsychotic with combined dopamine and serotonin receptor antagonist activity. *J. Pharmacol. Exp. Ther.*, **275**, 101–113.

Seeman, P. and Tallerico, T. (1999). Rapid release of antipsychotic drugs from dopamine D_2 receptors: an explanation for low receptor occupancy and early clinical relapse upon withdrawal of clozapine or quetiapine. *Am. J. Psychiatry*, **156**, 876–884.

Simpson, G.M. and Varga, E. (1974). Clozapine – a new antipsychotic agent. *Curr. Ther. Res. Clin. Exp.*, **16**, 679–686.

Warner, R., Laugharne, J., Peet, M., *et al.* (1999). Retinal function as a marker for cell membrane omega-3 fatty acid depletion in schizophrenia: a pilot study. *Biol. Psychiatry*, **45**, 1138–1142.

Depression and Mania

8

Synaptic effects of antidepressants: relationships to their therapeutic and adverse effects

Brian Leonard and Elliott Richelson

Key points

- In attempting to explain the delayed onset of antidepressant efficacy, emphasis is now being placed on adaptive changes in pre- and post-synaptic receptor-mediated processes.
- Following chronic antidepressant treatment, changes in cortical β, $\alpha_{1/2}$, DA autoreceptor, $GABA_B$, and $5\text{-}HT_{1A/2}$ receptor function have been reported.
- Additional neurochemical changes may modulate amine neurotransmission: glucocorticoid$_2$ receptors, PGE_2 concentration and possibly COX_2 activity, reduction in release of interleukins 1, 2 and 6 from brain macrophages, and changes in cytoskeletal structure of nerve cells.
- Information on the affinity of antidepressants for blocking monoamine transporters and neurotransmitter receptors can explain certain of their side effects and some of their drug interactions.
- Many new antidepressants have synaptic effects which distinguish them from older compounds; these effects may relate to therapeutic efficacy and/or to differences in adverse effect profiles.

Theories of the mechanism of action of antidepressants: is there a common mechanism of action of antidepressants

In an attempt to explain the reason for the delay in the onset of the therapeutic effect of antidepressants, which clearly is unrelated to the acute actions of these drugs on monoamine reuptake transporters or intracellular metabolizing enzymes, emphasis has moved away from the presynaptic mechanism governing the release of the monoamine transmitters to the adaptive changes that occur in pre- and post-synaptic receptors. These adaptive changes govern the physiological expression of neurotransmitter function.

Changes in neurotransmitter receptors with chronic treatment

Antidepressant therapy is usually associated with a delay of 2–3 weeks before the onset of a beneficial effect. Much of the improvement seen early in the treatment with antidepressants is probably associated with a reduction in anxiety that often occurs in the depressed patient and improvement in sleep caused by the sedative action of many of these drugs. The delay in the onset of the therapeutic response cannot be easily explained by the pharmacokinetic profile of the drugs as peak plasma (and presumably brain) concentrations are usually reached in 7–10 days. Furthermore, the 2–3 weeks delay is seen in many, though not all, patients given electroconvulsive therapy (ECT). Table 8.1 summarizes some of the changes in neurotransmitter receptors that occur in the cortex of rat brain following the chronic administration of antidepressants. It can be seen that, irrespective of the nature of the treatment, adaptational changes occur in adrenoceptors, serotonin, dopamine and gamma-aminobutyric acid (GABA)$_B$ receptors (Leonard, 1994).

In addition to these changes in GABA$_B$ and biogenic amine receptors, recent evidence has shown that a decrease in cortical muscarinic receptors occurs in the bulbectomized rat model of depression that, like most of the changes in biogenic amine receptors, returns to control values following treatment with either typical or atypical antidepressants.

Effects on muscarinic receptors are of particular interest as the anticholinergic activity of the tricyclic antidepressants is usually associated with their unacceptable central and peripheral side effects (as discussed below) and most second-generation antidepressants have gained in therapeutic popularity because they lack such side effects, due to their lack of effects on muscarinic receptors (see Tables 8.4 and 8.5). Nevertheless, support for the cholinergic hypothesis of depression is provided by the finding that the short-acting, reversible cholinesterase inhibitor pyridostigmine, when administered to drug-free, depressed patients, causes an enhanced activation of the anterior pituitary gland as shown by the release of growth hormone secretion (O'Keane et al., 1992). This suggests that the muscarinic receptors are supersensitive in the depressed patient. However, the mechanisms whereby the receptors are normalized by chronic (but not acute) antidepressant treatment vary and in most cases are unlikely to be due to a direct anticholinergic action.

Janowsky et al. (1986), for example, have postulated that depression arises as the result of an imbalance between the central noradrenergic and cholinergic systems; in depression the activity of the former system is decreased and, conversely, in mania it is increased. As most antidepressants, irrespective of the presumed specificity of their action on the noradrenergic and serotonergic systems, have been shown to enhance noradrenergic function, it is hypothesized that the functional reduction in cholinergic activity arises as a consequence of the increase in central noradrenergic activity.

Table 8.1 Changes in neurotransmitter receptors that occur in the cortex of rat brain following chronic antidepressant treatment

Cortical β-adrenoceptors	Decreased functional activity and density
Cortical α_1-adrenoceptors	Increased density
Cortical α_2-adrenoceptors	Decreased functional activity
Dopamine autoreceptors	Decreased functional activity
Cortical GABA$_B$ receptors	Decreased density
Limbic 5-HT$_{1A}$ receptors	Increased density and decreased functional activity
Cortical 5-HT$_2$ receptors	Decreased density and functional activity

Thus, irrespective of the specificity of the antidepressant following its acute administration, it would appear that a common feature of all of these drugs is to correct the abnormality in neurotransmitter receptor function. Such an effect of chronic antidepressant treatment largely parallels the time of onset of the therapeutic response and forms the basis of the receptor sensitivity hypothesis of depression and the common mode of action of antidepressants.

Considerable attention has recently been focused on the interaction between serotonergic and beta-adrenergic receptors, which may be of particular relevance to our understanding of the therapeutic effect of antidepressants. Thus the chronic administration of antidepressants enhances inhibitory responses of forebrain neurons to microiontophoretically applied 5-HT (Blier *et al.*, 1990). This enhanced response is blocked by lesions of the noradrenergic projections to the cortex. This dual effect could help to explain enhanced serotonergic function that arises after chronic administration of antidepressants or ECT. Thus most antidepressants decrease the functional activity of the beta-adrenoceptors that normally have an inhibitory role on the cortical 5-HT system. This decrease results in a disinhibition (or facilitation) of serotonergic and dopaminergic-mediated behaviours.

Conversely, impairment of the serotonergic system by use of a selective neurotoxin or a 5-HT synthesis inhibitor largely prevents the decrease in functional activity of cortical beta-adrenoceptors that usually arises following chronic antidepressant treatment (Aston-Jones *et al.*, 1991). Although there are approximately 15 molecularly cloned subtypes of the serotonin receptor and selective drugs are not yet available, experimental evidence suggests that these apparent changes in beta-adrenoceptors are more likely to be due to an increase in the density of 5-HT_{1B} receptor sites that are also labelled by the beta-adrenoceptor antagonist dihydroalprenolol, a ligand conventionally used to identify beta-adrenoceptors. The 5-HT_{1B} receptors are located on serotonergic nerve terminals that act as autoreceptors and, on stimulation by serotonin, decrease the further release of this amine. It has been hypothesized that the chronic administration of selective serotonin reuptake inhibition antidepressants (such as fluoxetine, paroxetine, sertraline, citalopram and fluvoxamine) desensitizes the inhibitory 5-HT_{1B} receptors and thereby enhances serotonin release.

In addition to the importance of the 5-HT_{1B} autoreceptors in the regulation of serotonergic function, there is experimental and clinical evidence that the 5-HT_{1A} receptors play a fundamental role in both anxiety and depression. In brief, the 5-HT_{1A} somatodendritic receptors inhibit the release of serotonin and it is postulated that enhanced release of the transmitter following the chronic administration of the selective serotonin reuptake inhibitors (SSRI) is a consequence of the desensitization of the inhibitory 5-HT_{1A} receptors (Blier *et al.*, 1990). The validity of this hypothesis is supported by the pharmacological effect of 5-HT_{1A} antagonists. Thus the beta-adrenoceptor antagonist and 5-HT_{1A} antagonist pindolol, in combination with fluoxetine or paroxetine, enhanced the therapeutic efficacy of the SSRI and, in some studies, reduced the time of onset of the peak therapeutic effect (Tome *et al.*, 1997).

Both clinical and experimental studies have provided evidence that 5-HT can also regulate dopamine turnover. Thus several investigators have shown that a positive correlation exists in depressed patients between homovanillic acid (HVA), a major metabolite of dopamine, and 5-hydroxyindole acetic acid (5-HIAA) concentrations in the CSF (Agren, 1980). In experimental studies, stimulation of the 5-HT cell bodies in the median raphé causes reduced firing of the substantia nigra where dopamine is the main neurotransmitter. There is thus convincing evidence that 5-HT plays an important role in modulating dopaminergic function in many regions of the brain, including the mesolimbic system. Sertraline has been shown to be particularly effective in enhancing dopaminergic function (possibly in part because of its effects on the dopamine transporter, as discussed below). Such findings imply that the effects of antidepressants that show an apparent selectivity for the serotonergic system could be equally ascribed to a change in dopaminergic function in mesolimbic and mesocortical regions of the brain. It has been postulated that the hedonic effect of antidepressants may be ascribed to enhanced dopaminergic function in the mesocortex.

Whereas much emphasis has been placed on the monoamine neurotransmitters with respect to the mechanism of action of antidepressants, little attention has been paid to changes in the glutamate system, the primary excitatory neurotransmitter pathway in the brain. Experimental evidence shows that tricyclic antidepressants inhibit the binding of dizolcipine (MK801) to the ion channel of the main glutamate receptor, the N-methyl-D-aspartate (NMDA) receptor, in the brain (Reynolds and Miller, 1988). The initial studies have more recently been extended to show that both typical and atypical antidepressants have a qualitatively similar effect by reducing the binding of MK801 to the NMDA receptors (Kitamura et al., 1991). Whether this is due to direct action of antidepressants on the ion channel receptor sites, or an indirect effect possibly involving the modulation of the glycine receptor site, is uncertain. However, there is evidence that glycine and drugs modulating the glycine site have antidepressant-like activity in animal models of depression.

These results suggest that antidepressants act as functional NMDA receptor antagonists. By acting in this way, it seems possible that antidepressants could prevent neuronal injury which arises in the brain of the depressed patient as a result of increased glucocorticoid receptor function combined with an increase in proinflammatory cytokines and inflammatory mediators (for example, prostaglandin E_2, nitric oxide (Hedqvist and Brundin, 1969; Piani et al., 1991)).

Effects of antidepressants on secondary messenger systems

Recent advances in molecular neurobiology have demonstrated how information is passed from the neurotransmitter receptors on the outer side of the neuronal membrane to the secondary messenger system on the inside. The coupling of this receptor to the secondary messenger is brought about by a member of the G-protein family. Beta-adrenoceptors are linked to adenylate cyclase and, depending on the type of receptor, 5-HT is linked to either adenylate cyclase (5-HT_{1A}, 5-HT_{1B}) or phospholipase (5-HT_{2A}, 5-HT_{2C}). Activation of phospholipase results in an intracellular increase in the secondary messengers diacylglycerol and inositol trisphosphate (IP_3), the IP_3 then mobilizing intraneuronal calcium.

The net result of activation of secondary messenger systems is to increase the activity of various protein kinases that phosphorylate membrane bound proteins to produce a physiological response. Racagni and co-workers (1991) have investigated the effect of chronic antidepressant treatment on the phosphorylation of proteins associated with the cytoskeletal structure of the nerve cell. These investigators suggested that antidepressants could affect the function of the cytoskeleton by changing the component of the associated protein phosphorylation system. In support of their hypothesis, they showed that both typical (e.g. desipramine) and atypical (e.g. (+) oxaprotiline, a specific noradrenaline reuptake inhibitor, and fluoxetine, a selective 5-HT uptake inhibitor) antidepressants increased the synthesis of a microtubule fraction, possibly by affecting the regulatory subunit of protein kinase type II. These changes in cytoskeletal protein synthesis occurred only after chronic antidepressant treatments and suggest that antidepressants, besides their well-established effects on pre- and post-synaptic receptors and amine uptake systems, might change neuronal signal transduction processes distal to the receptor.

Antidepressants, gene regulation, and stress hormones

Interest in the possible association of glucocorticoids with central neurotransmitter function arose from the observation that such receptors have been identified in the nuclei of catecholamine and 5-HT-containing cell bodies in the brain. Experimental studies have shown that glucocorticoid receptors function as DNA binding proteins that can modify the transcription of genes. Chronic imipramine treatment increases glucocorticoid receptor immunoreactivity in rat brain, the changes being particularly pronounced in noradrenergic and serotonergic cell body regions. Preliminary clinical studies have also shown that lymphocyte glucocorticoid receptors are abnormal in depressed patients. Such findings lend support to the hypothesis that changes in central neurotransmission occurring in depression are a reflection of the effects of chronic glucocorticoids on the transcription of proteins that play a crucial role in neuronal structure and function. Sulser and Sanders-Bush (1987) have formulated a 5-HT-noradrenaline-glucocorticoid-like hypothesis of affective disorders based on such findings. If the pituitary–adrenal axis plays such an important role in central neurotransmission, it may be speculated that glucocorticoid synthesis inhibitors (e.g. metyrapone) could reduce the abnormality in neurotransmitter function by decreasing cortisol concentration.

Adaptation of central glucocorticoid-type 2 receptors to the decrease in the concentration of corticoids caused by antidepressants would appear to require chronic drug treatment. Recent *in situ* hybridization studies in the rat have demonstrated that typical antidepressants increase the density of glucocorticoid receptors. Such an effect could increase the negative feedback mechanism and thereby reduce the synthesis and release of cortisol. In support of this hypothesis, there is preliminary clinical evidence that metyrapone (and the steroid synthesis inhibitor ketoconazole) may produce a beneficial effect in depressed patients more rapidly than typical antidepressants (O'Dwyer *et al.*, 1995; Sovner and Fogelman, 1996). Recently, several lipophilic antagonists of corticotrophin-releasing factor (CRF) type 1 receptors, which appear to be hyperactive in the brain of depressed patients, have been shown to be active in animal models of depression. Clearly this is a potentially important area for antidepressant development (Mansbach *et al.*, 1997).

Stress is frequently a predisposing factor for depression in vulnerable patients. There is clinical evidence to show that CRF is elevated in the cerebrospinal fluid of untreated depressed patients. This elevation presumably leads to the hypercortisolaemia that usually accompanies the condition. One of the consequences of elevated plasma glucocorticoids is a suppression of some aspects of cellular immunity. It is now established that many aspects of both cellular (e.g. natural killer cell activity, T-cell replication) and non-cellular (e.g. acute phase proteins) are abnormal in the untreated depressed patient (Song and Leonard, 1995). Such observations could help to explain the susceptibility of depressed patients to physical ill health.

A link between CRF, the cytokines which orchestrate many aspects of cellular immunity, and prostaglandins of the E series has been the subject of considerable research in recent years. There is clinical evidence to show that prostaglandin E_2 (PGE_2) concentrations are raised in the plasma of untreated depressed patients and are normalized following effective antidepressant treatment. Raised PGE_2 concentrations in the brain and periphery reflect increased cytokines (particularly interleukins 1, 6 and TNF-alpha), which occur as a consequence of increased macrophage activity in the blood and brain. In the brain, the microglia function as macrophages and produce cytokines locally. The increased synthesis of PGE_2 may contribute to the reduction in amine release in the brain that appears to underlie the pathology of depression. It has recently been postulated that many effective antidepressants normalize central neurotransmission by reducing brain concentrations of both the proinflammatory cytokines and PGE_2. This is achieved by inhibiting central and peripheral macrophage activity together with cyclo-oxygenase type 2 activity in the brain. Cyclo-oxygenase is the key enzyme in the synthesis of the prostaglandins. It is not without interest that the use of tricyclic antidepressants in severe rheumatoid arthritis can now be explained by the inhibitory action of such drugs on cyclo-oxygenase activity in both the periphery and brain. Such changes, together with those in glucocorticoid receptor function, may therefore, incrementally bring about the normalization of defective central neurotransmission as a consequence of antidepressant treatment.

Table 8.2 Some biochemical changes that may indirectly modulate amine neurotransmitters in depressed patients

- Normalization of hypofunctional central glucocorticoid type 2 receptors in limbic regions of the brain
- Decrease in the elevated concentration of PGE_2 in the brain and blood possibly due to an inhibition of cyclo-oxygenase type 2 activity
- Reduction in the release of interleukins (1, 2, 6) from macrophages in the brain (e.g. microglia, astrocytes)
- Changes in cytoskeletal structure of nerve cells

Another possible mechanism whereby antidepressants may change the physical relationship between neurons in the brain is by inhibiting neurite outgrowth from nerve cells. In support of this view, it has been shown that the tricyclic antidepressant amitriptyline, at therapeutically relevant concentrations, inhibited neurite outgrowth from chick embryonic cerebral explants in vitro (Wong et al., 1991). Presumably the reduction in the rate of synthesis of cyclic AMP caused by amitriptyline is responsible for the reduced neurite growth. While the relevance of such findings to the therapeutic effects of amitriptyline in man is unclear, they do suggest that a common mode of action of all antidepressants could be to modify the actual structure of nerve cells and possibly eliminate inappropriate synaptic contacts that are responsible for behavioural and psychological changes associated with depression.

There are several mechanisms whereby antidepressants can modify intracellular events that occur proximal to the post-synaptic receptor sites. Most attention has been paid to the actions of antidepressants on those pathways that are controlled by receptor coupled second messengers (such as cyclic AMP, inositol trisphosphate, nitric oxide, and calcium binding). However, it is also possible that chronic antidepressant treatment may affect those pathways that involve receptor interactions with protein tyrosine kinases, by increasing specific growth factor synthesis or by regulating the activity of proinflammatory cytokines (Duman et al., 1997). These pathways are particularly important because they control many aspects of neuronal function that ultimately underlie the ability of the brain to adapt and respond to pharmacological and environmental stimuli. It is known, for example, that learning and memory lead to changes in synaptic efficiency, which are related to physical changes in neuronal structure associated with neuronal atrophy or sprouting (Levine et al., 1995). One mechanism whereby antidepressants could increase the synthesis of trophic factors is by the activation of cyclic AMP-dependent protein kinase which, by activating calcium dependent protein kinases, increases the formation of the transcription factor CREB (cyclic AMP response element binding protein). The increase in CREB stimulates the target gene, brain-derived neurotrophic factor (BDNF) thereby linking the chronic administration of antidepressants with changes in neuronal plasticity which, presumably, underlies recovery from depression.

There is experimental evidence to show that the infusion of BDNF into the midbrain of rats results in antidepressant-like activity (Siuciak et al., 1997). This action of BDNF has been associated with an increase in the synthesis of tryptophan hydroxylase, the rate-limiting enzyme in the synthesis of serotonin. There is also experimental evidence to show that chronic stress causes a degeneration of noradrenergic axons in the frontal cortex of the rat brain and that chronic imipramine treatment attenuates this degenerative change (Kitayama et al., 1997).

Hypercortisolism occurs commonly in depression, and the relative insensitivity of the pituitary–adrenal axis to the inhibitory feedback effect of the glucocorticoid dexamethasone has been used as a biochemical marker of the disease. One possible explanation for this insensitivity to dexamethasone may lie in the hypersensitivity of central glucocorticoid receptors (Dinan, 1994).

Glucocorticoid receptors are present at a high density in the amygdala. Neuroimaging studies have shown that the amygdala is the only structure in which regional blood flow and glucose metabolism consistently correlate positively with the severity of depression (Lesser et al., 1994). This hypermetabolism appears to reflect an underlying pathological process as it also occurs in asymptomatic patients and in the close relatives of patients. Antidepressants have been shown not only to correct the symptoms of depression, but also to normalize the hypermetabolism of the amygdala (Drevets, 1998). While the precise mechanism for this action is uncertain, one possibility is that antidepressants decrease the density of glucocorticoid receptors in the amygdala and return their activity to control values. This could account for the link between glucocorticoid receptor function, hyperactivity of the amygdala and the therapeutic action of antidepressants (Drevets, 1994, 1998).

Acute synaptic effects of antidepressants predicting certain adverse effects and drug interactions

Theories about the presumed mechanism of action of antidepressants have led to many hypotheses to be tested in clinical studies. However, most, if not all, of these theories are based on animal studies. On the other hand, information from in vitro studies on the potency of antidepressants at blocking monoamine transporters and certain neurotransmitter receptors can explain certain of their side effects and some of their drug interactions.

Antidepressant blockade of neurotransmitter transport

More than one-half of the antidepressants available in the USA and Europe are more potent at blocking transport of serotonin than transport of norepinephrine at the molecularly cloned, human transporters (Table 8.3) (Tatsumi et al., 1997). Newer antidepressants are generally more selective and more potent than the older compounds at blocking transport of serotonin over norepinephrine (selective serotonin reuptake inhibitors or SSRIs). In addition, some antidepressants (e.g. mirtazapine) very weakly block transport of norepinephrine, serotonin, and dopamine. Bupropion, which is presently available solely in the USA, is the only antidepressant more selective for blocking transport of dopamine (Table 8.3) than for other neurotransmitters. However, bupropion may be more noradrenergic than dopaminergic, due to the effects of a metabolite which is present in much higher concentrations than in the parent compound (Ascher et al., 1995). Sertraline is the most potent of the antidepressants at blocking transport of dopamine, being about as potent as methylphenidate. Paroxetine is the most potent blocker of transport of serotonin, while citalopram is by far the most selective. While venlafaxine has been called a serotonin and norepinephrine reuptake inhibitor (SNRI) based on animal data (Bolden-Watson and Richelson, 1993), it is much weaker at the human norepinephrine transporter than at the rat homologue. It is, therefore, an SSRI. However, effects on the norepinephrine transporter can be achieved at higher dosages.

Table 8.3 Antidepressant affinities for human transporters of biogenic amine neurotransmitters norepinephrine (NE), serotonin (5-HT, SERT), and dopamine (DA) and selectivity for 5-HT over NE[a]

	Affinity for blocking transporter[b]			
	hNET	*hSERT*	*hDAT*	*Selectivity of 5-HT over NE*
amitriptyline	2.9	23	0.031	8.1[c]
amoxapine	6.2	1.7	0.023	0.28
bupropion	0.0019	0.011	0.19	5.7
butriptyline[d]	0.020	0.073	0.025	3.7
carbamazepine[d]	0.0010	0.0033	0.0010	3.3
citalopram	0.025	86	0.0036	3500
clomipramine	2.7	362	0.045	140
desipramine	120	5.7	0.031	0.047
dothiepin[d]	2.2	12	0.019	5.3
doxepin	3.4	1.5	0.0082	0.43
etoperidone[d]	0.0049	0.11	0.0019	23
femoxetine[d]	0.13	9.1	0.049	70
fluoxetine	0.41	123	0.028	300
fluvoxamine[d]	0.077	45	0.011	580
imipramine	2.7	71	0.012	27
iprindole[d]	0.079	0.062	0.015	0.78
iproniazid[d]	0.0020	0.0010	0.0010	0.49
lithium carbonate[d]	0.0010	0.0010	0.0010	1.0
lofepramine[d]	19	1.4	0.0054	0.077
maprotiline	9.0	0.017	0.10	0.0019
mianserin[d]	1.4	0.025	0.011	0.018
milnacipran[d]	1.2	11	0.0014	9.2
mirtazepine	0.021	0.0010	0.0010	0.047
nefazodone	0.28	0.50	0.28	1.8
nomifensine[d]	6.4	0.10	1.8	0.016
nortriptyline	23	5.4	0.088	0.24
oxaprotiline[d]	20	0.025	0.023	0.0012
paroxetine	2.5	798	0.20	320
phenelzine	0.0020	0.0010	0.012	0.49
protriptyline	71	5.1	0.047	0.072
reboxetine[d]	14	1.7	0.0087	0.12
sertraline	0.24	341	4.0	1400
tomoxetine[d]	49	11	0.092	0.23
tranylcypromine	0.017	0.0025	0.020	0.15
trazodone	0.012	0.63	0.014	53
trimipramine	0.041	0.67	0.026	16
venlafaxine	0.094	11	0.011	120
viloxazine[d]	0.64	0.0058	0.0010	0.0090
zimelidine[d]	0.011	0.66	0.0085	60

[a]Data from Tatsumi *et al.*, 1997 and unpublished data of E. Richelson.
[b]$10^{-7} \times 1/K_d$, where K_d = equilibrium dissociation constant in molarity.
[c]Indicates that amitriptyline is about 8.1 (23/2.9) times more potent at blocking transport of serotonin than transport of norepinephrine.
[d]Not marketed in the USA as an antidepressant or not available in the USA.
Data can be compared both vertically and across Tables 8.3 and 8.4 to find the most potent drug for a specific property and to find the most potent property for a specific drug.

Selectivity cannot be equated with potency since selectivity is derived from a ratio of potencies. Thus, although citalopram is by far more selective at blocking transport of serotonin than is paroxetine, it is only about one-tenth as potent as paroxetine at this blockade (Table 8.3).

Over the past 11 years in the USA, drug companies have introduced with FDA approval eight newer, second-generation antidepressants: fluoxetine, bupropion, sertraline, paroxetine, venlafaxine, nefazodone, mirtazapine, and citalopram. Also marketed during this time were clomipramine (Anafranil) and fluvoxamine (Luvox). Each of these latter compounds is approved in the USA for treatment of obsessive-compulsive disorder and each has efficacy for treating depression. Of all these compounds, only bupropion is not potent or selective for blocking transport of serotonin (Table 8.3). That is, citalopram, clomipramine, fluoxetine, fluvoxamine, nefazodone, sertraline, paroxetine, and venlafaxine are SSRIs and bupropion is not.

Blockade of neurotransmitter receptors by antidepressants

Most of the newer, second-generation antidepressants have lower potency (affinity) than the older compounds (especially, tricyclic antidepressants) at blocking receptors for certain neurotransmitters. As mentioned earlier, this has led to the more widespread use of the newer generation compounds, because of a more favourable side-effect profile.

Overall, the most potent interaction of antidepressants as receptor blockers, especially among the classical tricyclic drugs, is at the histamine H_1 receptor (Table 8.4). Histamine is a neurotransmitter in the brain (Schwartz et al., 1995) where, as elsewhere in the body, it works by its action at three types of receptors, histamine H_1, H_2, and H_3 (Richelson, 1992). The newest histamine receptor, H_3, affects the presynaptic synthesis and release of histamine and other neurotransmitters. Histamine H_2 receptors are present in brain, but classically these receptors are involved with gastric acid secretion. In addition, histamine H_1 receptors are traditionally involved with allergic reactions outside the nervous system. However, in brain this subtype is involved with arousal and appetite mechanisms, among others. Some antidepressants are exceedingly potent histamine H_1 antagonists (Table 8.4) and more potent than any of the histamine H_1 antagonists marketed in recent years in the USA. As a result clinicians are also using antidepressants to treat allergic and dermatological problems (Drake et al., 1994). Interestingly, a topical antipruritic agent with the active ingredient of doxepin was reported to cause a tricyclic antidepressant overdose in a child with eczema (Vo et al., 1995), even though the child never ingested the drug. It was readily absorbed through the skin.

The next most potent receptor blocking effect of antidepressants that is of certain clinical relevance is at the muscarinic acetylcholine receptor. These receptors are the predominant type of cholinergic receptor in brain. In that organ they are involved with memory and learning, among other functions (Richelson, 1995). In addition, as mentioned previously, there is some evidence to suggest that these brain receptors are involved with affective illness (Janowksky et al., 1986, 1994). Antidepressants have a broad range of affinities for human brain muscarinic receptors (Table 8.4). The most potent is

Table 8.4 Antidepressant affinities for neurotransmitter receptors of human brain[a]

	Histamine H_1	Muscarinic	α_1-adrenergic	α_2-adrenergic	Dopamine D_2	5-HT_{2A}
amitriptyline	91	5.6	3.7	0.11	0.10	3.4
amoxapine	4.0	0.10	2.0	0.038	5.6	97
bupropion	0.015	0.0021	0.022	0.0012	0.00048	0.0011
citalopram	0.21	0.045	0.053	0.0065	na[c]	0.042
clomipramine[d]	3.2	2.70	2.6	0.031	0.53	3.7
desipramine	0.91	0.51	0.77	0.014	0.030	0.36
dothiepin[d]	28	4.0	0.21	0.042	na	0.39
doxepin	420	1.2	4.2	0.091	0.042	4.0
etoperidone[d]	0.032	0	2.6	1.7	0.043	2.8
femoxetine[d]	0.024	0.54	0.15	0	0.17	0.76
fluoxetine	0.016	0.050	0.017	0.0077	0.015	0.48
fluvoxamine[d]	0.00092	0.0042	0.013	0.0067		0.018
imipramine	9.1	1.1	1.1	0.031	0.050	1.3
iprindole[d]	0.77	0.048	0.043	0.012	na	0.36
lofepramine[d]	0.28	1.5	1.0	0	0.050	0.49
maprotiline	50	0.18	1.1	0.011	0.29	0.83
mianserin[d]	250	0.12	2.9	1.4	0.048	14
milnacipran[d]	0.0082	0.0019	0.0065	na	na	0.012
mirtazapine	700	0.15	0.20	0.71	0.10	6.1
nefazodone	4.7	0.0091	3.9	0.015	0.11	30
nortriptyline	10	0.67	1.7	0.040	0.083	2.3
paroxetine	0.0045	0.93	0	0.0059	0.0031	0.0052
protriptyline	4.0	4.00	0.77	0.015	0.043	1.5
reboxetine[d]	0.32	0.015	0.0084	na	na	0.016
sertraline	0.0042	0.16	0.27	0.025	0.0093	0.010
tomoxetine[d]	0.018	0.048	0.026	0	0	0.11
trazodone	0.29	0.00031	2.8	0.20	0.026	13
trimipramine	370	1.7	4.2	0.15	0.56	3.1
venlafaxine	0	0	0	0	0	0
viloxazine[d]	0.0056	0.0019	0.0071	0.0023	na	0.0032
zimelidine[d]	0.025	0.0077	0.067	0.13	na	0.12

[a] Data from Richelson and Nelson, 1984; Wander et al., 1986; Cusack et al., 1994 and unpublished data of E. Richelson.
[b] $10^{-7} \times 1/K_d$, where K_d = equilibrium dissociation constant in molarity.
[c] na = data not available.
[d] Not marketed in the USA as an antidepressant or not available in the USA.
Data can be compared both vertically and across Tables 8.3 and 8.4 to find the most potent drug for a specific property and to find the most potent property for a specific drug.

amitriptyline. The SSRI paroxetine is unique among the newer compounds for having appreciable antimuscarinic potency, similar to that for imipramine (Table 8.4). Studies with the molecularly cloned human muscarinic receptors, of which there are five, show that paroxetine has highest affinity for the m3 subtype of this receptor (Stanton et al., 1993). This subtype is found predominantly in brain, glandular tissue, and smooth muscle. Overall, any given antidepressant varies little in its affinities for the five subtypes of the human muscarinic receptor (Stanton et al., 1993).

At the α_1-adrenoceptor, the most potent compounds, although a little weaker than the antihypertensive drug phentolamine (affinity = 5.6), are likely to have effects clinically at these receptors (Tables 8.4 and 8.5).

Antidepressants are also weak competitive antagonists of dopamine (D_2) receptors (Table 8.4).

Antidepressants also antagonize the 5-HT$_{2A}$ receptor, which, as mentioned previously, is one of approximately 15 molecularly cloned subtypes of the serotonin receptor. In general, antidepressants are weak at this blockade; however, exceptions are amoxapine, nefazodone, and mianserin (Table 8.4). It has been suggested that because of its ratio for blockade of 5-HT$_{2A}$ over dopamine D_2 receptors, that amoxapine is an atypical antipsychotic (Kapur et al., 1998).

The clinical relevance of blockade of 5-HT$_{2A}$ receptors is otherwise uncertain. Many of the clinical effects ascribed to 5-HT$_{2A}$ receptors may actually involve 5-HT$_{2C}$ receptors or a combination of both. However, activation of 5-HT$_{2A}$ receptors may cause anxiety, sleep disturbances, and sexual dysfunction. Blockade of these receptors may reduce anxiety, promote deep sleep, prevent migraine headaches, and alleviate psychosis. In addition, both 5-HT$_{2A}$ and 5-HT$_{2C}$ receptors may be involved in the alleviation of psychosis.

Monoamine oxidase inhibitors have very weak direct effects on neurotransmitter receptors and are practically without clinically significant pharmacological activity on them (data not shown).

Clinical importance of the synaptic effects of antidepressant drugs

The pharmacological effects of the drugs discussed above occur shortly after a patient has ingested a dose of the medication. Thus, most of the possible clinical effects to be discussed below occur early in the treatment of patients. However, with chronic administration of the drug, adaptive changes may occur which can result in an adjustment to certain side effects, the development of new side effects, and the onset of therapeutic effects. Table 8.5 lists the pharmacological properties and their possible clinical consequences. The clinician should keep in mind that the drugs most potent at the properties discussed are more likely to cause side effects than the drugs that are weak at these properties (Tables 8.3 and 8.4).

Evidence to date suggests that the efficacy of antidepressants is not related to selectivity or potency for norepinephrine, serotonin, or dopamine transport blockade. These data are from clinical studies (Nystrom and Hallstrom, 1985, 1987) and basic studies that show the wide range of potencies of antidepressants at blocking this transport (Table 8.3). On the other hand, clinical data suggest that potent transport blockade of serotonin is necessary for treatment of certain anxiety disorders as well as obsessive-compulsive disorder.

Transport blockade of neurotransmitters likely relates to certain adverse effects of these drugs and to some of their drug interactions (Table 8.5). For example, serotonin transport blockade is most likely the property that causes sexual side effects, seen more commonly with the SSRIs, and is the property that causes serious results when a monoamine oxidase inhibitor is combined with an antidepressant (serotonergic syndrome). In addition, researchers have reported adverse interactions between L-tryptophan, the precursor of serotonin, and fluoxetine (Steiner and Fontaine, 1986). An interaction between fenfluramine, which increases synaptic levels of seroto-

Table 8.5 Synaptic effects of antidepressants and their possible clinical consequences

Property	Possible clinical consequences
Blockade of norepinephrine transport at nerve endings	Alleviation of depression Tremors Tachycardia Erectile and ejaculatory dysfunction Blockade of the antihypertensive effects of guanethidine and guanadrel Augmentation of pressor effects of sympathomimetic amines
Blockade of serotonin transport at nerve endings	Alleviation of depression Gastrointestinal disturbances Increase or decrease in anxiety (dose-dependent) Sexual dysfunction Extrapyramidal side effects Interactions with L-tryptophan and monoamine oxidase inhibitors (serotonergic syndrome)
Blockade of dopamine transport at nerve endings	Psychomotor activation Antiparkinsonian effect Precipitation or aggravation of psychosis
Blockade of histamine H_1 receptors	Potentiation of central depressant drugs Sedation drowsiness Weight gain
Blockade of muscarinic receptors	Blurred vision Dry mouth Sinus tachycardia Constipation Urinary retention Memory dysfunction
Blockade of α_1-adrenoceptors	Potentiation of antihypertensives that block these receptors (e.g., prazosin, terazosin, doxazosin, labetalol) Postural hypotension, dizziness Reflex tachycardia
Blockade of serotonin 5-HT_{2A} receptors	Alleviation of depression Reduction of anxiety Promotion of deep sleep Prophylaxis of migraine headaches Alleviation of psychosis Alleviation or prevention of sexual side effects of SSRIs
Blockade of dopamine D_2 receptors	Extrapyramidal movement disorders Endocrine changes (including hyperprolactinemia, which can lead to impotence)

nin, and antidepressants that are serotonin transport inhibitors can be predicted. However, the combination of fenfluramine with an SSRI has been used in patients without the development of adverse effects (Coplan *et al.*, 1993).

There are reports about adverse effects of fluoxetine and other SSRIs that include extrapyramidal side effects (Bouchard *et al.*, 1989; Shihabuddin and

Rapport, 1994; Coulter and Pillans, 1995), anorgasmia and other sexual problems (Kline, 1989; Stein and Hollander, 1994; Modell *et al.*, 1997), paranoid reaction (Mandalos and Szarek, 1990), and intense suicidal preoccupation (Teicher *et al.*, 1990). These extrapyramidal side effects are not due to blockade of dopamine receptors, because these SSRIs are very weak at this binding site (Table 8.4). One can only speculate that these reactions involve serotonin, since serotonin transport blockade is the most potent property possessed by these compounds. In support of the hypothesis relating serotonin to anorgasmia is the use of serotonin receptor antagonists to treat this problem (Silverman, 1991; Aizenberg *et al.*, 1995). In addition, as discussed before, SSRIs can modulate dopaminergic function in many regions of the brain and probably cause extrapyramidal side effects by functionally reducing dopaminergic neurotransmission in the nigro-striatal region.

Potentiation of the effects of central depressant drugs, which cause sedation and drowsiness, is a drug interaction of antidepressants related to histamine H_1 receptor antagonism. This antagonism is probably responsible for side effects of sedation, drowsiness and weight gain. Sedation, however, may be a wanted effect in patients who are agitated and also depressed.

Trazodone frequently causes sedation and drowsiness in patients. As a result it is presently used in the USA as a hypnotic (Nierenberg *et al.*, 1994). Its relatively low affinity for the histamine H_1 receptor (Table 8.4) suggests that this drug causes these side effects by other mechanisms. However, data showing that, in clinical practice, trazodone achieves high blood levels (which relate to brain receptor site levels), are consistent with the idea that trazodone causes sedation and drowsiness by blocking the histamine H_1 receptor (Caccia *et al.*, 1982; Abernethy *et al.*, 1984).

Although effects of antidepressants on muscarinic receptors may relate to therapeutic effects (Janowsky *et al.*, 1986, 1994), their blockade by these antidepressants can be responsible for several adverse effects (Table 8.5). The relatively high affinity of paroxetine for these receptors distinguishes it from the other newer, second-generation compounds. In addition, it may explain the common complaint of dry mouth and constipation reported in some published clinical trials with paroxetine (Boyer, 1992). We need to be especially vigilant with the elderly patient to avoid or reduce these antimuscarinic effects of antidepressants.

Alpha$_1$-adrenoceptor receptor blockade by antidepressants may be responsible for orthostatic hypotension, the most serious common cardiovascular effect of these drugs. This side effect can cause dizziness and a reflex tachycardia. In addition, this property of antidepressants will result in the potentiation of several antihypertensive drugs that potently block α_1-adrenoceptors (Table 8.5).

Antidepressants are weak competitive antagonists of dopamine (D_2) receptors (Table 8.4). The most potent compound, amoxapine, is a demethylated derivative of the neuroleptic, loxapine. It is very likely that this *in vitro* activity of amoxapine explains its extrapyramidal side effects (Steele, 1982) and its ability to elevate prolactin levels in patients (Cooper *et al.*, 1981). Because of the dopamine receptor blocking property of amoxapine, this drug should be reserved for patients with psychotic depressions.

Antidepressants also block α_2-adrenoceptors, 5-HT$_{1A}$ and 5-HT$_2$ receptors (Richelson and Nelson, 1984; Wander *et al.*, 1986; Cusack *et al.*, 1994).

Antidepressants are usually weak at this blockade with the exception of trazodone and nefazodone, which are relatively potent at these three receptors. Trazodone's potent blockade of these serotonin receptors may explain why, despite its ability to block transport of serotonin, it can be used without serious results (serotonergic syndrome) in combination with monoamine oxidase inhibitors (Nierenberg and Keck, 1989).

Drug interactions not related to synaptic effects of antidepressants

Drug interactions for antidepressants can be divided into two groups – pharmacokinetic and pharmacodynamic. Pharmacokinetic interactions occur when one drug affects the metabolism or protein-binding of another drug. Pharmacodynamic interactions occur when one drug affects the mechanism of action of another drug. These pharmacodynamic drug interactions of antidepressants relate to their synaptic effects discussed above and are listed in Table 8.5.

Conclusions

This chapter has reviewed many of the current hypotheses about the mechanism of action of antidepressants. However, we still need much more research to know the mechanism of action of antidepressants in treating depression. Hypotheses derived from animal studies need to be tested in humans, although such research is always more difficult and often equivocal. From this clinical perspective, all antidepressants seem to be equally efficacious in treating major depressive disorder. Other characteristics of these agents serve to differentiate them from each other. Many of the antidepressants introduced within the last decade have synaptic effects that delineate them from the older compounds. These synaptic effects help to explain the advantages of newer compounds relative to the older compounds in terms of side-effect profiles and certain drug interactions. Clinically, these synaptic effects, especially as they involve some neurotransmitters, such as serotonin and norepinephrine, can be linked to therapeutic and certain adverse effects. The *in vitro* findings presented will help clinicians choose the most appropriate antidepressant for each patient and, potentially, will help to prevent or minimize the occurrence of certain side effects and drug interactions.

References

Abernethy, D.R., Greenblatt, D.J. and Shader, R.I. (1984). Plasma levels of trazodone: methodology and applications. *Pharmacology*, **28**, 42–46.

Agren, H. (1980). Symptom patterns in unipolar and bipolar depression correlating with monoamine metabolites in the cerebrospinal fluid: II. Suicide. *Psychiatry Res.*, **3**, 225–236.

Aizenberg, D., Zemishlany, Z. and Weizman, A. (1995). Cyproheptadine treatment of sexual dysfunction induced by serotonin reuptake inhibitors. *Clin. Neuropharmacol.*, **18**, 320–324.

Ascher, J.A., Cole, J.O., Colin, J.N., *et al.* (1995). Bupropion: a review of its mechanism of antidepressant activity. *J. Clin. Psychiatry*, **56**, 395–401.

Aston-Jones, G., Akaoka, H., Charlety, P., *et al.* (1991). Serotonin selectively attenuates gluat-mate-evoked activation of noradrenergic locus coeruleus neurons. *J. Neurosci.*, **11**, 760–769.

Blier, P., de Montigny, C. and Chaput, Y. (1990). A role for the serotonin system in the mechanism of action of antidepressant treatments: preclinical evidence. *J. Clin. Psychiatry*, **51** (Suppl.), 14–20; discussion 21.

Bolden-Watson, C. and Richelson, E. (1993). Blockade by newly-developed antidepressants of biogenic amine uptake into rat brain synaptosomes. *Life Sci.*, **52**, 1023–1029.

Bouchard, R.H., Pourcher, E. and Vincent, P. (1989). Fluoxetine and extrapyramidal side effects. *Am. J. Psychiatry*, **146**, 1352–1353.

Boyer, W.F.B.C.L. (1992). The safety profile of paroxetine. *J. Clin. Psychiatry*, **53**, 61–66.

Caccia, S., Fong, M.H., Garattini, S., *et al.* (1982). Plasma concentrations of trazodone and 1-(3-chlorophenyl)piperazine in man after a single oral dose of trazodone. *J. Pharm. Pharmacol.*, **34**, 605–606.

Cooper, D.S., Gelenberg, A.J., Wojcik, J.C., *et al.* (1981). The effect of amoxapine and imipramine on serum prolactin levels. *Arch. Intern. Med.*, **141**, 1023–1025.

Coplan, J.D., Tiffon, L. and Gorman, J.M. (1993). Therapeutic strategies for the patient with treatment-resistant anxiety. *J. Clin. Psychiatry*, **54** (Suppl.), 69–74.

Coulter, D.M. and Pillans, P.I. (1995). Fluoxetine and extrapyramidal side effects. *Am. J. Psychiatry*, **152**, 122–125.

Cusack, B., Nelson, A. and Richelson, E. (1994). Binding of antidepressants to human brain receptors: focus on newer generation compounds. *Psychopharmacology*, **114**, 559–565.

Dinan, T.G. (1994). Glucocorticoids and the genesis of depressive illness. A psychobiological model. *Br. J. Psychiatry*, **164**, 365–371.

Drake, L.A., Fallon, J.D., Sober, A., *et al.* (1994). Relief of pruritus in patients with atopic dermatitis after treatment with topical doxepin cream. *J. Am. Acad. Dermatol.*, **31**, 613–616.

Drevets, W.C. (1994). Geriatric depression: brain imaging correlates and pharmacologic considerations. *J. Clin. Psychiatry*, **55** (Suppl. A), 71–81.

Drevets, W.C. (1998). Functional neuroimaging studies of depression: the anatomy of melancholia. *Annu. Rev. Med.*, **49**, 341.

Duman, R.S., Heninger, G.R. and Nestler, E.J. (1997). A molecular and cellular theory of depression. *Arch. Gen. Psychiatry*, **54**, 597–606.

Hedqvist, P. and Brundin, J. (1969). Inhibition by prostaglandin E1 of noradrenaline release and of effector response to nerve stimulation in the cat spleen. *Life Sci.*, **8**, 389–395.

Janowsky, D.S., Risch, S.C., Kennedy, B., *et al.* (1986). Central muscarinic effects of physostigmine on mood, cardiovascular function, pituitary and adrenal neuroendocrine release. *Psychopharmacology (Berl.)*, **89**, 150–154.

Janowsky, D.S., Overstreet, D.H. and Nurnberger, J.I. (1994). Is cholinergic sensitivity a genetic marker for the affective disorders? *Am. J. Med. Genet.*, **54**, 335–344.

Kapur, S., Cho, R., Jones, C. *et al.* (1988). Is amoxapine an atypical antipsychotic? Supportive PET evidence [abstract.] *Biol. Psychiatry*, **43**, 185.

Kitamura, Y., Zhao, X.-H., Takei, M., *et al.* (1991). Effects of antidepressants on the glutamatergic system in mouse brain. *Neurochem. Int.*, **19**, 247–253.

Kitayama, I., Yaga, T., Kayahara, T., *et al.* (1997). Long-term stress degenerates, but imipramine regenerates, noradrenergic axons in the rat cerebral cortex. *Biol. Psychiatry*, **42**, 687–696.

Kline, M.D. (1989). Fluoxetine and anorgasmia. *Am. J. Psychiatry*, **146**, 804–805.

Leonard, B.E. (1994). Biochemical strategies for the development of antidepressants. *CNS Drugs*, **1**, 285–304.

Lesser, I.M., Mena, I., Boone, K.B., *et al.* (1994). Reduction of cerebral blood flow in older depressed patients. *Arch. Gen. Psychiatry*, **51**, 677–686.

Levine, E.S., Dreyfus, C.F., Black, I.B., *et al.* (1995). Brain-derived neurotrophic factor rapidly enhances synaptic transmission in hippocampal neurons via postsynaptic tyrosine kinase receptors. *Proc. Natl. Acad. Sci. USA*, **92**, 8074–8077.

Mandalos, G.E. and Szarek, B.L. (1990). Dose-related paranoid reaction associated with fluoxetine. *J. Nerv. Ment. Dis.*, **178**, 57–58.

Mansbach, R.S., Brooks, E.N. and Chen, Y.L. (1997). Antidepressant-like effects of CP-154,526, a selective CRF1 receptor antagonist. *Eur. J. Pharmacol.*, **323**, 21–26.

Modell, J.G., Katholi, C.R., Modell, J.D., *et al.* (1997). Comparative sexual side effects of bupropion, fluoxetine, paroxetine, and sertraline. *Clin. Pharmacol. Ther.*, **61**, 476–487.

Nierenberg, A.A. and Keck, P.E., Jr. (1989). Management of monoamine oxidase inhibitor-associated insomnia with trazodone. *J. Clin. Psychopharmacol.*, **9**, 42–45.

Nierenberg, A.A., Adler, L.A., Peselow, E., *et al.* (1994). Trazodone for antidepressant-associated insomnia. *Am. J. Psychiatry*, **151**, 1069–1072.

Nystrom, C. and Hallstrom, T. (1985). Double-blind comparison between a serotonin and a noradrenaline reuptake blocker in the treatment of depressed outpatients. *Acta Psychiatr. Scand.*, **72**, 6–15.

Nystrom, C. and Hallstrom, T. (1987). Comparison between a serotonin and a noradrenaline reuptake blocker in the treatment of depressed outpatients – a cross-over study. *Acta Psychiatr. Scand.*, **75**, 377–382.

O'Dwyer, A.M., Lightman, S.L., Marks, M.N., *et al.* (1995). Treatment of major depression with metyrapone and hydrocortisone. *J. Affect. Disord.*, **33**, 123–128.

O'Keane, V., O'Flynn, K., Lucey, J., *et al.* (1992). Pyridostigmine-induced growth hormone responses in healthy and depressed subjects: evidence for cholinergic supersensitivity in depression. *Psychol. Med.*, **22**, 55–60.

Piani, D., Frei, K., Do, K.Q., *et al.* (1991). Murine brain macrophages induced NMDA receptor mediated neurotoxicity in vitro by secreting glutamate. *Neurosci. Lett.*, **133**, 159–162.

Racagni, G., Tinelli, D. and Bianchi, E. (1991). cAMP dependent binding proteins and endogenous phosphorylation after antidepressant treatment. In: *5-Hydroxytryptamine in Psychiatry* (M. Sandler, A. Coppen and S. Hartnet, eds). Oxford, Oxford Medical Publication, pp. 116–123.

Reynolds, I.J. and Miller, R.J. (1988). Tricyclic antidepressants block N-methyl-D-aspartate receptors: similarities to the action of zinc. *Br. J. Pharmacol.*, **95**, 95–102.

Richelson, E. (1992). Histamine receptors in the central nervous system. In: *The Histamine Receptor* (J.-C. Schwartz and H.L. Haas, eds). Alan R. Liss Inc.: New York, pp. 271–295.

Richelson, E. (1995). Cholinergic transduction. In: *Psychopharmacology: Fourth Generation of Progress* (F.B. Bloom and D.J. Cooper, eds). Raven Press: New York, pp. 125–134.

Richelson, E. and Nelson, A. (1984). Antagonism by antidepressants of neurotransmitter receptors of normal human brain in vitro. *J. Pharmacol. Exp. Ther.*, **230**, 94–102.

Schwartz, J.C., Arrang, J.M., Garbarg, M., *et al.* (1995). Histamine. In: *Psychopharmacology: the Fourth Generation of Progress* (D. Kupfer and F. Bloom, eds), Raven Press: New York, pp. 397–405.

Shihabuddin, L. and Rapport, D. (1994). Sertraline and extrapyramidal side effects. *Am. J. Psychiatry*, **151**, 288.

Silverman, J.S. (1991). Reversing anorgasmia associated with serotonin uptake inhibitors. *J. Am. Med. Assoc.*, **266**, 2279.

Siuciak, J.A., Lewis, D.R., Wiegand, S.J., *et al.* (1997). Antidepressant-like effect of brain-derived neurotrophic factor (BDNF). *Pharmacol. Biochem. Behav.*, **56**, 131–137.

Song, C. and Leonard, B.E. (1995). The effect of olfactory bulbectomy in the rat, alone or in combination with antidepressants on immune function. *Hum. Psychopharmacol.*, **10**, 7–18.

Sovner, R. and Fogelman, S. (1996). Ketoconazole therapy for atypical depression [letter]. *J. Clin. Psychiatry*, **57**, 227–228.

Stanton, T., Bolden-Watson, C., Cusack, B., *et al.* (1993). Antagonism of the five cloned human muscarinic cholinergic receptors expressed in CHO-K1 cells by antidepressants and antihistaminics. *Biochem. Pharmacol.*, **45**, 2352–2354.

Steele, T.E. (1982). Adverse reactions suggesting amoxapine-induced dopamine blockade. *Am. J. Psychiatry*, **139**, 1500–1501.

Stein, D.J. and Hollander, E. (1994). Sexual dysfunction associated with the drug treatment of psychiatric disorders – incidence and treatment. *CNS Drugs*, **2**, 78–86.

Steiner, W. and Fontaine, R. (1986). Toxic reaction following the combined administration of fluoxetine and L-tryptophan: five case reports. *Biol. Psychiatry*, **21**, 1067–1071.

Sulser, F. and Sanders-Bush, E. (1987). The serotonin norepinephrine link hypothesis of affective disorders: receptor interactions in the brain. In: *Molecular Basis of Neuronal Responsiveness* (R.H. Erlich, E. Lennox and E. Kornecki, eds). Plenum Press: New York, pp. 489–502.

Tatsumi, M., Groshan, K., Blakely, R.D., *et al.* (1997). Pharmacological profile of antidepressants and related compounds at human monoamine transporters. *Eur. J. Pharmacol.*, **340**, 249–258.

Teicher, M.H., Glod, C. and Cole, J.O. (1990). Emergence of intense suicidal preoccupation during fluoxetine treatment. *Am. J. Psychiatry*, **147**, 207–210.

Tome, M.B., Isaac, M.T., Harte, R., *et al.* (1997). Paroxetine and pindolol: a randomized trial of serotonergic autoreceptor blockade in the reduction of antidepressant latency. *Int. Clin. Psychopharmacol.*, **12**, 81–89.

Vo, M.Y., Williamsen, A.R., Wasserman, G.S., *et al.* (1995). Toxic reaction from topically applied doxepin in a child with eczema. *Arch. Dermatol.*, **131**, 1467–1468.

Wander, T.J., Nelson, A., Okazaki, H., *et al.* (1986). Antagonism by antidepressants of serotonin S_1 and S_2 receptors of normal human brain in vitro. *Eur. J. Pharmacol.*, **132**, 115–121.

Wong, K.L., Bruch, R.C. and Farbman, A.I. (1991). Amitriptyline-mediated inhibition of neurite outgrowth from chick embryonic cerebral explants involves a reduction in adenylate cyclase activity. *J. Neurochem.*, **57**, 1223–1230.

9

Tricyclic antidepressants and classical monoamine oxidase inhibitors: contemporary clinical use

Michael Thase and Willem Nolen

Key points

- Tricyclic antidepressants (TCAs), once the mainstay of treatment, are now used as second-or-third-line medications for SSRI non-responders.
- MAOIs continue to be used as third-or-fourth-line treatments for depression.
- Side effects and lethality in overdose are the major drawbacks of the TCAs.
- Side effects, diet restrictions and drug interactions are the major drawbacks of the MAOIs.

Introduction

The classes of medication known as the tricyclic antidepressants (TCAs) and monoamine oxidase inhibitors (MAOIs) were introduced more than 40 years ago. Mainly by this historical difference they can be separated from the antidepressants introduced since 1988 (Table 9.1). Although neither class of medication is now considered to be on the 'cutting edge' of psychopharmacology, both are still used across the world and continue to be taken by millions of patients. This chapter will briefly review the clinical pharmacology of the TCAs and MAOIs, summarize the extensive evidence about their effectiveness, and discuss their current indications for use within modern treatment algorithms for depressive disorders.

Tricyclic antidepressants

The TCAs are derived from iminodibenzyl, a 3-ring structure discovered almost a century ago. Iminodibenzyl derivatives were researched in the 1940s as antihistamines and, following the discovery that the phenothiazines had antipsychotic effects, the psychotropic profiles of iminodibenzyls were examined. Although these compounds were not good antipsychotics, they did appear to have mood elevating effects. Kuhn (1958) was the first to study imipramine, conducting an open label trial of more than 100 patients that suggested antidepressant activity. This finding was subsequently replicated and confirmed by dozens of double-blind studies (see the comprehensive review by Depression Guideline Panel, 1993). The second TCA,

Table 9.1 Classes of antidepressants and specific agents in current use in the USA and The Netherlands

Generic names	Available in the USA Brand names®	Available in The Netherlands Brand names®
Tricyclic antidepressants		
amitriptyline	Elavil	Sarotex/Tryptizol
clomipramine	Anafranil[a]	Anafranil
desipramine	Norpramin	Pertrofan
dosulepine/dothiepine	—	Prothiaden
doxepin	Sinequan	Sinequan
imipramine	Tofranil	Tofranil
maprotiline	Ludiomil	Ludiomil
nortriptyline	Aventyl	Nortrilen
protrityline	Vivactil	—
trimipramine	Surmontil	Surmontil
Monoamine oxidase inhibitors		
isocarboxazid phenelzine	Marplan	—
tranylcypromine	Nardil	Nardil[b]
	Parnate	Parnate[b]
Newer antidepressants		
SSRIs		
citalopram	Celexa	Cipramil
fluoxetine	Prozac	Prozac
fluvoxamine	Luvox	Fevarin
paroxetine	Paxil	Seroxat
sertraline	Zoloft	Zoloft
SNRI		
venlafaxine	Effexor	Efexor
Reversible Inhibitor of MAO (RIMA)		
moclobemide	—	Aurorix
Other		
mianserin	—	Tolvon
mirtazapine	Remeron	Remeron
nefazodone	Serzone	Dutonin
trazodone	Desyrel	Trazolan

[a] Approved in the USA only for treatment of obsessive-compulsive disorder
[b] Available in The Netherlands only as an 'orphan drug'

amitriptyline, was introduced in 1961 and gained even broader acceptance world-wide. The remaining members of the TCA class were screened, tested, and introduced over the next 15 years.

The TCAs are now typically divided into two subclasses. The tertiary amine TCAs, typified by imipramine, amitriptyline, clomipramine, and doxepin, have two terminal methyl groups on the side chain (Figure 9.1). The secondary amine TCAs desipramine and nortriptyline are the des-methylated metabolites of imipramine and amitriptyline, respectively. Whereas the tertiary amine TCAs can be quite sedating, the des-methylated metabolites are significantly less so and they also tend to have more potent antidepressant effects on a milligram-to-milligram basis.

The TCAs, long the cornerstone of pharmacological treatment of severe depression, are either predominantly inhibitors of noradrenaline reuptake (i.e. nortriptyline, protriptyline, desipramine and maprotiline) or inhibitors

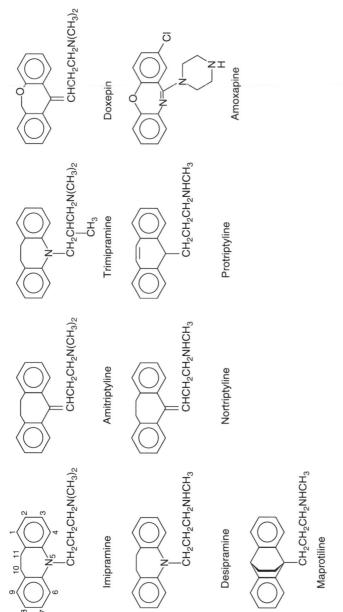

Figure 9.1 Structure of typical heterocyclic antidepressants currently available in the USA. (*Note:* These nine agents have many pharmacological characteristics in common with the original member of the series, imipramine, including an ability to interfere with the reuptake-inactivation of monoamines, especially norepinephrine. Trimipramine may be less active than other agents against norepinephrine uptake; doxepin is only slightly less active in clinically effective doses, and both may form desmethylated metabolites, which should be active. Amoxapine is the desmethyl derivative of a typical agent, loxapine, and has some neuroleptic-like as well as antidepressant properties, including antagonism of dopamine receptors, as well as ability to inhibit uptake of norepinephrine. (Reprinted from: Baldessarini, R.J. (1983). *Biomedical Aspects of Depression And Its Treatment,* American Psychiatric Press.)

of the reuptake of both noradrenaline and serotonin (e.g. clomipramine, imipramine, and amitriptyline) (Baldessarini, 1983). Early impressions that clomipramine, imipramine, and amitriptyline were selectively seroto-nergic were revised on the basis of knowledge of the noradrenergic actions of their secondary amine metabolites (Baldessarini, 1983). Nevertheless, the potency of clomipramine for inhibiting the reuptake of serotonin is much stronger than that of the other TCAs and therefore clomipramine is the only TCA that is classified as a potent serotonin reuptake inhibitor. It is also the only TCA with a documented efficacy in obsessive-compulsive disorder, a disorder for which a number of other serotoninergic antidepressants are also efficacious (Griest et al., 1995).

Treatment with TCAs is typically initiated at low dosages and titrated upward in relation to response and side effects. The typical daily doses of the more commonly prescribed TCAs are summarized in Table 9.2. The TCAs tend to show either linear or curvilinear dose–response characteristics (Preskorn and Fast, 1991; Perry et al., 1994). Plasma levels of imipramine, amitriptyline, desipramine, nortriptyline, and clomipramine can be mea-sured reliably and are available widely through commercial laboratories (Perry et al., 1994). Their measurement can be helpful in cases of exquisite sensitivity or non-response to apparently adequate dosages (Preskorn and Fast, 1991). Nortriptyline has the best-documented 'window' of therapeutic action, and there is some evidence that efficacy may lessen when plasma levels exceed 150–200 ng/ml. Central nervous system (e.g. seizures) and cardiovascular (e.g. conduction delays) toxicities have clear dose–response relationships that, fortunately, usually exceed therapeutic blood levels (Preskorn and Fast, 1991).

Side effects and potential lethality in overdose are the major drawbacks of the TCAs. About 20% of TCA trials end prematurely because of intolerable side effects (Depression Guideline Panel, 1993). Many TCA side effects are caused by blockade of cholinergic, histaminic, and α_1-adrenergic receptors

Table 9.2 Typical and usual maximum dosages of selected tricyclic and monoamine oxidase inhibiting antidepressants

Tricyclic antidepressant drugs	Typical dose range (mg/day)	Comment
Amitriptyline	150–250	Usual maximum: 300 mg/day
Clomipramine	100–250	Manufacturer warns not to exceed 250 mg/day
Desipramine	75–200	Usual maximum: 300 mg/day
Imipramine	150–250	Usual maximum: 300 mg/day
Maprotiline	150–250	Increased risk of seizures above 250 mg/day
Nortriptyline	50–150	Probably loss of therapeutic effect as plasma levels above 200 ng/ml
Monoamine oxidase inhibitors		
Isocarboxazid	15–30	Usual maximum: 45 mg/day
Phenelzine	45–75	Usual maximum: 90 mg/day
Tranylcypromine	30–50	Usual maximum: 60 mg/day

(Preskorn and Burke, 1992). For example, α_1-adrenergic blockade may cause fainting because of orthostatic hypotension, a particular problem for the elderly (Roose, 1992). The side effects commonly associated with anticholinergic effects include dry mouth, blurry vision, constipation, and urinary hesitancy and urinary retention. Cognitive dysfunction and delirium also can be problematic anticholinergic effects for the elderly treated with TCAs. Antihistaminic effects include sedation or drowsiness and weight gain. The secondary amine TCAs, e.g. nortriptyline and desipramine, and maprotiline are generally associated with fewer complaints of antihistaminic and anticholinergic side effects than tertiary amine agents like clomipramine, amitriptyline, and imipramine (Preskorn and Burke, 1992). A relatively high incidence of seizures and a rather late introduction have limited use of maprotiline in the USA.

The TCAs also have a quinidine-like effect on sodium fast channels that may cause cardiac problems, especially arrhythmias. Therefore TCAs must be used with caution for treatment of patients with existing cardiac conduction abnormalities (Roose, 1992). An electrocardiogram (ECG) should be obtained prior to treatment with a TCA for all children and patients over age 40, as well as younger patients with a history of heart problems. Periodic ECGs also may be indicated to monitor treatment effects. Nortriptyline has become the favoured TCA for treatment of elderly patients and/or patients with significant heart disease, in part because of more extensive studies in these patient groups and in part because of more narrowly defined dose/plasma level/response relationships (Roose, 1992).

The TCAs are the most extensively researched treatment in psychopharmacology. The weight of accumulated evidence is impressive, although about one-third of the published studies of TCAs in depression have failed to show an effect greater than placebo (Depression Guideline Panel, 1993). This is because the average drug–placebo difference ranges from 20% to 28% in meta-analyses, i.e. 60% vs 40% or 52% vs 24% (Depression Guideline Panel, 1993). These differences are considered to be moderate-sized effects, and studies need to be rather large (i.e. cell sizes ≥ 100 subjects) to have adequate statistical power to detect such effects reliably.

There appear to be certain patient subgroups that are less responsive to TCAs. For example, patients with atypical depression (Quitkin et al., 1993), recurrent depression with reversed neurovegetative features (Thase et al., 1991), and anergic, bipolar depressions (Himmelhoch et al., 1991; Thase et al., 1992) are less responsive to TCAs than to MAOIs. Younger women (Thase et al., in press) and adolescents of both sexes (see, for example, the studies reviewed by Emslie et al., 1997) also may be less responsive to TCAs than selective serotonin reuptake inhibitors (SSRIs).

It has also been more difficult to demonstrate TCA–placebo differences in studies of mild depression (e.g. Elkin et al., 1989) or in depressed patients treated in primary care settings (Paykel et al., 1988). Nevertheless, there is evidence that TCAs have therapeutic effects for patients with dysthymia (Thase et al., 1996) and chronicity per se does not mitigate against TCA efficacy when compared to SSRIs (Thase et al., 1996; Keller et al., 1998).

The efficacy of TCAs in psychotic depression is still somewhat controversial. Most studies have found TCAs to be less effective in psychotic than in non-psychotic depression when prescribed monotherapy. Antidepressant plus antipsychotic combinations or electroconvulsive therapy are thus recommended in treatment guidelines (American Psychiatric Association, 1993; Depression Guideline Panel, 1993). In contrast, however, Bruijn *et al.* (1999) found imipramine more effective in psychotic depressed patients (69.2%) than in non-psychotic patients (43.8%) in a well-designed study of hospitalized patients. Spiker *et al.* (1985) conducted the only prospective, double-blind study in psychotic depression, comparing amitriptyline and the phenothiazine antipsychotic perphenazine, alone and in combination, in a double-blind study of hospitalized patients. They found a better response to the combination than to amitriptyline alone, while perphenazine alone did worst. It must be noted, however, that they did not mention how many patients in their study had already received treatment with a tricyclic antidepressant prior to randomization.

Some experienced clinical investigators are convinced that the TCAs are more effective than the SSRIs for treatment of severe depressions, particularly the melancholic subtype (Potter *et al.*, 1991; Nelson, 1994; Nobler and Roose, 1998). Two well-designed studies among depressed inpatients have found clomipramine to be more effective than the SSRIs citalopram and paroxetine (Danish University Antidepressant Group, 1986, 1990). Another retrospective study of elderly patients with severe cardiovascular disease found a similar advantage for nortriptyline relative to fluoxetine (Roose *et al.*, 1994). However, not all studies are in agreement (Pande and Sayler, 1993; Stuppaeck *et al.*, 1994). If there is indeed differential efficacy, the inhibition of both serotonin and noradrenaline reuptake may be particularly important for the treatment of severe or melancholic depression (Nolen, 1995; Thase, 1997). The combined serotonin and noradrenaline reuptake inhibitor (SNRI) venlafaxine may offer similar advantages over the SSRIs for severe depression with better safety characteristics than a TCA (Clerc *et al.*, 1994). The place of other newer antidepressants with multiple actions for treatment of severe depression remains unclear. For instance mirtazapine was found to be more effective than fluoxetine in one inpatient study (Wheatley *et al.*, 1998), but less effective than imipramine in another (Bruijn *et al.*, 1996).

TCAs are now more commonly prescribed as second- or third-line medications for SSRI non-responders. Although tolerability may still be problematic, TCAs appear to have a 40–60% chance of working even after one or more SSRI failure (Thase and Rush, 1997). TCAs are also used in combination with SSRIs for treatment of more refractory patients (Nelson *et al.*, 1991). This strategy warrants some caution, however, because most of the SSRIs inhibit TCA metabolism, increasing blood levels unpredictably. Generally, secondary amine TCAs are preferred for co-therapy and TCA doses of one-third to one-half of the normal amounts are used. Monitoring of blood levels and electrocardiograms are often useful during combined therapy to lessen risks of drug–drug interactions.

A strong rationale for continued use of the TCAs is their relative inexpense when prescribed generically (Song *et al.*, 1993; Hotopf *et al.*, 1996). Although simple comparisons of pharmacy costs clearly favour the generic TCAs over the SSRIs, the actual savings is reduced when the costs of blood tests, electrocardiograms, more frequent pharmacy visits, ancillary medications (e.g. stool softeners), and non-compliance are tallied (Henry, 1993;

Burke *et al.*, 1994; Simon *et al.*, 1996). If decreased prescription of the TCAs results in lower rates of completed suicide, accidental poisonings, and ICU admissions after overdoses, the apparent cost savings of the TCAs disappear (Henry, 1993).

Finally, the TCAs have a continued, albeit secondary, role for treatment of panic disorder, generalized anxiety disorder, obsessive compulsive disorder (clomipramine only), eneuresis, attention deficit hyperactivity disorder, and several other childhood mental disorders. The TCAs are also widely used in general medicine for management of chronic pain syndromes.

Classical monoamine oxidase inhibitors

The classical monoamine oxidase inhibitors (MAOI) have been in use for more than 40 years (Ayd, 1957; Crane, 1957; Kline, 1958; West and Dally, 1959; Sargant, 1961), during which time their popularity has waxed and waned (e.g. Quitkin *et al.*, 1979; Paykel and White, 1989). Recently, the older MAOIs have been largely viewed as third- or fourth-line antidepressant medications (Paykel and White, 1989; Clary *et al.*, 1990; Thase *et al.*, 1995; Nolen, 1997) for reasons pertaining to both efficacy and safety.

Currently three of the older FDA-approved MAOIs are available in the USA (Figure 9.2). The two most commonly prescribed are phenelzine sulphate (PHZ) (Nardil) and tranylcypromine sulphate (TRP) (Parnate). A third older compound, isocarboxazid (Marplan), has recently been reintroduced after several years off the market. In The Netherlands none of the classical MAOIs is on the regular market. Nevertheless, both tranylcypromine and to a lesser extent phenelzine are prescribed as 'orphan drugs' for refractory patients. In contrast, moclobemide, a new reversible inhibitor of monoamine oxidase A, is on the market in The Netherlands, elsewhere throughout Europe, Canada, and Mexico, but it is not available on the USA market (see Table 9.1).

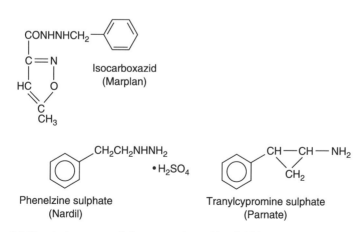

Figure 9.2 Chemical structure of the monoamine oxidase inhibitors isocarboxazid, phenelzine sulphate, and tranylcypromine sulphate.

Monoamine oxidase inhibitors are classified by their chemical structure (hydrazine versus non-hydrazine), by their relative selectivity for subforms of MAO (i.e. selective for Type A or Type B, or non-selective), and by the degree of affinity to enzyme inhibition sites (i.e. reversible versus functionally irreversible) (Klein and Davis, 1969; Mann et al., 1984; Murphy et al., 1984). The Type B MAO is found principally in the brain and blood platelets and has substrate specificity for phenethylamine and dopamine. The Type A MAO is found in the brain, gut, and liver and is relatively substrate-specific for noradrenaline, serotonin, and tyramine (Mann et al., 1984; Murphy et al., 1984).

Tranylcypromine, isocarboxazid and phenelzine are classified as irreversible enzyme inhibitors because they bind tightly to monoamine oxidase, essentially for the life of the enzyme. A minimum period of 7–14 days off medication is needed adequately to 'wash out' MAO inhibition caused by these agents. Thus, the clinical effects of the irreversible MAOIs may persist for several weeks after discontinuation (Murphy et al., 1987; Robinson and Kurtz, 1987; Mallinger and Smith, 1991). Plasma level monitoring of the irreversible MAOIs does not appear to be of clinical value, perhaps because of the short half-lives of these medications in relation to their pharmacodynamic effects (e.g. Mallinger et al., 1990). Available evidence suggests that plasma levels are not useful for the prediction of response (Thase et al., 1995).

Both phenelzine and tranylcypromine have some structural resemblance to amphetamine. However, neither agent is habit-forming nor are they euphoriogenic for the vast majority of patients (Mallinger and Smith, 1991; Thase et al., 1995). The structure of TRP, which may be viewed as a cyclized form of amphetamine, probably precludes its metabolism to amphetamine except under unusual circumstances, such as following a massive overdose (Youdim et al., 1979).

Phenelzine and isocarboxazid are further classified as hydrazine compounds, because they have a nitrogen-to-nitrogen bond in their side chains (Klein and Davis, 1969; Murphy et al., 1984). Considerable clinical evidence indicates that the hydrazine MAOIs have greater hepatotoxicity than TRP, a non-hydrazine compound (Klein and Davis, 1969; Timbrell, 1979). The hepatotoxicity of the hydrazine MAOIs was greatest for iproniazid, which was removed from the market despite considerable evidence of antidepressant efficacy (Timbrell, 1979).

All three non-selective MAOIs are absorbed rapidly following oral dosing and have elimination half-lives of the order of 1–4 hours (Murphy et al., 1987). These drugs are tightly protein bound and are excreted after hepatic metabolism. None has clinically important metabolites (Murphy et al., 1987; Robinson and Kurtz, 1987).

All three MAOIs are usually prescribed in divided doses, i.e. bid or tid. Phenelzine is available as 15 mg tablets and its therapeutic range extends between 45 mg/day and 90 mg/day; 60 mg/day would be considered an 'average' dose. Tranylcypromine is available as 10 mg tablets and therapeutic doses range between 30 mg/day and 60 mg/day, with 40 mg/day considered 'average' (Thase et al., 1995). Isocarboxazid is available as a 5 mg tablet and is usually prescribed in doses ranging from 15 mg to 30 mg per day. Some treatment-resistant patients respond to trials of higher doses of the MAOI, such as TRP up to 100 mg/day (Nolen *et al.*, 1988). Lower doses are typically used when a MAOI is added to a TCA and many experts opt for use of phenelzine over isocarboxazid or tranylcypromine in combination (Thase *et al.*, 1995). Generally, amitriptyline and doxepin are preferred for this combined therapy and clomipramine is specifically avoided (Thase *et al.*, 1995).

It was initially believed that the antidepressant effectiveness of MAOIs was the *direct* result of MAO inhibition. This acute effect decreases enzymatic degradation of monoamines (e.g. noradrenaline, serotonin, or dopamine); thereby resulting in an increased amount of these neurotransmitters available at the synapse (e.g. Schildkraut, 1965; Klein and Davis, 1969). The best evidence for a direct relationship came from an early study correlating therapeutic response with the percentage of platelet MAO-B inhibition during phenelzine therapy (Robinson *et al.*, 1973). Response to phenelzine was uncommon when platelet MAO-B was inhibited to values of <80% of pretreatment and significantly more likely at higher levels of inhibition. More recent research indicates that this simple mechanism cannot account for the efficacy of the MAOIs (Mann *et al.*, 1984; Murphy *et al.*, 1987). For example, MAO-B platelet inhibition is not correlated with response to tranylcypromine (Mallinger *et al.*, 1990) and selegiline, a potent and selective MAO-B inhibitor, is ineffective as an antidepressant until its dose is increased to non-selective level, i.e. > 20 mg/per day (Mann *et al.*, 1984). Moreover, moclobemide, as previously mentioned a selective MAO-A inhibitor, is effective at doses that do not significantly inhibit MAO-B.

The positive (+) stereo-isomer of TRP is a poor antidepressant despite inhibiting MAO-B (Escobar *et al.*, 1974). The main pharmacological difference between the negative (−) and + isomers of TRP is that the former has much weaker effects as a noradrenaline reuptake inhibitor in relation to its potency as a MAOI (Hendley and Snyder, 1968).

How do the MAOIs work?

More consistent with the 2- to 4-week lag in therapeutic effect, chronic treatment with a MAOI has been shown to reduce the number of α_2 and β-adrenergic and serotonin (5-HT$_2$) post-synaptic binding sites in the brain (e.g. Murphy *et al.*, 1987; de Montigny and Blier, 1988). It thus seems likely that inhibition of MAO in the brain only initiates a cascade-like neurochemical process that leads to therapeutic response. It remains to be seen if the effects of MAOIs, TCAs, and SSRIs ultimately converge on a final common pathway (Duman *et al.*, 1997).

There is no doubt that the MAOIs are effective antidepressants (Depression Guideline Panel, 1993; Thase *et al.*, 1995; Nolen, 1997). What has been controversial is the utility of MAOIs for treatment of severe depression. A recent meta-analysis, largely based on older studies, found phenelzine and isocarboxazid to be less effective than TCAs for hospitalized depressed patients (Thase *et al.*, 1995). However, it is presumed that many of these studies were flawed by use of MAOI doses that were too low (e.g. Quitkin *et al.*, 1979; Nolen, 1997). It is our impression that TRP is at least as effective as TCAs, especially when prescribed at higher doses. Moreover, in a study of hospitalized patients TRP was found effective in patients who had not responded to sequential trials of selective serotonin as well as selective noradrenaline reuptake inhibitors (Nolen *et al.*, 1988).

Another suggestion based on early studies is that MAOIs were superior to TCAs for the treatment of the so-called atypical depressions, including both anxious depressions and depressions characterized by reverse neurovegetative features (West and Dally, 1959; Sargant, 1961). Subsequent research has confirmed the latter impression (Himmelhoch *et al.*, 1991; Thase *et al.*, 1992; McGrath *et al.*, 1993; Quitkin *et al.*, 1993), although there is not strong evidence of differential efficacy (relative to imipramine) among patients with pronounced anxiety (Quitkin *et al.*, 1993). There is one study suggesting that phenelzine and the selective serotonin reuptake inhibitor fluoxetine are comparably effective treatments of atypical depression (Pande *et al.*, 1996).

How do the older MAOIs compare to moclobemide?

A meta-analysis of European, Canadian, South American, and Australian studies demonstrated that the older MAOIs were significantly more effective than the MAO type A selective compound moclobemide (Lotufo-Neto *et al.*, 1999). Additionally, Vink *et al.* (1994) studied the effects of switching patients from TRP to moclobemide after the latter drug became available in The Netherlands. All 28 patients had been suffering from major depression, and were resistant to TCAs and in many cases also the combination of TCA and lithium. Subsequently, all had responded to tranylcypromine and remained well for at least 2 months, with a mean duration of maintenance therapy of 4.3 years. After the switch from TRP to moclobemide, 16 of these patients (57.1%) relapsed within 2 months. The results of this study tend to reinforce the conclusion that moclobemide is not an effective alternative to TRP in resistant depression.

The MAOIs' perennial problems with 'image' stem largely from two qualities: the potential for hypertensive crises and the tendency to cause a small proportion of patients a large number of annoying side effects (Thase *et al.*, 1995). The hypertensive crisis, a sudden and dramatic increase in blood pressure, is caused by ingestion of foodstuffs that are rich in the amino acid tyramine or drugs with sympathomimetic effects, including a number of over-the-counter drugs. Inhibition of MAO in the gut and liver prevents the deactivation of these substrates, triggering pressor effects. A reasonably easy-to-follow diet and avoidance of hazardous concurrent drugs can virtually eliminate the risk of this problem, although dietary non-compliance is an endemic problem during longer-term treatment and about three to five patients per 100 will experience a hypertensive crisis during each year of therapy (Thase *et al.*, 1995). The irreversible MAOIs also have the potential for pharmacodynamic interactions with SSRIs and other serotoninergic drugs, including TCAs (especially clomipramine) and *perhaps* the herbal remedy St. John's Wort. The interaction is most commonly manifest as a 'serotonin syndrome', which is evident by fever, hyperthermia, rigidity, and hyperreflexia. The potential interaction of tranylcypromine with clomipramine or SSRIs appears to be particularly dangerous (Beasley *et al.*, 1993; Thase *et al.*, 1995).

There are a number of less acutely worrisome side effects that more frequently compromise long-term treatment. These include weight gain, daytime sedation, orthostatic hypotension, insomnia, sexual dysfunction and neuromuscular syndromes (Thase *et al.*, 1995; Nolen, 1997). Overall, the MAOIs and TCAs have comparable overall tolerability, although there are striking individual differences and poor tolerability to one class does not predict a subsequent experience with the other (Thase *et al.*, 1995).

Most experts nowadays place MAOIs as third- or fourth-line treatments (American Psychiatric Association, 1993; Depression Guideline Panel, 1993; De Groot, 1995; Nolen, 1997; Thase and Rush, 1997). The MAOIs would generally be placed after TCAs in treatment algorithms (Table 9.3), with several important exceptions. For example, most experts would rank MAOIs ahead of TCAs for depression with atypical features and many would recommend the MAOIs before the TCAs for treatment of bipolar depression. The use of MAOIs in these specific indications has nevertheless been curtailed by the introduction of SSRIs, bupropion, venlafaxine, and moclobemide.

Conclusion

The TCAs and MAOIs were the standard antidepressant therapies for more than 30 years. They are decidedly different classes of medication that, both historically and currently, offer distinct advantages for some difficult-to-treat patients. Although more potentially toxic than most of the antidepressants introduced after 1985, their use continues to be warranted for selected patients.

The TCAs are a second-line treatment for patients with major depression after one or more of the newer antidepressants therapies such as the SSRIs

Table 9.3 Place of different classes of antidepressants in the treatment of depression (De Groot, 1995; Thase and Rush, 1997; Nolen *et al.*, 1998)

	Newer ADs (SSRIs, SNRI, moclobemide)	*TCAs*	*TCAs + lithium*	*Classical MAOIs*
Major depression				
NL	1	2	3	4
US	1	2	—	3
Major depression, hospitalized				
NL	—	1	2	3
US	1	2	3	4
Atypical depression				
NL	1	3	4	2
US	1	3	4	2
Bipolar depression*				
NL	1*	2*	—	3*
US	1	3*	—	2

*With concomitant mood stabilizer

has failed. Moreover, they should remain a first choice treatment for hospitalized patients with severe major depression.

In contrast the older MAOIs are almost never first choice treatments, because of their adverse-effects profile and especially their risk for hypertensive crisis when combined with tyramine and sympathomimetic medications. Yet they are still indicated as second choice treatment in patients evidencing major depression with atypical features who have failed with newer antidepressants such as the SSRIs, bupropion, or moclobemide. Additionally they need to be considered for all depressed patients who have failed to respond to newer medications, TCAs, and ECT.

References

American Psychiatric Association (1993). Practice guideline for major depressive disorder in adults. *Am. J. Psychiatry*, **150**, 1–26.

Ayd, F.J. Jr. (1957). A preliminary report on Marsilid. *Am. J. Psychiatry*, **114**, 459.

Baldessarini, R.J. (1983). *Biomedical Aspects of Depression and its Treatment*. American Psychiatric Press: Washington DC.

Beasley, C.M., Masica, D.N., Heiligenstein, J.H., *et al.* (1993). Possible monoamine oxidase inhibitor-serotonin reuptake inhibitor interaction: fluoxetine clinical data and preclinical findings. *J. Clin. Psychopharmacol.*, **13**, 312–320.

Bruijn, J.A., Moleman, P., Mulder, P.G.H., *et al.*, (1996). A double-blind, fixed blood-level study comparing mirtazapine with imipramine in depressed in-patients. *Psychopharmacology*, **127**, 231–237.

Bruijn, J.A., Moleman, P., Mulder, P.G.H. and van den Broeck, W.W. (1998). Comparison of two treatment strategies for depressed inpatients: imipramine and lithium addiction or mirtazapine and lithium addiction: *J. Clin. Psychiatry*, **59**, 657–663.

Burke, M.J., Silkey, B. and Preskorn, S.H. (1994). Pharmacoeconomic considerations when evaluation treatment options for major depressive disorder. *J. Clin. Psychiatry*, **55**, 42–52.

Clary, C., Mandos, L.A. and Schweizer, E. (1990). Results of a brief survey on the prescribing practices for monoamine oxidase inhibitor antidepressants. *J. Clin. Psychiatry*, **51**, 226–231.

Clerc, G.E., Ruimy, P. and Verdeau-Pilles, J. (1994). A double-blind comparison of venlafaxine and fluoxetine in patients hospitalized for major depression and melancholia. *Int. Clin. Psychopharmacol.*, **9**, 139–143.

Crane, G.E. (1957). Iproniazid (Marsilid) phosphate, a therapeutic agent for mental disorder and debilitating disease. *Psychiatr. Res. Rep.*, **8**, 142–152.

Danish University Antidepressant Group (1986). Citalopram: clinical effect profile in comparison with clomipramine: a controlled multicenter study. *Psychopharmacology*, **90**, 131–138.

Danish University Antidepressant Group (1990). Paroxetine: a selective serotonin reuptake inhibitor showing better tolerance but weaker antidepressant effect than clomipramine in a controlled multicenter study. *J. Affect. Dis.*, **18**, 289–299.

De Groot, P. (1995). Consensus depressie bij volwassenen. *Ned. T. Geneesk.*, **139**, 1237–1241.

de Montigny, C. and Blier, P. (1988). Modifications of monoaminergic system properties by MAOIs: basis for their therapeutic effect? In: *MAOI Therapy* (R.I. Shader, ed.), Audio Visual Medical Marketing, Inc., pp. 5–12.

Depression Guideline Panel (1993). *Depression in Primary Care: Vol. 2. Treatment of Major Depression* (AHCPR Publication No. 93-0551). U.S. Department of Health and Human Services, Agency for Health Care Policy and Research, Rockville, MD.

Duman, R.S., Heninger, G.R. and Nestler, E.J. (1997). A molecular and cellular theory of depression. *Arch. Gen. Psychiatry*, **54**, 597–606.

Elkin, I., Shea, M.T., Watkins, J.T., *et al.* (1989). National Institute of Mental Health Treatment of Depression Collaborative Research Program: general effectiveness and treatments. *Arch. Gen. Psychiatry*, **46**, 971–982.

Emslie, G.J., Rush, A.J., Weinberg, W.A., *et al.* (1997). A double-blind, placebo-controlled trial of fluoxetine in children and adolescents with depression. *Arch. Gen. Psychiatry*, **54**, 1031–1037.

Escobar, J.I., Schiele, B.C. and Zimmermann, R. (1974). The tranylcypromine isomers: a controlled clinical trial. *Am. J. Psychiatry*, **131**, 1025–1026.

Griest, J.H., Jefferson, J.W., Kobak, K.A., *et al.* (1995). Efficacy and tolerability of serotonin transport inhibitors in obsessive-compulsive disorder. *Arch. Gen. Psychiatry*, **52**, 53–60.

Hendley, E.D. and Snyder, S.H. (1968). Relationship between the action of monoamine oxidase inhibitors on the noradrenaline uptake system and their antidepressant efficacy. *Nature*, **220**, 1330–1331.

Henry, J.A. (1993). Debits and credits in the management of depression. *Br. J. Psychiatry*, **163**, 33–39.

Himmelhoch, J.M., Thase, M.E., Mallinger, A.G., *et al.* (1991). Tranylcypromine versus imipramine in anergic bipolar depression. *Am. J. Psychiatry*, **148**, 910–916.

Hotopf, M., Lewis, G. and Normand, C. (1996). Are SSRIs a cost-effective alternative to tricyclics? *Br. J. Psychiatry*, **168**, 404–409.

Keller, M.B., Gelenberg, A.J., Hirschfeld, R.M.A., *et al.* (1998). The treatment of chronic depression, part 2: a double-blind, randomized trial of sertraline and imipramine. *J. Clin. Psychiatry*, **59**, 598–607.

Klein, D.F. and Davis, J.M. (1969). *Diagnosis and Drug Treatment of Psychiatric Disorders.* New York: Williams & Wilkins.

Kline, N.S. (1958). Clinical experience with iproniazid (marsilid). *J. Clin. Exp. Psychophathol.*, **19**, 72–78.

Kuhn, R. (1958). The treatment of depressive states with G-22355 (imipramine hydrochloride). *Am. J. Psychiatry*, **115**, 459–464.

Lotufo-Neto, F., Trivedi, M. and Thase, M.E. (1999). Metaanalysis of the reversible inhibitors of monoamine oxidase type A moclobemide and brofaromine in the treatment of depression. *Neuropsychopharmacology*, **20**, 226–247.

Mallinger, A.G., Himmelhoch, J.M., Thase, M.E., *et al.* (1990). Plasma tranylcypromine: relationship to pharmacokinetic variables and clinical antidepressant actions. *J. Clin. Psychopharmacol.*, **10**, 176–183.

Mallinger, A.G. and Smith, E. (1991). Pharmacokinetics of monoamine oxidase inhibitors. *Psychopharmacol. Bull.*, **27**, 493–502.

Mann, J.J., Aarons, S.F., Frances, A.J. and Brown, R.D. (1984). Studies of selective and reversible monoamine oxidase inhibitors. *J. Clin. Psychiatry*, **45**, 62–66.

McGrath, P.J., Stewart, J.W., Nunes, E.V., *et al.* (1993). A double-blind crossover trial of imipramine and phenelzine for outpatients with treatment-refractory depression. *Am. J. Psychiatry*, **250**, 118–123.

Murphy, D.L., Garrick, N.A., Aulakh, C.S. and Cohen, R.M. (1984). New contributions from basic science to understanding the effects of monoamine oxidase inhibiting antidepressants. *J. Clin. Psychiatry*, **45**, 37–43.

Murphy, D.L., Aulakh, C.S., Garrick, N.A., *et al.* (1987). Monoamine oxidase inhibitors as antidepressants: implications for the mechanism of action of antidepressants and the psychobiology of the affective disorders and some related disorders. In *Psychopharmacology: The Third Generation of Progress* (H.Y. Meltzer, ed.), New York: Raven Press, pp. 545–552.

Nelson, J.C. (1994). Are the SSRIs really better tolerated than the TCAs for treatment of major depression? *Psychiatr. Ann.*, **24**, 628–631.

Nelson, J.C., Mazure, C.M., Bowers, M.B., *et al.* (1991). A preliminary open study of the combination of fluoxetine and desipramine for rapid treatment of major depression. *Arch. Gen. Psychiatry*, **48**, 303–307.

Nobler, M.S. and Roose, S.P. (1998). Differential response to antidepressants in melancholic and severe depression. *Psychiatr. Ann.*, **28**, 84–88.

Nolen, W.A. (1995). The clinical relevance of treatment with antidepressants. *Acta Neuropsychiatrica*, **7**, 52–54.

Nolen, W.A. (1997). Classical and selective monoamine oxidase inhibitors in the treatment of depression. In: *Depression, Neurobiological, Psychopathological and Therapeutic Advances* (A. Honig and H.G.M. van Praag, eds), London: John Wiley & Sons, pp. 385–395.

Nolen, W.A., Van de Putte, J.J., Dijken, W.A., *et al.* (1988). Treatment strategy in depression; II: MAO inhibitors in depression resistant to cyclic antidepressants: two controlled studies with tranylcypromine versus l-5-hydroxytryptophan and nomifensine. *Acta Psychiatr. Scand.*, **78**, 676–683.

Nolen, W.A., Knoppert-van der Klein, E.A.M., Bouvy, P.F., *et al.* (1998). *Richtlijn Farmacotherapie Bipolaire Stoornissen*. Meppel (NL): Uitgeverij Boom.

Pande, A. and Sayler, M.E. (1993). Severity of depression and response to fluoxetine. *Int. Clin. Psychopharmacol.*, **8**, 243–245.

Pande, A., Birkett, M., Fechner-Bates, S., *et al.* (1996). Fluoxetine versus phenelzine in atypical depression. *Biol. Psychiatry*, **40**, 1017–1020.

Paykel, E.S. and White, J.L. (1989). A European study of views on the use of monoamine oxidase inhibitors. *Br. J. Psychiatry*, **155**, 9–17.

Paykel, E.S., Hollyman, J.A., Freeling, P., *et al.* (1988). Predictors of therapeutic benefit from amitriptyline in mild depression: a general practice placebo-controlled trial. *J. Affect. Dis.*, **14**, 83–95.

Perry, P.J., Zeilmann, C. and Arndt, S. (1994). Tricyclic antidepressant concentrations in plasma: an estimate of their sensitivity and specificity as a predictor of response. *J. Clin. Psychopharmacol.*, **14**, 230–240.

Potter, W., Rudorfer, M. and Manji, H. (1991). The pharmacologic treatment of depression. *N. Eng. J. Med.*, **325**, 633–642.

Preskorn, S.H. and Burke, M. (1992). Somatic therapy for major depressive disorder: selection of an antidepressant. *J. Clin. Psychiatry*, **52**, 5–18.

Preskorn, S.H. and Fast, G.A. (1991). Therapeutic drug monitoring for antidepressants: efficacy, safety, and cost effectiveness. *J. Clin. Psychiatry*, **52**, 23–33.

Quitkin, F.M., Rifkin, A. and Klein, D.F. (1979). Monoamine oxidase inhibitors. *Arch. Gen. Psychiatry*, **35**, 749–760.

Quitkin, F.M., Stewart, J.W., McGrath, P.J., *et al.* (1993). Columbia atypical depression. A subgroup of depressives with better response to MAOI than to tricyclic antidepressants or placebo. *Br. J. Psychiatry*, **163**, 30–34.

Robinson, D.S. and Kurtz, N.M. (1987). Monoamine oxidase inhibiting drugs: pharmacologic and therapeutic issues. In: *Psychopharmacology: The Third Generation of Progress* (H.Y. Meltzer, ed.), New York: Raven Press, pp. 1297–1304.

Robinson, D.S., Nies, A., Ravaris, C.L., *et al.* (1973). The monoamine oxidase inhibitor, phenelzine, in the treatment of depressive-anxiety states. *Arch. Gen. Psychiatry*, **29**, 407–413.

Roose, S.P. (1992). Modern cardiovascular standards for psychotropic drugs. *Psychopharmacol. Bull.*, **28**, 35–43.

Roose, S.P., Glassman, A.H., Attia, E., *et al.* (1994). Comparative efficacy of selective serotonin reuptake inhibitors and tricyclics in the treatment of melancholia. *Am. J. Psychiatry*, **151**, 1735–1739.

Sargant, W. (1961). Drugs in the treatment of depression. *Br. Med. J.*, **1**, 225–227.

Schildkraut, J.J. (1965). The catecholamine hypothesis of affective disorder. A review of supporting evidence. *Am. J. Psychiatry*, **122**, 509–522.

Simon, G.E., VonKorff, M., Heiligenstein, J.H., *et al.* (1996). Initial antidepressant choice in primary care. Effectiveness and cost of fluoxetine vs tricyclic antidepressants. *J. Am. Med. Assoc.*, **275**, 1897–1902.

Song, F., Freemantle, N. and Sheldon, T.A. (1993). Selective serotonin reuptake inhibitors: meta-analysis of efficacy and acceptability. *Br. J. Med.*, **306**, 683–687.

Spiker, D.G., Weiss, J.C., Dealy, R.S., *et al.* (1985). The pharmacological treatment of delusional depression. *Am. J. Psychiatry*, **142**, 430–436.

Stuppaeck, C.H., Geretsegger, C. and Whitworth, A.B. (1994). A multicenter double-blind trial of paroxetine versus amitriptyline in depressed inpatients. *J. Clin. Psychopharmacol.*, **14**, 241–246.

Thase, M.E. (1997). Do we really need all these new antidepressants? Weighing the options. *J. Practical Psychiatry Behav. Health*, **3**, 3–17.

Thase, M.E. and Rush, A.J. (1997). When at first you don't succeed...sequential strategies for antidepressant nonresponders. *J. Clin. Psychiatry*, **58**, 23–29.

Thase, M.E., Carpenter, L., Kupfer, D.J., *et al.* (1991). Clinical significance of reversed vegetative subtypes of recurrent major depression. *Psychopharmacol. Bull.*, **27**, 17–22.

Thase, M.E., Fava, M., Halbreich, U., *et al.* (1996). A placebo-controlled, randomized clinical trial comparing sertraline and imipramine for the treatment of dysthymia. *Arch. Gen. Psychiatry*, **53**, 777–784.

Thase, M.E., Frank, E., Kornstein, S., *et al.* (in press). Sex-related differences in response to treatment of depression. In: *Sex, Society, and Madness: Gender and Psychopathology* (E. Frank, ed.), American Psychiatric Press.

Thase, M.E., Trivedi, M.H. and Rush, A.J. (1995). MAOIs in the contemporary treatment of depression. *Neuropsychopharmacology*, **12**, 185–219.

Timbrell, J.A. (1979). The role of metabolism in the hepatotoxicity of isoniazid and iproniazid. *Drug Metab. Rev.*, **10**, 125–147.

Vink, J., Nolen, W.A. and Verbraak, M. (1994). Is moclobemide bij therapieresistente depressie een alternatief voor tranylcypromine? enige ervaringen. *Tijdschrift voor Psychiatrie*, **36**, 639–646.

West, E.D. and Dally, P.J. (1959). Effects of iproniazid in depressive syndromes. *Br. Med. J.*, **1**, 1491–1494.

Wheatley, D.P., Van Moffaert, M., Timmerman, L., *et al.* (1998). Mirtazapine: efficacy and tolerability in comparison with fluoxetine in patients with moderate to severe major depressive disorder. *J. Clin. Psychiatry*, **59**, 306–312.

Youdim, M.B.H., Aronson, J.K., Blau, K., *et al.* (1979). Tranylcypromine ('Parnate') overdose: measurement of tranylcypromine concentrations and MAO inhibitory activity and identification of amphetamines in plasma. *Psychol. Med.*, **9**, 377–382.

10

Selective serotonin reuptake inhibitors: clinical use and experience

Ted Dinan, Jeffrey Kelsey and Charles Nemeroff

Key points

- SSRIs are a safe and effective group of antidepressants.
- Dosing is less complicated than with tricyclic antidepressants; the initial dose is usually the therapeutic dose.
- The most common side effects of SSRIs are nausea/vomiting, sexual dysfunction, headache, insomnia, tremor, increased perspiration, sedation and dizziness.
- The half-life and the time to reach steady state vary from one SSRI to the next. Fluoxetine requires a long washout period but, unlike the short half-life SSRIs, is less likely to cause withdrawal problems when abruptly discontinued.

Introduction

The development of the selective serotonin reuptake inhibitors (SSRIs) is a major landmark in the pharmacological management of depression. In contrast to the tricyclic antidepressants and monoamine oxidase inhibitors, the SSRIs have a highly favourable tolerability and safety profile. As a result they are far more widely prescribed than any of their predecessors. Fluoxetine, the first SSRI to be launched in the USA, is now the second most commonly prescribed medication with a brand name widely recognized by the general public. Zimelidine, produced by the Swedish company Astra was the first SSRI launched in Europe, but it was withdrawn after a short time because of toxicity problems. It was followed in most European countries by fluvoxamine, a drug now licensed for the treatment of obsessive-compulsive disorder in the USA. Because nausea is a significant problem with this drug, its use as an antidepressant has been limited. Apart from fluoxetine, the other SSRIs available in the USA for treating depression are sertraline, citalopram and paroxetine (Tables 10.1 and 10.2).

Millions of patients world-wide have benefited from SSRI therapy. The fact that for most patients the starting dose is the therapeutic dose, has removed one of the great problems of the tricyclic medications, namely the necessity to escalate significantly from the starting dose, with many patients, especially in primary care, never achieving a proper therapeutic level. The SSRIs do not act as fast sodium channel blockers and therefore are not associated with the cardiotoxicity displayed by the tricyclics. Neither do they act on alpha-adrenoceptors producing the postural hypotension

Table 10.1 Pharmacokinetic profile of the SSRIs

Drug	Half-life	Metabolite half-life	Time to steady state	Degree of protein binding (%)
Fluoxetine	4–6 days	4–16 days	28–35 days	95
Sertraline	26 h	60–100h	4–7 days	95
Paroxetine	21 h	—	5–10 days	95
Fluvoxamine	15 h	—	5–7 days	80
Citalopram	33 h	—	7–14 days	50

Table 10.2 Relative merits of SSRIs

Drug	Advantage	Drawbacks
Fluoxetine	Low risk of withdrawal symptoms	Theoretical risk of drug interactions Lengthy washout required
Paroxetine	May be more effective in anxiety	Withdrawal symptoms pronounced
Sertraline	Flexible dose schedule	May require higher doses in a psychiatric setting
Citalopram	Favourable side-effects profile	Efficacy at 20 mg has been questioned
Fluvoxamine	Effective when anxiety present	Nausea is a significant side effect

seen with older compounds. The most common side effect of the class is nausea, which occurs in around one in three patients treated and generally decreases after a few days. Administration with meals helps to minimize this problem.

Sexual dysfunction was initially poorly recognized but is now regarded as an important side effect which affects a significant number of patients, both men and women.

Drug interactions, both among the SSRIs and between the SSRIs and other drugs, have been the subject of considerable debate recently and no clear guidelines are available. There are two broad categories of drug interactions involving SSRIs, protein binding and enzyme inhibition. SSRIs show a very high degree of protein binding and there is a theoretical risk that such a high degree of binding will result in the displacement of drugs, such as warfarin. In clinical practice it seems prudent to monitor other compounds with a high protein binding and low therapeutic indices when coprescribed with an SSRI.

The capacity of SSRIs to inhibit the cytochrome P450 system is now well recognized. Due to genetic polymorphism of certain isoenzymes, some individuals are either relatively deficient or totally deficient of a specific isoenzyme. The 2D6 isoenzyme has received particular scrutiny as tricyclics, fluoxetine, sertraline and paroxetine are all metabolized by this enzyme, while at the same time these SSRIs are all inhibitors of this enzyme.

Fluoxetine

Meta-analysis of fluoxetine efficacy studies conclude that there are no significant differences in efficacy between fluoxetine and tricyclics or between fluoxetine and other SSRIs (Bech and Ciadella, 1992; Anderson and Tomenson, 1994; Bech et al., 1994). That fluoxetine is efficacious and safe in the treatment of major depressive disorder is beyond doubt. What has been called into question has been its efficacy at the severe melancholic end of the depressive spectrum. Pande and Sayler (1993) compared the efficacy of fluoxetine, tricyclics and placebo in 3183 patients with mild, moderate or severe depression. Patients were assigned to one of these categories on the basis of their Hamilton depression scale scores. Fluoxetine was found to be significantly superior to placebo in all three severity subgroups. In an 8-week multicentre, double-blind study of 89 outpatients with DSM-IIIR major depression, 52 of whom were of the melancholic subtype, fluoxetine was found to be significantly superior to placebo (Heiligenstein et al., 1994). A comparison study of fluoxetine and clomipramine in the treatment of melancholically depressed inpatients revealed no differences between the two drugs (Ginestet, 1989).

A number of studies have evaluated the efficacy of fluoxetine in the treatment of atypical depression. Fluoxetine and imipramine were equally effective in 32 randomly assigned patients (Stratta et al., 1991). Pande and colleagues (1992) treated 40 patients diagnosed as having atypical depression with either fluoxetine (20–60 mg/day) or phenelzine (45–90 mg/day). They reported that fluoxetine was as effective as phenelzine but was better tolerated.

Fluoxetine has been found to be especially well tolerated in the elderly. The rate of discontinuation for adverse events in these studies has been similar for fluoxetine and placebo, indicating its favourable therapeutic index in this population. Comparison studies show it to have similar efficacy to amitriptyline, mianserin and superior efficacy to trazodone (Scott, 1997).

It is now well established that a period of continuation treatment is required following apparent response to an antidepressant and it is recommended in different consensus guidelines that all courses of antidepressant treatment continue for at least 6 months (WHO Mental Health Collaborating Centres, 1995). Montgomery et al. (1988) examined the long-term efficacy of fluoxetine in a group with recurrent depression who had at least two episodes in 5 years. Following response to fluoxetine, each individual was randomly assigned to placebo or fluoxetine 40 mg/day for the subsequent year and the number of relapses in each treatment group was documented. There was a highly significant reduction in the number of new episodes in the fluoxetine-treated group.

Messiha (1993) has provided the most comprehensive review of adverse effects and drug–drug interactions with fluoxetine. The common side effects reported in therapeutic studies of fluoxetine are primarily those of nausea, headache, insomnia and nervousness with a prevalence of 15–23%, followed to a lesser degree by tremors, sweating, dry mouth, anxiety, drowsiness and diarrhoea reported by 10–14% of patients.

Fluoxetine is well established as improving both the sleep disturbance and the anxiety components of depression. Studies clearly indicate its tendency to normalize sleep architecture (von Bardeleben *et al.*, 1989) and, although some patients show an increase in anxiety in the first few weeks of fluoxetine treatment, overall anxiety decreases as the depressive syndrome responds to treatment (Tollefson *et al.*, 1994). In general, the effects of fluoxetine on the cardiovascular system are minimal compared to the tricyclic antidepressants, but there are a small number of case reports of atrial fibrillation and bradycardia occurring in patients on fluoxetine. The presence of pre-existing cardiovascular disease in these patients cannot be excluded. Hyponatraemia and/or syndrome of inappropriate antidiuretic hormone secretion (SIADH) has been reported with fluoxetine (Blacksten and Birt, 1993) as well as with the tricyclics. In general the hyponatraemia resolves upon cessation of the drug. Fluoxetine has been associated with haematological complications most notably increased bleeding tendencies (Humphries *et al.*, 1990). This is not thought to be due to increased bleeding time but rather to abnormalities of platelet aggregation, presumably due to the role of 5-HT in the platelet.

Because of its relatively long half-life, 8 days for fluoxetine and 19 days for its active metabolite norfluoxetine, withdrawal effects are not a problem when the drug is suddenly stopped, unlike other SSRIs with relatively short half-lives. As a potent inhibitor of cytochrome P450 2D6, caution should be observed when the drug is coprescribed with tricyclic antidepressants, antipsychotics such as thioridazine, fluphenazine or clozapine, beta-blockers, antiarrhythmic agents, carbamazepine and antitussives.

Paroxetine

Paroxetine has been demonstrated superior to placebo in several controlled trials in patients with major depression (Nemeroff, 1993). In a pooled analysis of four trials involving 273 patients with major depression, paroxetine was found to be superior to placebo in treating both measures of anxiety and depression. Paroxetine separated from placebo by week 2 and sustained this difference throughout the 6-week trial period.

A number of different trials have compared paroxetine to imipramine (Corby and Dunne, 1997). Pooling six studies of similar design of outpatients with major depression in which patients were randomized to treatment with paroxetine, imipramine, or placebo, both active treatments showed superiority compared to placebo. Both drugs were equal in efficacy and superior to placebo by week 2, but paroxetine was much better tolerated than imipramine.

Paroxetine has been compared to clomipramine in a large multicentre study involving 1019 patients with major depression and associated anxiety. After 12 weeks of treatment similar responses were noted in both treatment groups. This is in contrast to the results of the Danish study of inpatients with major depression who received either 40 mg/day of paroxetine or 150 mg/day of clomipramine (Danish University Antidepressant Group, 1990). Clomipramine was found to have greater efficacy than paroxetine as measured by changes in Hamilton depression scale scores.

Paroxetine is reported to have similar efficacy to fluoxetine in a study investigating the treatment of 178 inpatients with major depression (De Wilde *et al.*, 1993). At the end of 6 weeks the response rates were 67% in the paroxetine group and 64% in the fluoxetine group.

Paroxetine and fluoxetine were compared in a study of depression in the elderly (Schone and Ludwig, 1993). Patients were randomly assigned to treatment with paroxetine (20–40 mg/day) or fluoxetine (20–60 mg/day). At week 3 the paroxetine group showed greater improvement than did the fluoxetine group; however, the two groups showed no difference in efficacy by week 6. In general paroxetine is very well tolerated in the elderly.

The side effects reported for paroxetine are very similar to those described above for fluoxetine. As in the case of other SSRIs, paroxetine is highly protein bound and may potentially displace drugs such as warfarin. The manufacturer warns that there may be a pharmacokinetic interaction between paroxetine and warfarin. Like fluoxetine, it is a relatively potent inhibitor of P450 2D6 so that drugs metabolized by this isoenzyme system should be coprescribed with paroxetine cautiously. Several reports of a paroxetine withdrawal syndrome have emerged recently (Frost and Lal, 1995; Debattista and Schatzberg, 1995). Both physical and psychological symptoms have been described, most notably severe anxiety and dizziness. The manufacturers recommend gradual withdrawal of paroxetine.

Sertraline

Sertraline has been extensively compared both with placebo and other active antidepressant medication. Three hundred and sixty-nine outpatients with major depression were randomly assigned to treatment either with sertraline 50 mg, 100 mg, 200 mg/day or placebo. All three doses of sertraline were found to be superior to placebo (Fabre *et al.*, 1995). There was a trend for greater improvement in the 100–200 mg/day group, though this did not attain statistical significance. One hundred and sixty-eight outpatients with major depression were treated either with sertraline or amitriptyline (50–150 mg/day). Overall sertraline was found to be as efficacious as amitriptyline but better tolerated (Reimherr *et al.*, 1990). In a double-blind 6-week study of 286 outpatients with DSM IIIR major depression, sertraline was found to be as effective as fluoxetine (Aguglia *et al.*, 1993). Several other comparative studies against tricyclics and SSRIs have now been reported in the literature. It is clear that sertraline is an effective antidepressant with a favourable side-effect profile. The recommended starting dose for sertraline is 50 mg/day but the dose can be escalated to a maximum of 200 mg/day, depending upon response.

Sertraline appears to be well tolerated with only 15% of over 2500 patients in premarketing trials discontinuing due to adverse events. It does not significantly alter cardiac rhythm or blood pressure. Individuals with existing cardiac disease in general tolerate the drug well. As with other SSRIs there has been reporting of abnormal bleeding or bruising in patients taking the drug. The incidence of nausea in controlled trials is 26% for sertraline as opposed to 12% for placebo. A higher incidence of diarrhoea is also reported in these trials. Insomnia, somnolence, agitation, nervousness, anxiety, and impaired concentration are all reported more often in sertraline-treated patients than in those treated with placebo. The reported incidence of sexual dysfunction in controlled trials is 15.5% for male and 1.7% for females. These figures are much lower than those reported in routine clinical practice. As with other SSRIs, the drug tightly binds to serum proteins. The manufacturer warns against a potential interaction between sertraline and other tightly protein bound drugs such as digoxin and warfarin. It is a less potent inhibitor of cytochrome P450 2D6 than fluoxetine or paroxetine. It weakly inhibits the 2C isoenzyme system so that theoretically it could interfere with the metabolism of tolbutamide, the oral hypoglycaemic agent.

Fluvoxamine

This is currently licensed in the USA for the treatment of obsessive-compulsive disorder, but it has been available in Europe for many years for the treatment of depression. The effective dose of fluvoxamine in the treatment of depression is usually between 100–300 mg/day. Placebo-controlled studies indicate its superiority over placebo (Dominguez et al., 1985), while in a comparison study with desipramine it was found to have similar efficacy. It has also been compared to fluoxetine in a trial of 100 patients with major depression (Rapaport et al., 1996). Fluvoxamine (100–150 mg/day) and fluoxetine (20–80 mg/day) produced similar changes in Hamilton depression scale scores over a 7-week period. While the side-effects profile for fluvoxamine is similar to that of other SSRIs, the incidence of nausea in post-marketing studies is higher than that of its competitors. This side effect has limited its usefulness as an antidepressant in most European countries. In a comparative trial with sertraline, it had equal efficacy but was associated with less sexual dysfunction (Nemeroff et al., 1996).

Fluvoxamine is less tightly protein bound than the other SSRIs and may be less likely to produce displacement of tightly protein bound drugs. In the P450 system fluvoxamine is an inhibitor of the 1A2, 2C9 and 3A4 isoenzymes. Aminophylline, warfarin, propranolol and caffeine are all metabolized through the 1A2 isoenzyme system. In the presence of fluvoxamine, warfarin metabolism may be inhibited through the 2C9 isoenzyme system. As benzodiazepines undergo hepatic oxidation by the 3A4 isoenzyme, significant increases in serum concentrations may be found in the presence of fluvoxamine. The manufacturer warns against the coadministration of fluvoxamine with terfenidine, astemizole or cisapride. These compounds are all inactive upon ingestion and require 3A4 activity to produce an active metabolite. Smokers demonstrated a 25% increase in fluvoxamine metabolism compared to non-smokers, probably due to an induction of 1A2 enzymes.

Citalopram

This is the most selective of the SSRIs currently available. It is usually commenced at 20 mg/day and increased to a maximum of 60 mg/day if required. Two studies conducted in the USA have compared citalopram

20–80 mg/day (flexible dosing) or 10–60 mg/day (fixed dosing) with placebo over a 4- and 6-week period. Both studies demonstrated evidence of efficacy with greatest response seen for the 40–60 mg doses.

Two UK studies both carried out for 10 weeks compared 20–40 mg of citalopram with placebo. The first was a hospital-based study in which 199 patients took part, all with moderate to severe depression and high scores on the Hamilton depression rating scale. Significant advantage was demonstrated for 40 mg citalopram at weeks 3, 4 and 6. No significant effect was seen in the 20 mg group. The second of these studies involved 274 patients who were treated with 20 mg or 40 mg of citalopram or placebo. Though the outcome showed quite a high placebo response rate, there was significant advantage for citalopram 20 mg over placebo.

A meta-analysis of nine placebo-controlled studies involving a total of 949 patients treated with either citalopram or placebo showed the benefit of citalopram compared with placebo (Montgomery et al., 1994). A similar meta-analysis was conducted by Bech and Ciadella (1992). In five trials doses of citalopram ranged from 20 to 80 mg and a total of 396 patients took part. Response, defined as a 50% reduction in Hamilton depression scores, showed a significant advantage of citalopram over placebo and equal efficacy to tricyclics.

Studies in the elderly demonstrate the drug to be effective and well tolerated. A 24-week study of citalopram 20 mg, 40 mg and placebo in the treatment and prevention of relapse of major depression has been reported (Montgomery et al., 1993). A total of 147 patients who had responded in a placebo study to 6 weeks' treatment of an episode of major depression with either 20 mg or 40 mg citalopram were randomized double blind to continue on the same dose of citalopram or to receive placebo. The citalopram 20 mg and 40 mg groups showed a significant advantage compared to placebo in relapse prevention.

Citalopram has been shown to have relatively few adverse effects and to be relatively safe in overdose. The adverse events that can be attributed to citalopram are generally considered to be of mild to moderate severity and in placebo-controlled studies the most frequently reported events are nausea, dry mouth, somnolence, sweating, tremor, diarrhoea and sexual dysfunction. The excess in incidence of these adverse events over placebo has never exceeded 10% and the pattern of adverse events reported by patients does not seem to be dose-related.

Conclusions

The SSRIs (Table 10.2) are a well-tolerated class of antidepressant and offer major advantages over their predecessors, the tricyclics and monoamine oxidase inhibitors. They have a favourable side-effects profile which does not include the cardiotoxicity and profound anticholinergic problems of the tricyclics. In general they are relatively safe in overdose and well tolerated in the elderly. For most patients and most SSRIs the starting dose is the therapeutic dose, unlike the tricyclics where dose escalation is required. As is the case with older antidepressants, the therapeutic response is slow to emerge, usually 2–6 weeks after commencing the medication, and only approximately 70% of patients respond to treatment. Given the high protein binding and isoenzyme inhibition, a theoretical possibility of drug interactions exists. In reality fluoxetine, as the most widely prescribed psychotropic so far developed, has shown few significant adverse drug interactions. Nonetheless, such interactions should be borne in mind when a decision to prescribe an SSRI is made. Furthermore, a withdrawal syndrome is well established, especially in the case of short half-life SSRIs, and they therefore should always be gradually tapered prior to discontinuation.

References

Aguglia, E., Casacchia, M., Cassano, G.B., *et al.* (1993). Double-blind study of the efficacy and safety of sertraline versus fluoxetine in major depression. *Inter. Clin. Psychopharm.*, **8**, 197–203.

Anderson, I. and Tomerson, B. (1994). A meta-analysis of the selective serotonin reuptake inhibitors compared to tricyclic antidepressants in depression. XIX CINP Meeting: Washington DC.

Bech, P. and Ciadella, P. (1992). Citalopram in depression: meta-analysis of intended and unintended effects. *Inter. Clin. Psychopharm.*, **6** (Suppl. 5), 45–54.

Bech, P., Tollefson, G., Ciadella, P., *et al.* (1994). A meta-analysis of controlled fluoxetine trials. XIX CINP Meeting: Washington DC.

Blacksten, J.V. and Birt, J.A. (1993). Syndrome of inappropriate secretion of antidiuretic hormone secondary to fluoxetine. *Ann. Pharmacother.*, **27**, 723–724.

Corby, C.L. and Dunne, G. (1997). Paroxetine: a review. *J. Serotonin Res.*, **4**, 47–64.

Danish University Antidepressant Group (1990). Paroxetine: a selective serotonin reuptake inhibitor showing better tolerance, but weaker efficacy than clomipramine in a controlled multicenter study. *J. Affect. Dis.*, **18**, 289–295.

Debattista, C. and Schatzberg, A.F. (1995). Physical symptoms associated with paroxetine withdrawal. *Am. J. Psychiatry*, **152**, 1235–1236.

De Wilde, J., Spiers, R., Mertens, C., *et al.* (1993). A double-blind, comparative, multicentre study comparing paroxetine with fluoxetine in depressed patients. *Acta Psychiat. Scand.*, **87**, 141–145.

Dominguez, R.A., Goldstein, B.J., Jacobsen, A.F., *et al.* (1985). A double-blind placebo-controlled study of fluvoxamine and imipramine in depression. *J. Clin. Psychiatry*, **46**, 84–88.

Fabre, L.F., Abuzzahab, F.S., Amin, M., *et al.* (1995). Sertraline safety and efficacy in major depression: a double-blind fixed-dose comparison with placebo. *Biol. Psychiatry*, **38**, 592–597.

Frost, L. and Lal, S. (1995). Shock-like sensations after discontinuation of SSRIs. *Am. J. Psychiatry*, **152**, 810.

Ginestet, D. (1989). Fluoxetine in endogenous depression and melancholia versus clomipramine. *Inter. Clin. Psychopharm.*, **4** (Suppl. 10), 37–40.

Heiligenstein, D.J., Tollefson, G.D. and Fairies, D.E. (1994). Response patterns of depressed outpatients with and without melancholia: a double blind placebo-controlled trial of fluoxetine versus placebo. *J. Affect. Dis.*, **30**, 163–173.

Humphries, J.E., Wheby, M.S. and Van Den Berg, S.R. (1990). Fluoxetine and bleeding time. *Arch. Path. Lab. Med.*, **114**, 727–728.

Messiha, F.S. (1993). Fluoxetine: adverse effects and drug–drug interactions. *Clin. Toxicol.*, **31**, 603–630.

Montgomery, S.A., Dufour, H., Brion, S., *et al.* (1988). The prophylactic efficacy of fluoxetine in unipolar depression. *Br. J. Psychiatry*, **153** (Suppl. 3), 69–76.

Montgomery, S.A., Rasmussen, J.G.C. and Tanghoj, P. (1993). A 24 week study of 20 mg Citalopram, 40 mg Citalopram and placebo in the prevention of relapse in major depression. *Inter. Clin. Psychopharm.*, **4** (Suppl. 5), 65–70.

Montgomery, S.A., Pendersen, V., Tanghoj, P., *et al.* (1994). The optimal dosing regime for Citalopram – a meta analysis of placebo-controlled studies. *Inter. Clin. Psychopharm.*, **9** (Suppl. 1), 35–40.

Nemeroff, C.B. (1993). Paroxetine: an overview of the efficacy and safety of a new selective serotonin reuptake inhibitor in the treatment of depression. *J. Clin. Psychopharmacol.*, **13** (Suppl. 2), 10S.

Nemeroff, C.B., DeVane, C.L. and Pollock, B.G. (1996). Newer antidepressants and the cytochrome P450 system. *Am. J. Psychiatry*, **153**, 311.

Pande, A.C. and Sayler, M.E. (1993). Severity of depression and response to fluoxetine. *Inter. Clin. Psychopharm.*, **8**, 243–245.

Pande, A.C., Haskett, R.F. and Greden, J.F. (1992). Fluoxetine versus phenelzine in atypical depression. *Inter. Clin. Psychopharm.* **18** (Suppl. 31), 21.

Rapaport, M., Coccaro, E., Sheline, Y., *et al.* (1996). A comparison of fluvoxamine and fluoxetine in the treatment of major depression. *J. Clin. Psychopharmacol.*, **16**, 373–384.

Reimherr, F.W., Chouinard, G., Cohn, C.K., *et al.* (1990). Antidepressant efficacy of sertraline: a double-blind, placebo- and amitriptyline-controlled, multicenter comparison study in outpatients with major depression. *J. Clin. Psychiatry*, **51** (Suppl. B), 18–23.

Schone, W. and Ludwig, M. (1993). A double-blind study of paroxetine compared with fluoxetine in geriatric patients with major depression. *J. Clin. Psychopharm.*, **13**, 34S.

Scott, L.V. (1997). Fluoxetine: a review of its pharmacology and clinical applications. *J. Serotonin Res.*, **3**, 173–192.

Stratta, P., Bolino, F., Culillari, M., *et al.* (1991). A double blind parallel study comparing fluoxetine and imipramine in the treatment of atypical depression. *Inter. Clin. Psychopharm.*, **16**, 193–196.

Tollefson, G.D., Holman, S.L., Sayer, M.E., *et al.* (1994). Fluoxetine, placebo and tricyclic antidepressants in major depression with and without anxious features. *J. Clin. Psychiatry*, **55**, 50–59.

Von Bardeleben, U., Steiger, A., Gerken, A., *et al.* (1989). Effect of fluoxetine on pharmacoendocrine and sleep-EEG parameters in normal controls. *Inter. Clin. Psychopharm.*, **4** (Suppl. 1), 1–5.

WHO Mental Health Collaborating Centres (1995). Pharmacotherapy of depressive disorders. A consensus statement. *J. Affect. Dis.*, **17**, 197–198.

11

Nefazodone, mirtazapine and venlafaxine: clinical use and experience

Madhukar Trivedi and Trisha Suppes

Key points

- Nefazodone has also been found to improve symptoms of poor sleep quality, sleep disturbance, anxiety, and agitation in depressed patients.
- Mirtazapine has been shown to be effective for both the short- and long-term treatment of major depressive disorder.
- Venlafaxine is also an effective treatment for major depression and, like nefazodone, may also be of benefit in the treatment of anxiety disorders.

Introduction

Pharmacotherapy has profited in the past few years from the availability of several novel compounds for the treatment of various psychiatric disorders. However, the increase in medication options also carries the inherent complexity and challenge of incorporating the new information with existing knowledge in selecting a treatment for a particular patient or patient population. This chapter will focus on the treatment of mood disorders with the novel compounds – nefazodone, venlafaxine and mirtazapine – that have recently become available in the USA and Europe. Each drug has specific attributes that should be considered before choosing it for certain psychiatric disorders, combinations of disorders, or patient subgroups within disorders.

Clinical pharmacology

Nefazodone is an antidepressant for oral administration with a chemical structure unrelated to selective serotonin reuptake inhibitors (SSRIs), tricyclics, tetracyclics, or monoamine oxidase inhibitors (MAOIs). Nefazodone is a synthetically derived phenylpiperazine antidepressant (Greene and Barbhaiya, 1997). It inhibits neuronal uptake of serotonin and norepinephrine and has no significant affinity for alpha$_2$ and beta adrenergic, 5-HT$_{1A}$, cholinergic, dopaminergic, or benzodiazepine receptors (Table 11.1).

Mirtazapine, an oral antidepressant, has been available for the treatment of depression in the USA since 1996 and has been in use in Europe since 1994. Mirtazapine's efficacy is attributed to its novel dual neurotransmitter

Table 11.1 Mechanism of action of nefazodone, mirtazapine, and venlafaxine

	Nefazodone	Mirtazapine	Venlafaxine
5-HT reuptake	+ +	+ + +	−
Blockade 5-HT$_1$	+ + +	+−	−
Blockade 5-HT$_2$	+ + +	+−	+ + + +
NE reuptake	+ +	+ +	−
DA reuptake	+	+	−
Blockade ACh	+−	−	+
Blockade H$_1$	+−	−	+ + + + +
Blockade a$_1$	+ + +	−	+ +
Blockade a$_2$	+ +	+−	+ + +
Blockade D$_2$	+ +	−	+
Selectivity	NE < 5-HT	NE < 5-HT	−

(Bezchlibnyk-Butler and Jeffries, 1996)

action, enhancing both noradrenergic and 5-HT receptor-mediated seroto-nergic neurotransmission and blockade of 5-HT$_2$ and 5-HT$_3$ receptors (de Boer, 1995, 1996) (see Table 11.1).

Venlafaxine is a structurally novel agent belonging to a new generation of antidepressants known as serotonergic noradrenergic reuptake inhibitors (SNRIs). Venlafaxine is a phenylethylamine compound that inhibits the reuptake of serotonin and norepinephrine without significant effect on other neurotransmitter systems, including histamine or cholinergic receptors (see Table 11.1).

Pharmacokinetics and metabolism

Nefazodone is rapidly and completely absorbed, but is subject to extensive metabolism, so that its absolute bioavailability is low, about 20%, and variable (Greene and Barbhaiya, 1997).

- Peak plasma concentrations occur at about one hour.
- Half-life of nefazodone is 2–4 hours.
- Both nefazodone and its pharmacologically similar metabolite, hydroxy-nefazodone (HO-NEF), exhibit non-linear kinetics for both dose and time.
- Nefazodone is widely distributed in body tissues, including the central nervous system and myocardial tissue.
- At concentrations of 25–2500 ng/ml nefazodone is extensively (> 99%) bound to human plasma proteins in vitro.
- Food delays the absorption of nefazodone and decreases the bioavail-ability of nefazodone by approximately 20%.
- Metabolized primarily by the liver.

The pharmacology of mirtazapine is well described (Stimmel et al., 1997; Delbressine and Vos, 1997). It has an absolute bioavailability ~50%; food has little impact on rate or extent of absorption (Cohen et al., 1997).

- Peak plasma level within 2 hours of administration, independent of dose.
- Metabolized in the liver by cytochrome P450 D6 and P450 3A main iso-enzymes.

- Metabolized and eliminated in urine and faeces.
- Half-life of 20–40 hours.

Venlafaxine is well absorbed from the gastrointestinal tract (at least 92%) and extensively metabolized in the liver.

- O-desmethylvenlafaxine (ODV) is only major active metabolite.
- Food has no effect on absorption or formation of ODV.
- Less than 30% bound to plasma protein.
- Peak plasma level reached by venlafaxine IR in 2.3 hours, venlafaxine XR 6 hours, and ODV in 2–6 hours.
- Major elimination is via the urine, clearance decreased by 24% in renal disease and 50% in hepatic disease.
- Metabolized by cytochrome P450 IID6; weak inhibitor of this enzyme.
- The elimination half-lives of venlafaxine and ODV are 5 hours and 11 hours respectively (Ellingrod and Perry, 1994; Morton et al., 1995).

Indications and usage

Nefazodone is currently approved for the treatment of depression. Nefazodone has also been found to improve symptoms of poor sleep quality, sleep disturbance, anxiety, and agitation in depressed patients (Armitage et al., 1994; Fawcett et al., 1995; Armitage et al., 1997). Recent studies suggest that nefazodone may be effective in the treatment of panic disorder, migraine headache, and premenstrual syndrome (PMS).

Mirtazapine has been shown to be effective for both the short- and long-term treatment of major depressive disorder (MDD). It is at least as effective as other standard antidepressants given at comparable doses for the treatment of MDD, as demonstrated in several short-term, 6-week studies (Stahl et al., 1997; Montgomery, 1998).

Venlafaxine has been shown to be an effective treatment for major depression in a broad range of patients (Ellingrod and Perry, 1994; Morton et al., 1995; Ballenger, 1996). As with many other antidepressants, it is thought to possess significant antianxiety properties and have a place in the treatment of anxiety disorders. Clinical trials are currently being conducted on the use of venlafaxine for anxiety disorders such as social phobia, obsessive-compulsive disorder and panic disorder; however it has not yet gained approval for these disorders (Morton et al., 1995). An extended release formulation of venlafaxine (venlafaxine XR) has been developed that provides prolonged absorption, but the same total absorption of active drug as the immediate release formulation (Thase, 1997).

Dosage and administration

Nefazodone is supplied as hexagonal tablets containing 50 mg, 100 mg, 150 mg, 200 mg, or 250 mg of nefazodone (Robinson et al., 1996). The suggested initial dose is 100 mg bid, with increases in increments of 50–100 mg bid at intervals of no less than 1 week. The effective dose range is 300–600 mg/day, though possibly taking several weeks for full response. The suggested initial dose for elderly patients is 50 mg bid, followed by modifying the rate of subsequent dose titration as needed. Treatment of acute episodes should continue for up to 6 months or longer. Efficacy has been maintained for up to 36 weeks following 16 weeks of acute treatment at doses averaging 438 mg/day (Robinson *et al.*, 1996). The suggested maintenance dose will usually be that associated with response during acute treatment.

Based on clinical trials and the recommendations of the manufacturer, mirtazapine should be administered in the evening starting with 15 mg (Stimmel *et al.*, 1997). Onset of clinical effect is generally 2–4 weeks, with improvement in sleep and anxiety possible within the first week of treatment (Stimmel *et al.*, 1997). Increases may be made, based on response, up to a maximum dose of 45 mg. In order to give adequate time to gauge response, dose increments should not begin until after 1–2 weeks of treatment with the initial dose. The half-life of mirtazapine is 20–40 hours; therefore, once daily dosing is sufficient. No taper is necessary when discontinuing treatment with Remeron. Immediately switching from SSRIs to mirtazapine was shown to be safe and well tolerated (Fava abstract).

Mirtazapine has been shown to be effective and well tolerated in elderly patients with no differences in efficacy or adverse events (Hoyberg *et al.*, 1996; Richelson, 1997, 1998). However, it has a longer elimination half-life in these patients and, therefore, caution is recommended when increasing dose in this population.

Venlafaxine IR is available in 25, 37.5, 50, and 100 mg tablets. The recommended starting dose is 75 mg/day in two or three divided doses taken with food. The dosage can be increased in increments of up to 75 mg/day at intervals of no less than 4 days. The target dose is 150–225 mg/day and the maximum daily dose 375 mg/day (Ellingrod and Perry, 1994).

Venlafaxine XR is available in 37.5, 75, and 150 mg tablets. The recommended starting dose is 75 mg/day given in a single dose. However, for some patients, it may be desirable to start at 37.5 mg/day for 4–7 days, to allow new patients to adjust to the medication before increasing to 75 mg/day. The target dose is 75–150 mg/day, with the maximum daily dosage of 225 mg (Physician's Desk Reference, 1999). The potential advantages of the once daily dosing of venlafaxine XR are better patient compliance and convenience, improved patient tolerability and maintained or improved effectiveness (Thase, 1997).

Dosage adjustments for use in healthy elderly adults are not required; however it is necessary to decrease dose by 25% in patients with renal disease. The dosage for patients with hepatic impairment is dependent on the degree of impairment. Because abrupt withdrawal has been shown to cause symptoms such as asthenia, dizziness, headache, nausea and nervousness, tapering over a 2-week period is suggested (Ellingrod and Perry, 1994).

Adverse reactions/side effects

Nefazodone is generally well tolerated by most patients. The most common side effect is nausea. The side-effect profile of nefazodone is given in Table 11.2.

Table 11.2 Side effects of nefazodone

Nausea	Insomnia	Palpitations
Fatigue	Dyspepsia	Vomiting
Confusion	Diarrhoea	Anorexia
Dizziness	Increased appetite	Oedema
Blurred vision	Abnormal ejaculation/orgasm	Weight gain
Orthostatic hypotension	(men)	Delayed micturition
Dry mouth	Orgasm disturbance (women)	Tremor
Constipation	Sweating	Tachycardia
Drowsiness	Cardiac arrhythmia	Rash
Headache	Agitation	
GI distress	Anxiety	

Most side effects are alleviated after dosage is stabilized. Side effects that subsist are generally managed through appropriate countermeasures or discontinuation of the medication (Bezchlibnyk-Butler and Jeffries, 1996; Nelson, 1997).

The side effects associated with mirtazapine are very different from many other standard antidepressants, including SSRIs, SNRIs and tricyclics. Mirtazapine produces less nausea and sexual dysfunction than the SSRIs due to its blockade of the $5-HT_2$ and $5-HT_3$ receptors. Due to its pharmacological action, mirtazapine lacks significant cholinergic, adrenergic and serotonergic side effects. This is likely to present a clear advantage for some patients (Nutt, 1997). Overall, mirtazapine is well tolerated. In a meta-analysis conducted by Stahl and colleagues (1997), the attrition rate due to adverse events for mirtazapine was 10%. Somnolence and weight gain are the most commonly reported adverse events (Montgomery et al., 1998). (See Table 11.3 for a more complete list of associated side effects.)

Paradoxically, studies have shown that increasing the initial dose of mirtazapine may decrease somnolence. This conclusion is based on evidence from studies that note decreases in number of patients reporting sedation after titrated to a higher dose, and fewer number of patients overall reporting sedation in groups of patients receiving higher doses (van Moffaert et al., 1995; Burrows and Kremer, 1997).

Venlafaxine is well tolerated by most patients. Attrition rates due to adverse effects ranged from 7% to 16% in the literature reviewed (Schweizer et al., 1991; Ballenger, 1996; Lecrubier et al., 1997; Mahapatra

Table 11.3 Side effects of mirtazapine

Increased appetite	Constipation	Abnormal thinking
Somnolence	Dry mouth	Myalgia
Dizziness	Oedema	Tremor
Weight gain (secondary to increased appetite/increased intake)	Confusion	Agranulocytosis
	Abnormal dreams	

and Hackett, 1997; Thase, 1997; Feighner *et al.*, 1998); (See Table 11.4 for a list of side effects associated with venlafaxine).

Nausea appears to be the most commonly reported side effect with venlafaxine, with incidence ranging from 25% to 55% (Morton *et al.*, 1995). However, studies show that nausea decreases after the first 2–3 weeks (Lecrubier *et al.*, 1997). Administration with food often helps alleviate the nausea associated with venlafaxine. Most of the other side effects are manageable and can be treated with a decrease in dosage, change of administration times or adjunctive medication. Discontinuation of venlafaxine is necessary in the case of the more serious adverse effects, such as seizures or mania.

Contraindications

Nefazodone is contraindicated in patients with known hypersensitivity to nefazodone or other phenylpiperazine antidepressants. It should also be used with caution in patients with a cardiovascular disorder or seizure disorder.

Mirtazapine increases the effects of direct-acting sympathomimetics, alcohol, barbiturates, and CNS depressants. Benzodiazepines should be used with caution due to increased plasma concentrations when administered with mirtazapine. Coadministration with MAO inhibitors may cause hypertensive crisis, hyperpyretic crisis or convulsions. Care should be exercised in patients with severe renal or hepatic failure. Due to the side-effect profile, mirtazapine should not be a first choice for patients with atypical symptoms.

Venlafaxine is contraindicated in patients with a known hypersensitivity to it. Because venlafaxine is associated with sustained increases in blood pressure especially at increased doses, it should be used with caution in patients with hypertension. Venlafaxine should also be cautiously administered to patients with history of mania or seizure disorder (Ellingrod and Perry, 1994; Physician's Desk Reference, 1999).

Drug interactions

Concomitant use of nefazodone with benzodiazepines increases the plasma concentration of the benzodiazepines. Its concomitant use with non-sedating antihistamines, such as terfenadine or astemizole, can result in a possibly fatal reaction. Coadministration with MAOIs should be avoided, as it may cause a hypertensive crisis.

Table 11.4 Side effects of venlafaxine

Nausea (37%)	Hypertension (2%)	Seizures (0.3%)
Somnolence (23%)	Anxiety (6%)	Activation of mania (0.5%)
Dizziness (19%)	Sexual dysfunction (12%)	(Bezchlibnyk-Butler and
Constipation (15%)	Tachycardia (2%)	Jeffries, 1996)
Dry mouth (22%)	(Physician's Desk Reference,	
Insomnia (18%)	1999)	
(Morton *et al.*, 1994)		

Data thus far indicate that mirtazapine has a relatively low likelihood of causing drug interactions with drugs metabolized by the P450 enzymes. (Richelson, 1997, 1998; Owen and Nemeroff, 1998). Mirtazapine may be a preferred choice for use in elderly patients due to this advantage.

Concomitant use of venlafaxine with MAOIs should be avoided as it may cause serotonergic reaction, hypertensive crisis, hyperthermia, rigidity, and mental status changes. The use of cimetidine with venlafaxine decreases the clearance by 43%, increasing the plasma concentration by 60% (Ellingrod and Perry, 1994).

Clinical studies/efficacy

Nefazodone has been marketed since 1994 for the treatment of major depressive disorder. Six trials provide supportive data on efficacy. In the treatment of outpatient depression, nefazodone, at the appropriate dose, proved to be superior to placebo and as effective as imipramine, fluoxetine, sertraline, and paroxetine. A nefazodone dose–response relationship across studies employing a low-dose range and/or high-dose range dose titration schedule was established. Only studies that permitted the higher dose range of up to 500 or 600 mg/day demonstrated efficacy (Physician's Desk Reference, 1999).

In studies evaluating the effect of nefazodone (400–600 mg/day) on sleep architecture in depressed patients, nefazodone was associated with improvement in sleep disturbance and better sleep quality (Armitage et al., 1994, 1997). One study found that nefazodone increased sleep efficiency and reduced the number of awakenings and percent awake and movement time in comparison with fluoxetine, which increased the number of awakenings and did not significantly alter sleep efficiency or percent awake and movement time. This study also found that nefazodone increased REM sleep, decreased REM latency, and did not alter stage 1 sleep (Armitage et al., 1997).

Nefazodone treatment has also been associated with improvement of anxiety and agitation symptoms in depressed patients (Fawcett et al., 1995). A meta-analysis of six randomized, placebo-controlled, double-blind trials found that patients treated with nefazodone showed significantly greater improvement in somatic anxiety (HAM-D item 11) than patients on placebo (week 4 to end of treatment) or imipramine (Table 11.5). Patients taking nefazodone also showed more rapid improvement on agitation (HAM-D item 9) than those on placebo or imipramine.

There have been several double-blind trials that have demonstrated mirtazapine's effectiveness as an antidepressant (see Table 11.6).

It was shown to be superior in efficacy and tolerability to trazodone in a study by Montgomery et al., (1998). Of note in this study, starting doses of mirtazapine were 24 mg qd, with increases on days 4, 7, 10, and 13 based on tolerability, with a maximum dose of 56 mg, or of 72 mg at day 16 if there was inadequate response. Despite relatively high doses, mirtazapine was found to be better tolerated than trazodone, with only half as many reported incidences of somnolence (21% at day 14, 13% at day 42 for trazodone; 10% and 5% respectively for mirtazapine). These results are consistent with

Table 11.5 Studies of nefazodone

Author(s)	Study Design	Patient population	Length of tx	pts in each cell	Dose	Overall results
Armitage et al., 1997	Randomized, double-blind, parallel group investigation comparing effects of nefazodone and fluoxetine on sleep architecture and sleep measures in depressed patients	Outpatients with moderate to severe, non-psychotic major depressive disorder	8 weeks	43 nefazodone: n = 22 fluoxetine: n = 21	Nefazodone: 200–500 mg/day Fluoxetine: 20–40 mg/day	Nefazodone increased sleep efficiency and reduced number of awakenings and percent awake and movement time
Armitage et al., 1994	Polysomnographic study on depressed patients during 4–8 weeks of open-trial treatment with nefazodone	Outpatients with non-psychotic major depressive disorder	4–8 weeks	10	400–600 mg/day	Nefazodone was associated with significantly decreased wake and movement time and increased minutes and percentage of stage 2 sleep at the expense of light stage 1 sleep
Fawcett et al., 1995	Meta-analysis of six randomized, placebo-controlled, double-blind trials to evaluate effectiveness of nefazodone in relieving symptoms of anxiety and agitation in depressed patients	Outpatients with moderate to severe major depressive disorder	6–8 weeks	817 placebo: n = 345 imipramine: n = 288 nefazodone: n = 184	Imipramine: 25–300 mg/day Nefazodone: 100–600 mg/day	Nefazodone-treated patients showed improvement in somatic anxiety and improved more rapidly on agitation than patients on placebo or imipramine

Table 11.5 continued

Reference	Study	Duration	n	Dose	Outcome
DeMartinis et al., 1996	8-week trial of nefazodone in patients with panic disorder	Patients with panic disorder and concurrent diagnosis of major depression, dysthymia, generalized anxiety disorder, and depression NOS	8 weeks	14	200–600 mg/day	Preliminary evidence for efficacy and tolerability of nefazodone in panic disorder and panic disorder with comorbid depression or depressive symptoms
Zajecka, 1996	Retrospective analysis of two randomized, placebo-controlled trials evaluating effectiveness of nefazodone in relieving depression-associated anxiety symptoms	Outpatients with major depressive disorder	8 weeks	318 (MDD with comorbid panic disorder: n = 55) nefazodone: n = 92 placebo: n = 93 imipramine: n = 88	Nefazodone: 50–600 mg/day Imipramine: 50–300 mg/day	During nefazodone treatment, patients with comorbid panic disorder experienced marked global improvement compared with placebo, including relief of panic and phobic anxiety symptoms
Freeman et al., 1994	8-week, open-label nefazodone treatment	Women with well-defined PMS symptoms and women with concurrent PMS and major depressive disorder or dysthymia	8 weeks	47 PMS only: n = 23 PMS with MDD or dysthymia: n = 24	100–600 mg/day	Premenstrual symptoms improved significantly from pretreatment baseline values, with similar improvement in both groups

Table 11.6 Studies of mirtazapine

Author(s)	Study Design	Patient population	Length of Tx	pts in each cell	Dose	Overall results
Montgomery et al., 1998	Double-blind, mirtazapine vs. amitriptyline vs. placebo	MDD, responders to acute phase Tx	20 weeks; preliminary analyses of 2-year study	217; 74 mirtazapine, 86 amitriptyline, 57 placebo		Mirtazapine was effective in reducing relapse and recurrence of depression; there was also a significantly longer time to relapse
van Moffaert et al., 1995	Random, double-blind treatment with mirtazapine or trazodone	Hospitalized; moderate to severe MDD	6 weeks	200	24–72 mg/day mirtazapine; 150–450 mg/day trazodone	Mirtazapine was shown to have superior efficacy and tolerability compared to trazodone
Smith et al., 1990	Double-blind, mirtazapine vs. amitriptyline vs. placebo	MDD	6 weeks	150	Mean dose mirtazapine = 18 mg; mean dose of amitriptyline = 111 mg	Mirtazapine was as effective as amitriptyline, and superior to it regarding cardiovascular and anticholinergic side effects
Wheatley et al., 1998	Double-blind, mirtazapine vs. fluoxetine	Severe MDD	6 weeks	133; 66 mirtazapine, 67 fluoxetine	mirtazapine 5–60 mg (15–45 mg in USA), mean dose wks 1–4 = 36.5; fluoxetine 20–40 mg, mean dose wks 1–4 = 19.6;	Mirtazapine well-tolerated and significantly greater effectiveness than fluoxetine after 3–4 weeks of treatment
Hoyberg et al., 1996	Random, double-blind treatment with mirtazapine or amitriptyline	Elderly (60–80); MDD	6 weeks	115; 56 mirtazapine, 59 amitriptyline	15–45 mg/day mirtazapine – final mean dose 37.3 mg; 150–450 mg/day amitriptyline – final mean dose 73.8 mg	Both medications were well-tolerated and equally effective

other studies that indicate subjects frequently experience a reduction in the severity of somnolence when the dose of mirtazapine was higher. Mirtazapine was found to be equally effective, with superior tolerability to amitriptyline, and superior efficacy to placebo in a study by van Mofaert et al. (1995).

Higher doses of mirtazapine were shown to be more effective than lower doses in more severely symptomatic, hospitalized patients in randomized controlled trials by van Moffaert et al., 1995; Richou, 1995; Zivkov, 1995, according to a review by Kasper, 1995.

Patient subgroups for which mirtazapine was evaluated to be especially effective for were identified in a meta-analysis by Nutt (1998). These included patients with significant anxiety, agitation, retardation, or insomnia, as assessed by HAM-D factors of anxiety/somatization and sleep disturbance.

Mirtazapine was more effective than placebo in preventing relapse and recurrence of depression after responders from an acute phase trial continued on their treatment for a 20-week continuation phase. In this study by Montgomery et al. (1998), patients experienced a significantly longer period of remission before they relapsed, as compared to placebo.

Efficacy in major depression and the safety of venlafaxine has been extensively evaluated and documented in numerous double-blind trials (Table 11.7) A study by Schweizer et al. (1994) demonstrates venlafaxine's comparable efficacy to imipramine, while having a somewhat lower attrition rate due to adverse effects than imipramine. Another study examining the use of venlafaxine in general practice compared to imipramine and placebo showed that venlafaxine produced significantly superior improvement of depressive symptoms over placebo and over imipramine on a number of measures (Lecrubier et al., 1997). As shown in Table 11.7 the dosages ranged from 75 mg/day to 150 mg/day.

Venlafaxine has been shown to be a safe, effective choice for the long-term treatment of depression. In a study by Shrivastava et al. (1994), comparing the use of imipramine and venlafaxine for up to 1 year, fewer venlafaxine-treated patients withdrew due to adverse events and unsatisfactory response than those treated with imipramine. Additionally, a consistent trend of therapeutic response rates in favour of venlafaxine was present and statistically significant at 2, 6 and 12 months. In another study evaluating the long-term efficacy and safety of venlafaxine in depressed geriatric patients with a high probability of recurrence, only 20% of the patients had a single new episode with no significant side effects observed (Amore et al., 1997).

Expanding clinical indications

Nefazodone has been shown in uncontrolled clinical trials to be effective in the treatment of panic disorder. In some clinical anxiety trials, nefazodone reduced the number of panic attacks in patients with major depression and comorbid panic disorder. Patients who were treated with nefazodone or SSRIs (sertraline or fluoxetine) had the same mean reduction in the number of spontaneous and situational panic attacks from baseline. Overall, 87% of patients treated with nefazodone had no panic attacks at endpoint com-

Table 11.7 Studies of venlafaxine

Author(s)	Study Design	Patient population	Length of tx	pts in each cell	Dose	Overall results
Armitage et al., 1997	Random, double-blind, placebo-controlled treatment with 3 fixed doses of venlafaxine	Adult MDD outpatients	6 weeks	60, placebo $n = 16$ VLF low dose $n = 15$ VLF int dose $n = 15$ VLF high dose $n = 14$	60, placebo $n = 16$ VLF low dose $n = 15$ VLF int dose $n = 15$ VLF high dose $n = 14$	VLF low dose 25 mg/ TID VLF int dose 75 mg/TID VLF high dose 125 mg/TID
	Venlafaxine was shown to have superior efficacy over placebo at all three doses, with the high dose resulting in earlier improvement					
Schweizer et al., 1994	Random, double-blind, placebo- and imipramine-controlled, treatment with venlafaxine	Adult MDD outpatients	6 weeks	224, placebo $n = 78$ venlafaxine $n = 73$ imipramine $n = 73$	Flexible TID dosage Mean max daily dose: venlafaxine 182 mg imipramine 176 mg	Venlafaxine was shown to be similarly efficacious to imipramine and superior to placebo, with response rates of 90%, 79% and 53% respectively
Lecrubier et al., 1997	Random, double-blind, placebo- and imipramine-controlled, treatment with venlafaxine	Adults with major, minor, or intermittent depression in general practice	13 weeks	229, placebo $n = 76$ venlafaxine $n = 78$ imipramine $n = 75$	venlafaxine 75–150 mg/ day, imipramine 75–150 mg/day	Venlafaxine was shown to have superior efficacy compared to placebo and imipramine
Thase, 1997	Random, double-blind, placebo-controlled, treatment with venlafaxineXR	Adult MDD outpatients	8 weeks	191, placebo $n = 100$ venlafaxine $n = 91$	venlafaxine 75–225 mg/ day	Venlafaxine was shown to have superior efficacy over placebo
Mahapatra and Hackett, 1997	Random, double-blind treatment with venlafaxine or dothiepin in geriatric patients with MDD	Geriatric patients with MDD	10 weeks	92, venlafaxine $n = 44$ dothiepin $n = 48$	venlafaxine 50–150 mg/ day, dothiepin 50–150 mg/day	Venlafaxine was shown to be similarly efficacious to dothiepin in treatment of geriatric

Table 11.7 continued

			Duration	n	Dose	Results
Entsuah and Chitra, 1997	Random, double-blind, placebo-controlled, comparing risk/benefit ratio of treatment with venlafaxineIR and venlafaxineXR	Adult MDD outpatients	12 weeks	298, placebo $n = 99$ venlafaxineXR $n = 92$ venlafaxineIR $n = 87$	venlafaxineIR 75–150 mg/day venlafaxineXR 75–150 mg/day	VenlafaxineXR demonstrated a superior risk/benefit ratio compared with venlafaxine IR, with a statistically significant benefit to risk ratio of at least 2:1 over venlafaxineIR for nausea and dizziness
Nierenberg et al., 1994	Open label trial of venlafaxine in treatment-resistant unipolar depression	Adult outpatients and inpatients with MDD who had failed to respond to at least 3 adequate trials of antidepressants from at least 2 different classes	12 weeks	84	150–450 mg mean = 245.2 mg	Approximately one third of patients were judged to be full or partial responders after 12 weeks of treatment
Dunner et al., 1997	Open label trial of venlafaxine in treatment of dysthymic disorder	Adults with dysthymic disorder	9 weeks	17	venlafaxine 37.5–225 mg/day	All patients showed improvement over baseline

pared with 77% of patients treated with an SSRI (DeMartinis *et al.*, 1996; Zajecka, 1996).

In a preliminary study of nefazodone in the treatment of PMS, significant improvement was seen in patients with PMS only and in patients with PMS and comorbid major depression (Freeman *et al.*, 1994).

No controlled studies have been done using nefazodone for the treatment of bipolar depression. Anecdotally it appears to be efficacious, consistent with other antidepressant use for bipolar depression. The likelihood of switch into mania has not been defined. The clinical advantages and disadvantages of nefazodone are highlighted in Table 11.8.

Preliminary evidence (Fava abstract-98) indicates that mirtazapine may be a good choice for SSRI refractory or intolerant patients. Mirtazapine is currently being studied in open trials for the treatment of bipolar depression. Results from trials of mirtazapine in patients with bipolar disorder are not yet available, therefore caution is recommended for use in this population. To date, there is a lack of controlled studies for patients with psychiatric disorders other than mood disorders. The clinical advantages and disadvantages of mirtazapine are highlighted in Table 11.9.

Although venlafaxine is currently FDA approved only for the treatment of depression, many clinical trials have been conducted and are underway to evaluate its efficacy in the treatment of other psychiatric disorders, such as

Table 11.8 Clinical advantages and disadvantages of nefazodone

Advantages	Disadvantages
• Well-tolerated by most patients • May provide more rapid improvement than other antidepressants • Can treat a broad range of symptoms/disorders • May work for patients that have failed on TCAs, SSRIs, or MAOIs	• Contraindicated or cautioned usage with some medications • Cautioned for use on patients with cardiovascular or seizure disorders • Possible fatal reaction with MAOIs

Table 11.9 Clinical advantages and disadvantages of mirtazapine

Advantages	Disadvantages
• Sedative effect + for insomnia (studies show reduction of initial, middle and terminal insomnia per items 4–6 of HAM-D) • Overdose, less toxic (safer profile) (Bremner *et al.*, 1998; Hoes and Zijpveld, 1996; Stimmel *et al.*, 1997) • Absence of cholinergic, serotonergic (Nutt, 1997), and adrenergic adverse events (Pinder, 1997; Tulen *et al.*, 1996) • Less likely to cause pharmocokinetic drug interactions with drugs metabolized by cytochrome P450 enzymes (Richelson, 1997; Owen and Nemeroff, 1998) • QD dosing	• Side effects of weight gain and somnolence may make use prohibitive in some patients • Limited use in patients with atypical depression (usually, due to side effects) • Limited information for use in other disorders to date • No studies in children to date

Table 11.10 Clinical advantages and disadvantages of venlafaxine

Advantages	Disadvantages
• Dual mechanism of action • May be effective for use in treatment-resistant depression • Well tolerated by most patients • Available in extended release form • Low affinity for muscarinic, histaminergic and adrenergic receptors • May be effective for anxiety disorders	• May cause hypertension in some patients • May not be used concurrently with MAOI • Must be tapered due to symptoms with abrupt withdrawal

comorbid anxiety, panic disorder, social phobia and obsessive-compulsive disorder. In an open label study for the treatment of social phobia, eight of the nine patients had a marked improvement on venlafaxine (Kelsey, 1995). In a review on new treatments for panic disorder, Gorman reports two open label trials using venlafaxine that suggest that it is effective in the treatment of panic disorder (Gorman, 1997). In a study by Amsterdam (1998), venlafaxine was shown to be equally efficacious for use in bipolar II depressed patients as unipolar depressed patients. No episodes of mania induction were observed. Other areas of current research include obsessive-compulsive disorder and general anxiety disorder.

The clinical advantages and disadvantages of venlafaxine are highlighted in Table 11.10.

References

Amore, M., Ricci, M., Raffaella, Z., *et al.* (1997). Long-term treatment of geropsychiatric depressed patients with venlafaxine. *J. Affect. Dis.*, **46**, 293–296.

Amsterdam, J. (1998). Efficacy and safety of venlafaxine in the treatment of bipolar II major depressive episode. *J. Clin. Psychopharmacol.*, **18**, 414–417.

Armitage, R., Rush, A.J., Trivedi, M., *et al.* (1994). The effects of nefazodone on sleep architecture in depression. *Neuropsychopharmacology*, **10**, 123–127.

Armitage, R., Yonkers, K., Cole, D., *et al.* (1997). A multicenter, double-blind comparison of the effects of nefazodone and fluoxetine on sleep architecture and quality of sleep in depressed outpatients. *J. Clin. Psychopharmacol.*, **17**, 161–168.

Ballenger, J.C. (1996). Clinical evaluation of venlafaxine. *J. Clin. Psychopharmacol.*, **16** (Suppl. 2), 29S–36S.

Bezchlibnyk-Butler, K.Z. and Jeffries, J.J. (1996). *Clinical Handbook of Psychotropic Drugs*: sixth revised edition, Seattle, WA: Hogrefe & Huber.

Bremner, J.D., Wingard, P. and Walshe, T.A. (1998). Safety of mirtazapine in overdose. *J. Clin. Psychiatry*, **59**, 233–235.

Burrows, G.D. and Kremer, C.M. (1997). Mirtazapine: clinical advantages in the treatment of depression. *J. Clin. Psychopharmacol.*, **17**, 34S–39S.

Cohen, M., Panagides, J., Timmer, C.J., *et al.* (1997). Pharmacokinetics of mirtazapine from orally administered tablets: influence of a high-fat meal. *Eur. J. Drug Metab. Pharmacokinet.*, **22**, 103–110.

de Boer, T. (1995). The effects of mirtazapine on central noradrenergic and serotonergic neurotransmission. *Int. Clin. Psychopharmacol.*, **10** (Suppl. 4), 19–23. (Published erratum appears in *Int. Clin. Psychopharmacol.* (1996), **11**, 153.)

de Boer, T. (1996). The pharmacologic profile of mirtazapine. *J. Clin. Psychiatry*, **57** (Suppl. 4), 19–25.

Delbressine, L.P. and Vos, R.M. (1997). The clinical relevance of preclinical data: mirtazapine, a model compound. *J. Clin. Psychopharmacol.* **17**, 295–335.

DeMartinis, N.A., Schweizer, E. and Rickels, K. (1996). An open-label trial of nefazodone in high comorbidity panic disorder. *J. Clin. Psychiatry*, **57**, 245–248.

Dunner, D.L., Hendrickson, H.E., Bea, C., *et al.* (1997). Venlafaxine in dysthymic disorder. *J. Clin. Psychiatry*, **58**, 258–531.

Ellingrod, V.L. and Perry, P.J. (1994). Venlafaxine: A heterocyclic antidepressant. *Am. J. Hosp. Pharmacol.*, **51**, 3033–3046.

Entsuah, R. and Chitra, R. (1997). A benefit-risk analysis of once-daily venlafaxine extended release (XR) and venlafaxine immediate release (IR) in outpatients with major depression. *Psychopharmacol. Bull.*, **33**, 671–676.

Fava, M., Zajecka, J., Trivedi, M., *et al.* (1998). An open trial of mirtazapine in the treatment of depressed outpatients refractory to or intolerant of treatment with SSRIs: Preliminary report. Poster presentation, APA.

Fawcett, J., Marcus, R.N., Anton, S.F., *et al.* (1995). Response of anxiety and agitation symptoms during nefazodone treatment of major depression. *J. Clin. Psychiatry*, **56** (Suppl. 6), 37–42.

Feighner, J.P., Entsuah, A.R. and McPherson, M.K. (1998). Efficacy of once-daily venlafaxine extended release (XR) for symptoms of anxiety in depressed outpatients. *J. Affect. Dis.*, **47**, 55–62.

Freeman, E.W., Rickels, K., Sondheimer, S.J., *et al.* (1994). Nefazodone in the treatment of premenstrual syndrome: A preliminary study. *J. Clin. Psychopharmacol.*, **14**, 180–186.

Gorman, J.M. (1997). The use of newer antidepressants for panic disorder. *J. Clin. Psychiatry*, **58** (Suppl. 14), 54–58.

Greene, D.S. and Barbhaiya, R.H. (1997). Clinical pharmacokinetics of nefazodone. *Clin. Pharmacokinetics*, **33**, 260–275.

Hoes, M.J., Zeijpveld, J.H. (1996) First report of mirtazapine overdose. *Int. J. Clin. Psychopharmacol.* **11** (2), 147.

Hoyberg, O.J., Maragakis, B., Mullin, J., *et al.* (1996). A doubleblind multicentre comparison of mirtazapine and amitriptyline in elderly depressed patients. *Acta. Psychiatr. Scand.*, **93**, 184–190.

Kasper, S. (1995). Clinical efficacy of mirtazapine: a review of meta-analyses of pooled data. *Int. Clin. Psychopharmacol.*, **10** (Suppl. 4), 25–35. (Published erratum appears in *Int. Clin. Psychopharmacol.* (1996) **153** (2), 25–35.)

Kasper, S., PraschakRieder, N., Tauscher, J., *et al.* (1997a). A risk–benefit assessment of mirtazapine in the treatment of depression. *Drug Safety*, **17**, 251–264.

Kasper, S., Zivkov, M., Roes, K.C., *et al.* (1997). Pharmacological treatment of severely depressed patients: a meta-analysis comparing efficacy of mirtazapine and amitriptyline. *Eur. Neuropsychopharmacol.*, **7**, 115–124.

Kelsey, J.E. (1995). Venlafaxine in social phobia. *Psychopharmacol. Bull.*, **31**, 767–771.

Lecrubier, Y., Bourin, M., Moon, C.A.L., *et al.* (1997). Efficacy of venlafaxine in depressive illness in general practice. *Acta. Psychiatr. Scand.*, **95**, 485–493.

Mahapatra, S.N. and Hackett, D. (1997). A randomised, double-blind, parallel-group comparison of venlafaxine and dothiepin in geriatric patients with major depression. *Int. J. Clin. Pract.*, **51**, 209–213.

Montgomery, S.A., Reimitz, P.E. and Zivkov, M. (1998). Mirtazapine versus amitriptyline in the long-term treatment of depression: a double-blind placebo-controlled study. *Int. Clin. Psychopharmacol.*, **13**, 63–73.

Morton, W.A., Sonne, S.C. and Verga, M.A. (1995). Venlafaxine: a structurally unique and novel antidepressant. *Ann. Pharmacother.*, **29**, 387–395.

Nelson, J.C. (1997). Safety and tolerability of the new antidepressants. *J. Clin. Psychiatry*, **58** (Suppl. 6), 26–31.

Nierenberg, A.A., Feighner, J.P., Rudolph, R., *et al.* (1994). Venlafaxine for treatment resistant unipolar depression. *J. Clin. Psychopharmacol.*, **14**, 419–423.

Nutt, D. (1997). Mirtazapine: pharmacology in relation to adverse effects. *Acta Psychiatry Scand.* (Suppl.) **391**, 31–37.

Nutt, D.J. (1998). Efficacy of mirtazapine in clinically relevant subgroups of depressed patients. *Depress. Anxiety*, **7** (Suppl. 1), 710.

Owen, J.R. and Nemeroff, C.B. (1998). New antidepressants and the cytochrome P450 system: focus on venlafaxine, nefazodone, and mirtazapine. *Depress. Anxiety*, **7** (Suppl. 1), 24–32.

Physician's Desk Reference (1999). Medical Economics Company, Inc. Montvale, NJ.

Pinder, R.M. (1997). Designing a new generation of antidepressant drugs. *Acta Psychiatr. Scand.* (Suppl.) **391**, 7–13.

Richelson, E. (1997). Pharmacokinetic drug interactions of new antidepressants: a review of the effects on the metabolism of other drugs. *Mayo Clin. Proc.*, **72**, 835–847.

Richelson, E. (1998). Pharmacokinetic interactions of antidepressants. *J. Clin. Psychiatry*, **59** (Suppl. 10), 22–26.

Richou, H., Ruimy, P., Cherbaut, J., *et al.*, (1995). A multi-centre, double-blind, clomipramine controlled efficacy and safety study of Org 3770. *Human Psychopharmacol.*, 263–271.

Robinson, D.S., Marcus, R.N., Archibald, D.G., *et al.* (1996). Therapeutic dose range of nefazodone in the treatment of major depression. *J. Clin. Psychiatry*, **57** (Suppl. 2), 6–9.

Schweizer, E., Weise, C., Clary, C., *et al.* (1991). Placebo-controlled trial of venlafaxine for the treatment of major depression. *J. Clin. Psychopharmacol.*, **11**, 233–236.

Schweizer, E., Feighner, J., Mandas, L.A., *et al.* (1994). Comparison of venlafaxine and imipramine in the acute treatment of major depression in outpatients. *J. Clin. Psychiatry*, **55**, 104–108.

Shrivastava, R.K., Cohn, C., Crowder, J., *et al.* (1994). Long-term safety and clinical acceptability of venlafaxine and imipramine in outpatients with major depression. *J. Clin. Psychopharmacol.*, **14**, 322–329.

Smith, W.T., Glaudin, V., Panagides, J., *et al.* (1990). Mirtazapine vs. amitriptyline vs. placebo in the treatment of major depressive disorder. *Psychopharmacol. Bull* **26**, 191–196.

Stahl, S., Zivkov, M., Reimitz, P.E., *et al.* (1997). Meta-analysis of randomized, double-blind, placebo-controlled, efficacy and safety studies of mirtazapine versus amitriptyline in major depression. *Acta Psychiat. Scand. Suppl.*, **391**, 22–30.

Stahl, S.M. (1998). Basic psychopharmacology of antidepressants, part 1: antidepressants have seven distinct mechanisms of action. *J. Clin. Psychiatry*, **59** (Suppl. 4), 5–14.

Stimmel, G.L., Dopheide, J.A. and Stahl, S.M. (1997). Mirtazapine: an antidepressant with noradrenergic and specific serotonergic effects. *Pharmacotherapy*, **17**, 1021.

Thase, M.E. for the Venlafaxine XR 209 study group (1997). Efficacy and tolerability of once-daily venlafaxine extended release (SR) in outpatients with major depression. *J. Clin. Psychiatry*, **58**, 393–398.

Tulen, J.H., Bruijn, J.A., de Man, K.J., *et al.* (1996). Cardiovascular variability in major depressive disorder and effects of imipramine or mirtazapine (Org 3770). *J. Clin. Psychopharmacol.*, **16**, 135–145.

van Moffaert, M., de Wilde, J., Vereecken, A., *et al.* (1995). Mirtazapine is more effective than trazodone: a double-blind controlled study in hospitalized patients with major depression. *Int. Clin. Psychopharmacol.*, **10**, 39.

Wheatley, D.P., van Moffaert, M., Timmerman, L., *et al.* (1998). Mirtazapine: efficacy and tolerability in comparison with fluoxetine in patients with moderate to severe major depressive disorder. Mirtazapine Fluoxetine Study Group. *J. Clin. Psychiatry*, **59**, 306–312.

Zajecka, J.M. (1996). The effect of nefazodone on co-morbid anxiety symptoms associated with depression: Experience in family practice and psychiatric outpatient settings. *J. Clin. Psychiatry*, **57** (Suppl. 2), 10–14.

Zivkov, M. and Jongh, D. (1995). Org 3770 versus emitryptiline: a six week randomized double-blind, multi-centre trial in hospitalized depressed patients. *Human Psychopharmacol.*, **10**, 173–180.

12

Psychopharmacology of mood stabilizers

Robert Post

Key points

- Lithium has complex intracellular effects, including reduction in inositol, alterations in second messenger systems and induction of neurotrophic factors.
- Carbamazepine affects aminergic systems in addition to effects on sodium/ potassium cellular influx.
- Valproic acid reduces GABA catabolism and enhances GABA release, resulting in higher CNS GABA levels. Gabapentin has similar effects on the GABA-ergic system via different mechanisms. Lamotrigine appears to work through a different mechanism.

Introduction

It has long been hoped that understanding the mechanisms of action of lithium carbonate would not only help to reveal pathological processes in bipolar illness, but also enable one to find new drugs with a better therapeutic index. Until most recently, this hope has proven illusory, but now a series of potential new treatment approaches are emerging from an improved understanding of the comparative pharmacology of lithium and the other second-generation putative mood stabilizing anticonvulsants such as carbamazepine and valproate, as well as the putative third generation of newer agents including lamotrigine and, perhaps also, topiramate and gabapentin (Post *et al.*, 1996a, 1998a).

Moreover, the increasing evidence for lithium's acute antidepressant (Souza *et al.*, 1990) as well as antimanic effects and the clear cut prophylactic effects of lithium for both manic and depressive recurrences, has raised the therapeutic conundrum of how a single agent can be effective in both phases of bipolar illness. While it is possible that different actions of lithium and the other mood stabilizing anticonvulsants and calcium channel blockers are involved in the differential therapeutic effects in mania and depression, it is more parsimonious to assume that each of these agents possesses actions that may be of potential importance in both phases of the illness. To this extent, one may be assisted by a re-conceptualization of both phases of the illness as involving pathological increases in a given neurotransmitter system (Post and Chuang, 1991; Post *et al.*, 1992c) with either an excessive primary responsivity in a given system or deficient dampening mechanisms (Post and Weiss, 1992; Post *et al.*, 1998c). To the extent that this occurs in neurotransmitter systems mediating primarily excitatory or inhibitory behaviour, one can then more easily envision common effects of the mood stabilizers in dampening overactivated pathways in both manic and depressive phases of the illness. Given this perspective, intracellular signalling and transduction mechanisms then become important potential targets of the mechanism of the psychotropic action of the mood stabilizers (Figure 12.1). That is, excessive reactivity in the illness may be dampened by a common effect on G-protein transduction mechanisms or other second messenger systems such as those involved in calcium influx, adenylate cyclase regulation, the phosphoinositol (PI) cycle, and a whole host of kinases such as protein kinase C (PKC).

In contrast, more discrete aminergic receptor or reuptake effects on a given neurotransmitter system appear characteristic of the unimodal antidepressants, such as the tricyclic antidepressants, monoamine oxidase inhibitors, or now the second- and third-generation agents, as well as the unipolar antimanics such as the typical and atypical neuroleptics. The bimodal (mood stabilizing) agents appear to be characterized by a panoply of mechanisms, but increasingly prominent candidates have involved second-messenger and other downstream signal transduction mechanisms. Since approaches to these systems have already suggested a variety of new potential agents for therapeutics, these systems will be the primary focus of this chapter. Nonetheless, several of the major mood stabilizers also share aminergic effects on these neurotransmitter systems in common, and these will be mentioned briefly.

Aminergic effects of the mood stabilizers

Dopamine (DA)

As summarized by Maitre et al. (1984) and Post et al. (Post and Chuang, 1991; Post et al., 1992, 1994, 1999b), lithium, carbamazepine, and valproate all share the ability to decrease dopamine turnover. As such, this becomes a candidate mechanism for their mood stabilizing effects, but much work remains to be performed in order to clarify whether this is, in fact, related to their psychotropic effects.

Serotonin (5-HT)

Similarly, lithium, carbamazepine, and valproate all share some ability to enhance serotonergic tone (Post and Weiss, 1998). Lithium exerts complex effects on serotonin metabolism (Knapp and Mandell, 1973), as does valproate (Maes et al., 1997), and recently it has been demonstrated that carbamazepine increases serotonin levels in the hippocampus in proportion to its anticonvulsant effects (Dailey et al., 1996, 1997, 1998). Given the original formulation of the permissive hypothesis of Sourkes (1977), Prange et al. (1979), Coppen et al. (1972), and Curzon (1988), it is of some interest that these agents' ability to increase serotonergic tone could play a role in their common therapeutic effects. However, the lack of ability of the selective serotonin reuptake inhibitor (SSRI) antidepressants to exert antimanic effects makes this potential mechanism more unlikely. Yet, each

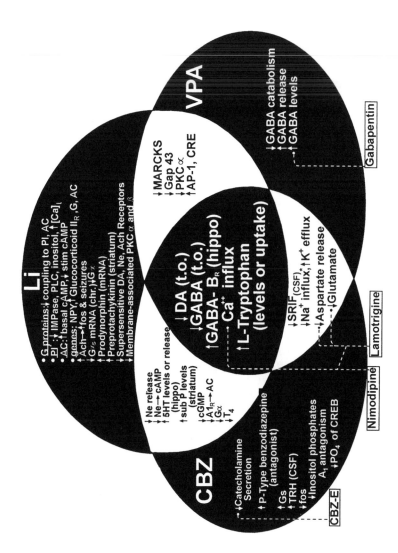

Figure 12.1 Common and differential mechanisms of mood stabilizers; PI = phosphoinositol; AC = adenylate cyclase; IMP = inositol monophosphate; cAMP = cyclic adenosine 3',5'-monophosphate; NPY = neuropeptide Y; Ach = acetylcholine; DA = dopamine; Ne = norepinephrine; PKC = protein kinase C; 5-HT = serotonin; sub P = substance P; T_4 = thyroxine; GABA = gamma-aminobutyric acid; Ca = calcium; MARCKS = myristoylated alanine-rich C kinase substrate'; SRIF = somatostatin; Na = sodium; TRH = thyrotrophin releasing hormone; CSF = cerebrospinal fluid; CREB = cyclic AMP-responsive element-binding protein; CBZ -E = carbamazepine epoxide; K = potassium; VPA = valproate; Li = lithium; CBZ = carbamazepine; PLC = phospholipase C; cGMP = cyclic guanosine 3',5'-monophosphate; AP-1 = activator protein-1; t.o. = turnover; PO_4 = phosphorylation.

of the mood stabilizers appears to exert its serotonergic action through a non-reuptake mechanism, still leaving other aspects of this neurotransmitter system viable candidate mechanisms for that of the mood stabilizers.

GABA$_B$ receptor upregulation

Interestingly, all three of the major mood stabilizers—lithium, carbamazepine, and valproate—increase gamma-aminobutyric acid (GABA)$_B$ receptors in the hippocampus upon chronic, but not acute, administration (Motohashi et al., 1989; Motohashi, 1992). In contrast to a variety of acute antidepressants which appear to exert this effect in the frontal cortex (Bernasconi, 1982; Lloyd et al., 1986), perhaps this action of the mood stabilizers at the level of the hippocampus is, in part, related to their common actions as mood stabilizers. An orally active GABA$_B$ antagonist, which should theoretically increase GABA$_B$ receptors in a number of brain areas, might provide a partial test of this GABA$_B$ hypothesis (Post et al., 1991).

Norepinephrine (Ne)

Lithium and carbamazepine share the ability to decrease synaptic norepinephrine, but by different actions. While lithium facilitates norepinephrine reuptake, carbamazepine decreases norepinephrine's stimulated-induced release (Post et al., 1985, 1994). Each exerts complex effects on norepinephrine turnover.

G-protein effects

While common effects of the three major mood stabilizers have been postulated and documented in some studies on G-proteins (Avissar et al., 1990; Avissar and Schreiber, 1992a,b), these have not always been replicated by all investigators and differential effects on G-protein levels have been reported by several investigative groups (Colin et al., 1991; Lesch et al., 1991; Schreiber et al., 1991; Li et al., 1991; Manji et al., 1995; Avissar et al., 1997). Nonetheless, there is considerable evidence for Gsα hyperactivity based on some studies in cellular elements and in autopsy studies of patients with bipolar illness (Young et al., 1991, 1993; Friedman and Wang, 1996; Mitchell et al., 1997). To the extent that lithium and other mood stabilizing anticonvulsants dampen this putative hyperactivity of Gsα, this could very clearly be linked to its possible psychotropic effects.

Inhibition of adenylate cyclase and cyclic-AMP formation

This has been a candidate mechanism of lithium's psychotropic effects for many years, since the initial demonstration that lithium, in both animals and in clinical studies, could inhibit noradrenergic-stimulated cyclase increases (Klein et al., 1985; Belmaker et al., 1991). That this effect is also shared by carbamazepine makes it an even more intriguing mechanism (Post et al., 1982). Attempts by Belmaker (1984) to document this as a potential mechanism of lithium's antimanic effects have been partially successful with the use of the antibiotic demeclocycline, which also inhibits adenylate cyclase. While other agents that also exert this effect should be investigated for their potential antimanic efficacy, the ability of the phosphodiesterase inhibitors such as rolopram (which enhance the actions of cyclic-AMP) to act as antidepressants (Fleischhacker *et al.*, 1992; Nibuya *et al.*, 1996) is also partially consistent with this formulation.

Effects on phosphoinositol (PI) turnover

Lithium has substantial potency in the inhibition of a variety of phosphatases which limits the ability of the PI cycle to regenerate membrane inositol. It is this depletion that has been postulated to account for lithium's mechanism of action (Sherman *et al.*, 1985; Berridge, 1989). However, at the same time, inositol has been reported to be depleted in the basal medication-free condition in brain and cerebrospinal fluid (CSF) (Benjamin *et al.*, 1995a) and, most recently, Manji and colleagues have reported decreased brain inositol by magnetic resonance spectroscopy (MRS) in proportion to the severity of depression (Manji *et al.*, 1998). Paradoxically, lithium treatment further decreased levels of this compound. Also paradoxically, the administration of inositol itself has been reported to be therapeutic in both depression and the anxiety disorders (panic and obsessive-compulsive disorders) (Benjamin *et al.*, 1995a,b; Levine, 1997), a profile closely related to that of the SSRIs. Inositol has been reported to have significant antidepressant effects in one study that included some bipolar patients (Levine *et al.*, 1995), and to show a trend for such effects in another study by Gershon and associates (1998).

In contrast to the effects of lithium on inositol phosphatase, carbamazepine has been reported in one study to enhance the effects of this enzyme, and valproate to be inactive (Vadnal and Parthasarathy, 1995). To the extent that this mechanism was involved in the psychotropic effects of these agents, it might provide a mechanism for the differential responsivity between lithium and valproate in some subgroups of affectively ill patients. It is also possible that other aspects of lithium's effects on the PI turnover cycle could be related to its psychotropic effects. Since the cycle involves the breakdown of phosphatidylinositol-4,5-biphosphate (PIP2) to inositol 1,4,5-triphosphate (IP3) (which releases intracellular stores of calcium) and diacyl glycerol (which facilitates the action of PKC), it is possible that these actions of lithium downstream to its ability to inhibit phosphatases could be relevant. In particular, as discussed below, the ability of lithium and valproate to share PKC inhibition has been extensively studied by Manji and associates (Manji *et al.*, 1996).

Intracellular calcium (Figure 12.2)

Blockade of calcium influx through the NMDA receptor

Either by effects on IP3 or through other mechanisms, lithium has been reported to enhance basal intracellular calcium in some systems, and alteration in calcium metabolism has been postulated in relation to lithium's action (Meltzer, 1990; Okamoto *et al.*, 1995). In fact, recent evidence

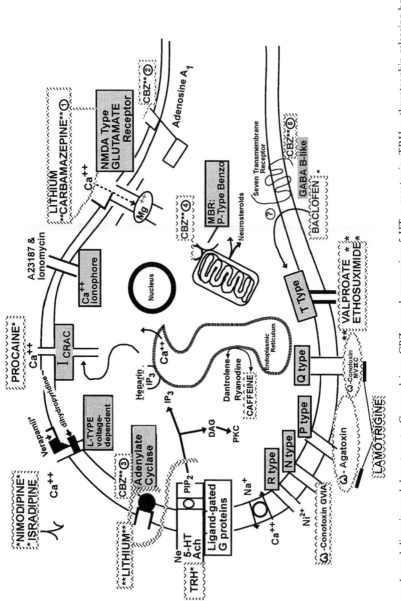

Figure 12.2 Calcium channel diversity and drug targets; Ca = calcium; CBZ = carbamazepine; 5-HT = serotonin; TRH = thyrotrophin-releasing hormone; Ach = acetylcholine; Na = sodium; Ni = nickel; PKC = protein kinase C; DA6 = diacylglycerol; IP_3 = inositol 1,4,5-triphosphate; MBR = mitochondrial or peripheral (P) type benzodiazepine receptor; NMDA = N-methyl-D-aspartate; Mg = magnesium; PIP_2 = phosphatidylinositol-4,5-biphosphate

from Drs Chuang and Hough in the Biological Psychiatry Branch, National Institute of Mental Health (NIMH), indicates that all of the mood stabilizers tested to date, including lithium, carbamazepine, valproate, and lamotrigine, share the common ability to inhibit calcium influx through the *N*-methyl-D-aspartate (NMDA) receptor (Hough *et al.*, 1996; 1998, unpublished data) (Figure 12.3). Whether this is occurring as an indirect effect of initial increases in intracellular calcium or via more direct effects on the NMDA receptor, remains to be investigated. Nevertheless, this may be a particularly important system for the modulatory effects of some compounds. For example, the blockade by carbamazepine of calcium influx to the NMDA receptor is glycine-dependent. At low levels of glycine concentration, carbamazepine actually facilitates calcium influx, while at high levels of glycine, it inhibits calcium influx (Hough *et al.*, 1996). Thus, the potential for activity-dependent modulation exists for this compound and the precise mechanisms of NMDA blockade by the other agents remain to be further examined.

Lithium is neuroprotective *in vivo* and *in vitro*

It is likely that the ability of lithium to block calcium influx at the NMDA receptor is clinically relevant. Calcium blockade through the NMDA receptor *in vitro* is linked to lithium's neuroprotective or antiapoptotic effects in cerebellar granule cells and hippocampal granule cells in culture (Nonaka *et al.*, 1998a,b). In order to test the potential physiological relevance of this effect *in vivo*, these investigators treated animals with lithium or a controlled diet for 16 days prior to ligation of the middle cerebral artery. Compared with controls, those treated with lithium had a 50% reduction in the size of the anoxic area produced by the stroke and had a highly significant reduction in the resulting neurological defect (Nonaka and Chuang, 1998). These effects occurred at clinically relevant levels of lithium in animals.

These preclinical findings are also of interest in relation to the fact that not only does lithium normalize the death rate by suicide in patients with bipolar illness (Crundwell, 1994; Tondo *et al.*, 1998), but it also helps normalize the excess death rate by other associated medical causes (Ahrens *et al.*, 1995). Given these preclinical and clinical data, it would appear important to ascertain further whether lithium's ability to diminish the size of cerebral infarct and associated neurological injury is a mechanism that is also clinically active in humans.

In addition to relevance in stroke, this ability shared by many of the mood stabilizing agents could be relevant to their psychotropic effects as well. Since glutamate is a prime candidate for modulating increases in neural excitability as the main excitatory neurotransmitter in the CNS, modulatory effects at this system could clearly be of importance. Moreover, Skolnick and associates (Nowak *et al.*, 1993a; Paul *et al.*, 1994) have postulated that the antidepressants acting at the glycine modulatory site of the NMDA receptor would all share the common ability to decrease glycine binding on chronic, but not acute, administration. Thus, it is possible to conceptualize both antimanic and antidepressant effects occurring through modulation of different aspects of the NMDA receptor and its associated calcium influx.

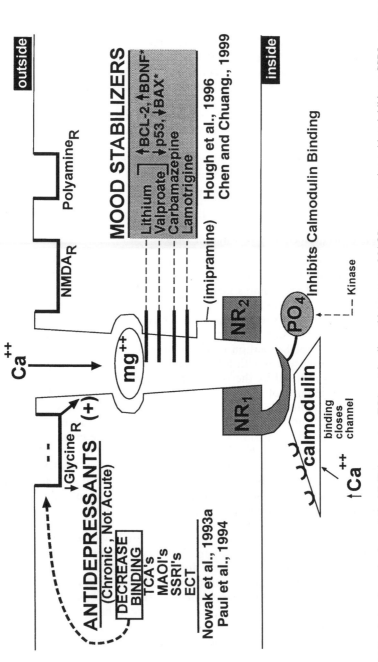

Figure 12.3 Psychotropic mechanisms at the NMDA receptor. TCA = tricyclic antidepressants; MAOI = monoamine oxidase inhibitors; SSRI = serotonin-selective reuptake inhibitors; ECT = electroconvulsive therapy; mg = magnesium; Ca = calcium; NMDA$_R$ = N-methyl-D-aspartate receptor; PO$_4$ = phosphorylation; * = Demonstrated for lithium only.

L-type voltage-dependent calcium channels

In addition to calcium influx of the NMDA receptor, calcium influx through L-type voltage-dependent calcium channels may also be relevant to psychotropic effects. The dihydropyridine L-type calcium channel blocker nimodipine appears capable of exerting both antimanic and antidepressant effects in a subgroup of lithium-refractory bipolar patients (Pazzaglia *et al.*, 1993, 1998). These data converge with and extend those of the initial observations of Dubovsky and associates (1992, 1994) who reported both increases in intracellular calcium in bipolar patients as well as the acute antimanic efficacy of verapamil (Dubovsky *et al.*, 1982, 1987).

Further examination has revealed that the phenylalkylamine calcium channel blocker verapamil has very different biological and behavioural properties from the dihydropyridines such as nimodipine, isradipine, and amlodipine (Post *et al.*, 1999a) (Tables 12.1 and 12.2). These latter com-

Table 12.1 Differential effects of dihydropyridine L-type calcium channel blockers vs verapamil

Effect	*Dihydropyridine Nimodipine/Isradipine*	*Phenylalkylamine Verapamil*	*Reference(s)*
Lipid Soluble	+ +	±	Freedman and Waters, 1987
Anticonvulsant:			
Animals:			
a. Kindling	+ +	±	Wurpel and Iyer, 1994 Vezzani *et al.*, 1988
b. Re-perfusion	+ +	0	Meyer *et al.*, 1986
c. Kainic acid	+	0	Vezzani *et al.*, 1988 Paczynski *et al.*, 1990
Patients	+ +	NA	Brandt *et al.*, 1988 Larkin *et al.*, 1991 de Falco *et al.*, 1992
Block cocaine-induced:			
a. Hyperactivity	+ +	0	Pani *et al.*, 1990 Rosetti *et al.*, 1990
b. Sensitization	+ +	NA	Weiss *et al.*, unpublished data
c. Dopamine overflow	+ +	0	Pani *et al.*, 1990 Rosetti *et al.*, 1990
Positive in forced swim model	+ +	0	Czyrak *et al.*, 1989 de Jonge *et al.*, 1993 Mogilnicka *et al.*, 1987, 1988
Positive in learned helplessness model	+ +	0	Geoffroy *et al.*, 1988 Martin *et al.*, 1989 de Jonge *et al.*, 1993
Like antidepressants: ↓Glycine inhibition of ^{3}[H] 5,7-DCKA binding	+ +	NA	Nowak *et al.*, 1993b
Rapid cycling affective illness	+ +	0, ±	Pazzaglia *et al.*, 1993, 1998

+ + = very effective; + = effective; ± = equivocal; 0 = none; NA = not applicable or studied

Table 12.2 Half-lives, dosages and effectiveness of L-type calcium channel inhibitors in mood disorders

	Phenylalkylamine (on outside of Ca^{++} channel)	Dihydropyridines (inside membrane and Ca^{++} channel)		
	Verapamil	Nimodipine	Isradipine	Amlodipine
Half-life	Short (5–12 hours)	Short (1–2 hours)	Short (8 hours)	Long (30–50 hours)
Starting dose	30 mg tid	30 mg tid	2.5 mg bid	5 mg hs
Peak daily dosage	480 mg	240–480 mg	15 mg	10–15 mg
Antimanic	+ +	+ +	(+ +)	( )*
Antidepressant	±	+	(+)	( )*
Antiultradian	±	+ +	(+ +)	( )*
Anticocaine (dopamine)	–	+ +	+ +	( )*

+ + = very effective; + = effective; I = equivocal; – = none
*No systematic studies; only case reports and clinical observation

pounds, for example, appear capable of blocking cocaine-induced hyperactivity and its associated dopamine overflow (Pani *et al.*, 1990), and were positive in animal models of depression in which verapamil was not (as reviewed elsewhere: Post *et al.*, 1999a; Post, 1999). Therefore, it was not entirely surprising that response to the dihydropyridines (nimodipine/isradipine) did not cross to the phenylalkylamine (verapamil) under double-blind conditions in several carefully studied patients (Pazzaglia *et al.*, 1998) (Figure 12.4). Nevertheless, the overall data suggest that inhibition of calcium influx through the voltage-dependent calcium channel could be another potential mechanism of mood stabilization.

This is an intriguing possibility in light of the now very well replicated evidence for increased intracellular calcium in the blood elements of patients with bipolar illness in more than a dozen studies, as summarized elsewhere (Post *et al.*, 1999a). Thus, it is possible to conceptualize that blockade of calcium influx, either through the NMDA receptor or through L-type calcium channels, could each be clinically relevant. The data also raise the theoretical possibility of combined effects on several different calcium mechanisms being more effective than treatment with either agent alone (Figure 12.5). A modicum of clinical data is supportive of this notion with Manna (1991) reporting that lithium and nimodipine in combination were more effective in prophylaxis than either agent alone, and a number of patients in the series of Pazzaglia *et al.* (1998) also showed better effects with nimodipine augmented by carbamazepine (which should inhibit calcium influx through the NMDA receptor as well).

T-type calcium channels

Valproate exerts effects on calcium at the level of the calcium T-type receptor (Macdonald and Kelly, 1995), which has been thought to be involved in the generation of absence seizures (Snead, 1995). To the extent that etho-

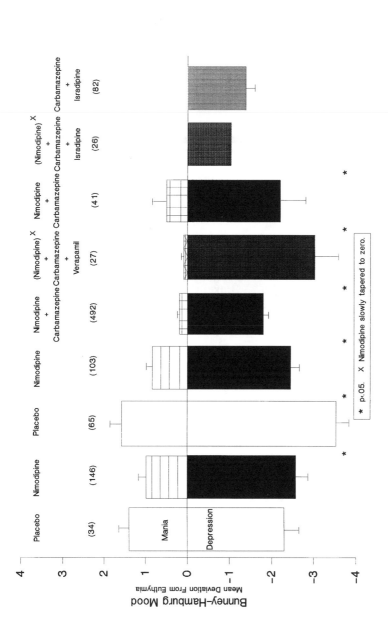

Figure 12.4 Efficacy of dihydropyridine L-type calcium channel blockers. Mean deviation from euthymia ratings; positive = mania; negative = depression; (number of days in parentheses) in a **BP II** ultra-rapid cycling patient showing the following: efficacy of nimodipine monotherapy; efficacy of nimodipine-carbamazepine combination therapy; unsuccessful transition from nimodipine to verapamil; successful reinstitution of nimodipine-carbamazepine combination therapy; and finally, successful transition to isradipine-carbamazepine combination therapy. *P < 0.05; [x]nimodipine slowly tapered to zero

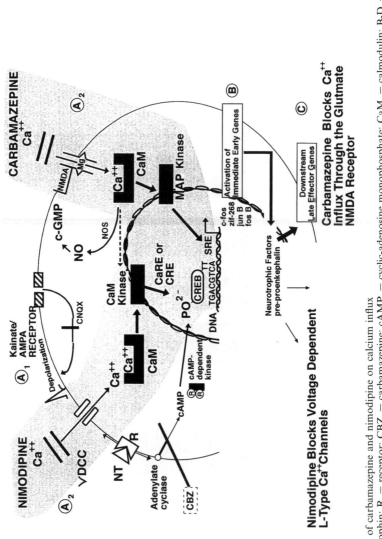

Figure 12.5 Differential effects of carbamazepine and nimodipine on calcium influx

Ca = calcium; NT = neurotrophin; R = receptor; CBZ = carbamazepine; cAMP = cyclic-adenosine monophosphate; CaM = calmodulin; B-D = brain-derived; CREB = cyclic AMP responsive element binding protein; NMDA = N-methyl-D-aspartate; Mg = magnesium; c-GMP = cyclic quanosine 3′,5′-monophosphate; NO = nitric oxide; NOS = nitric oxide synthase; PO = phosphate; CNQX = cyano,3-dihydro-7-nitrogluinoxaline-2,3-dione; SRE = serum response element; C_aRE = calcium response element; CRE = cyclic AMP response element suximide is also a blocker of the T-type calcium channel (Macdonald and Kelly, 1995), one would predict that it would have antimanic and potential mood stabilizing effects. This proposition, as well, remains to be directly tested.

N-type and P-type calcium channels

Recent data suggest that lamotrigine may block calcium influx through N-type calcium channels (Wang *et al.*, 1996, 1998). To the extent that lamotrigine emerges as a clinically useful mood stabilizer, as initial open (Calabrese *et al.*, 1998) and double-blind studies (Calabrese *et al.*, 1999; Frye *et al.*, 1998) appear to suggest, this mechanism of calcium influx also remains a candidate for further study.

Protein kinase C (PKC) inhibition – a new target of therapeutics with tamoxifen

In addition to lithium's effects on the PI turnover second-messenger system, one of the products of the generation of this cycle—diacylglycerol—activates PKC. Manji and associates (Manji *et al.*, 1996) have found that both lithium and valproate inhibit PKC activation and this has led to one of the first neurochemically guided, specifically-hypothesized interventions in mania, i.e. that with the PKC inhibitor tamoxifen. Initial data are positive (Bebchuk *et al.*, 1999) in six of the first nine manic patients studied, and it remains to be elucidated in further double-blind trials with more selective PKC antagonists whether this mechanism is effective in mania (and even whether it could also be effective in acute depression and prophylaxis) (see Figure 12.1).

Transcriptional regulatory effects

In a further series of elegant studies, Manji and associates have documented that both chronic lithium and valproate share other common transcriptional regulatory effects using differential display PCR techniques (Chen *et al.*, 1999). These include the ability to increase polyomavirus enhancer-binding protein 2β (PEBP2β) and Bcl-2 and thus likely affect one of its downstream targets, p53. Other data suggest that both lithium and valproate increase DNA binding activity at the activator protein-1 (AP-1) site (Manji *et al.*, 1996) and also increase brain-derived neurotrophic factor (BDNF) and decrease BAX, a putative cell death protein (Chen and Chuang, 1999). The effects of lithium in p53 and BDNF are of considerable interest in relationship to lithium's neurotrophic effects demonstrated in both *in vitro* and *in vivo* preparations.

In contrast with lithium and valproate's effects in enhancing AP-1 binding, carbamazepine appears to be able to suppress *c-fos* induction (Tolle *et al.*, 1995), although its effects on AP-1 binding have not been definitively dissected. Thus, it would appear that several of the major mood stabilizing agents have quite different effects, even at the level of DNA binding and their transcriptional regulatory activities. It remains a clinical hope that if the downstream targets of these transcriptional regulatory activities can be identified, they can be more precisely targeted in order to achieve both a greater therapeutic index and rapidity of onset. In this regard, the effects of carbamazepine on lithium, on substance P levels, and on sensitivity are of interest, particularly in light of recent reports of well-tolerated antidepressant effects of the substance P antagonist MK-869 (Kramer *et al.*, 1998).

Neuropeptide regulation

Substance P levels and sensitivity

As illustrated in Table 12.3, both lithium and carbamazepine upregulate substance P levels in the striatum with chronic administration (Le Douarin *et al.*, 1983; Hong *et al.*, 1983; Mitsushio *et al.*, 1988). In addition, carbamazepine, like a variety of other antidepressant modalities, increases substance P sensitivity (Jones *et al.*, 1985). This latter effect could be associated with a relative blockade of substance P receptors by this and a variety of other antidepressant modalities could account for the possible parallelism between the antidepressant effects of these agents and that of the specific substance P antagonist MK-869 (Kramer *et al.*, 1998).

Somatostatin

This neuropeptide is permanently decreased in Alzheimer's disease, often in proportion to the degree of cognitive defect (Minthon *et al.*, 1997). In contrast, it is transiently decreased in active multiple sclerosis (MS) and in acute depression with apparent normalization on recovery from each syndrome (Rubinow *et al.*, 1992). Thus, it is of interest that carbamazepine decreases somatostatin (Rubinow *et al.*, 1985) while the dihydropyridine L-type calcium channel blocker nimodipine increases it (Pazzaglia *et al.*, 1995). It is

Table 12.3. Effects of lithium and carbamazepine on substance P

	Lithium	*Carbamazepine*
Acute treatment		
↑Substance P levels	None[a,b]	None[c]
↑Substance P sensitivity	None[d]	None[d]
Chronic treatment		
Substance P levels	↑Striatum[a,b]	↑Striatum[c]
	↑Substantia nigra	↑Substantia nigra
	↑Nucleus accumbens	
	↑Frontal cortex	
↑Substance P is haloperidol-reversible	Yes[a,b]	Yes[c]
↑Substance P sensitivity	?	Yes[d]

[a]Hong *et al.*, 1983
[b]LeDouarin *et al.*, 1983
[c]Mitsushio *et al.*, 1988
[d]Jones *et al.*, 1985

noteworthy that, compared with non-responders, nimodipine responders have lower CSF somatostatin levels at baseline (Frye *et al.*, 1997) (perhaps indicative of a need for such somatostatin increases that are provided by nimodipine). Somatostatin decrements have also been functionally linked to the hypercortisolaemia of depression (Molchan *et al.*, 1993) and dysregulation of this system may provide a target for therapeutics.

Corticotrophin-releasing hormone (CRH)

CRH has been measured in the CSF of patients with depression and found to be increased in some (Risch *et al.*, 1984; Banki *et al.*, 1992), but not all studies (Roy, 1993; Gold *et al.*, 1995; Osuch *et al.*, 1998, unpublished data). CRH is a putative anxiogenic and proconvulsant compound (Ehlers *et al.*, 1983; Weiss *et al.*, 1992) with a spectrum of effects not dissimilar from those observed in classical depression syndromes such as sleep loss, anxiety, anorexia, and hypercortisolaemia. A series of proposed CRH antagonists in the clinical drug development pipeline are thus eagerly awaited so that they can be tested for their potential antidepressant and anxiolytic efficacy.

Thyrotrophin-releasing hormone (TRH)

TRH, in contrast, is a putative endogenous antidepressant, anxiolytic, and anticonvulsant neuropeptide (Loosen, 1988) that may deserve attempts at enhancement in order to achieve possible therapeutic effects (Marangell *et al.*, 1997). TRH itself, or longer-lasting analogues, clearly deserve further exploration for their possible clinical role in the affective disorders.

Neuromodulation of inhibitory neurotransmitter function

As outlined in Figure 12.6, valproate and gabapentin appear to increase brain and CSF GABA levels via a variety of effects on metabolism (valproate) (Bernasconi *et al.*, 1984; Macdonald and Kelly, 1995) and the L-amino acid transporter (gabapentin) (Taylor *et al.*, 1998). In contrast, the newly approved anticonvulsant tiagabine is a selective blocker of GABA reuptake (Dalby and Nielsen, 1997), thus enhancing GABAergic function via this mechanism. Valproate is now a well established and approved agent for its antimanic effects and is widely used for its mood-stabilizing properties.

Gabapentin appears to be more effective in combination treatment from the open add-on literature. In one study of monotherapy in refractory unipolar and bipolar affective disorders, it was not more effective than placebo and significantly less effective than lamotrigine (Frye *et al.*, 1998). Gabapentin has efficacy in a variety of pain syndromes (Attal *et al.*, 1998; Backonja *et al.*, 1998; Merren, 1998) and appears to be effective in the treatment of anxiety disorders such as social phobia (Pande *et al.*, 1999; Pollack *et al.*, 1998). Since it is well tolerated, has few potential serious side effects, is excreted by the kidney, and has few pharmacokinetic interactions with other psychotropic or anticonvulsant agents, it may have an adjunctive role in the treatment of bipolar illness, particularly given the high incidence of comorbid anxiety and pain syndromes.

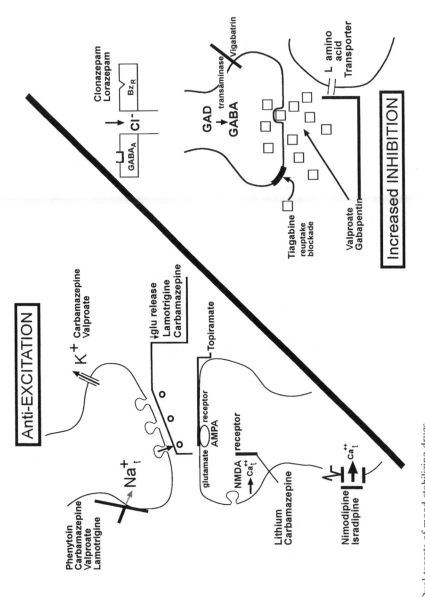

Figure 12.6 Dual targets of mood-stabilizing drugs

Na = sodium; K = potassium; NMDA = N-methyl-D-aspartate; Ca = calcium; GABA = gamma-aminobutyric acid; GAD = glutamate decarboxylase; Cl = chloride; BZ$_R$ = benzodiazepine receptor.

Excitatory amino acid targets

The recognized (lithium, carbamazepine, and valproate) and putative mood stabilizers appear to exert a variety of actions at sites that inhibit the function of excitatory amino acids, either in terms of inhibition of release or blockade of inhibition of calcium influx through the NMDA receptor (Dixon *et al.*, 1994; Waldmeier *et al.*, 1995; Hough *et al.*, 1996; Dixon and Hokin, 1997; White, 1997) or, uniquely in the case of topiramate, blockade of the AMPA-glutamate receptor (Rosenfeld, 1997), as shown in Figure 12.6. At a variety of sites in the CNS, dopaminergic and glutamatergic function appear to oppose each other and, as postulated in schizophrenia, relative decrements in glutamate function may thus enhance that of dopamine and potentially provide another mechanism for indirectly enhancing dopamine-related function (Coyle, 1996), which may be of importance for modulation of the mood disorders.

In addition, relative blockade of glutamate release or the NMDA receptor could be neuroprotective, as noted above. Influx of calcium through the NMDA receptor appears to be one regulator of preprogrammed cell death (apoptosis) as well as excitotoxicity (Nonaka *et al.*, 1998a). Lithium's ability to block calcium influx through the NMDA receptor has recently been linked to potentially physiologically relevant degrees of neuroprotection in the model of middle cerebral artery ligation (Nonaka and Chuang, 1998) as well as a variety of *in vitro* models (Nonaka *et al.*, 1998a). Recent data also suggest that lithium increases the relative ratio of a variety of neurotrophic versus putative cell death proteins such that it increases brain-derived neurotrophic factor (BDNF) and Bcl-2, and decreases BAX (Chen and Chuang, 1999).

The antidepressants have been reported to have effects on neurotrophic factor gene expression that are converse to those of stressors and, in some instances, show the ability to inhibit stress-induced changes in neurotrophic factor gene expression (Smith *et al.*, 1995; Duman *et al.*, 1997; Duman, 1998). Given the potential role of BDNF in animal models of depression (Siuciak *et al.*, 1997), this neurotrophic factor (important for CNS development, long-term potentiation, and cell survival) deserves further exploration. Similarly, it is also possible that the mood stabilizing agents, such as lithium, can directly interact with not only excitatory and inhibitory neurotransmitter balance, but via this mechanism affect synaptic formation, axonal and dendritic sprouting and retraction, and even cell life and death. Thus, they may be able to influence the microstructure of the brain which could be of substantial importance in relation to the increasing evidence for anatomical and cellular alterations in the affective disorders.

Overview

How this panoply of potential mechanisms of action (Figures 12.1 and 12.7) of the confirmed and putative mood-stabilizing agents relate to their profile of psychotropic effects or side effects (Table 12.4) remains to be carefully dissected and delineated. In the meantime, a whole new series of potential

Table 12.4 Comparative clinical and side-effect profiles of lithium, nimodipine, and the putative mood-stabilizing anticonvulsants (preliminary clinical impressions)

	Lithium (0.5–1.2 mEq/l)	Carbamazepine (4–12 μg/ml)	Valproate (50–120 μg/ml)	Nimodipine (12 ng/ml)	Lamotrigine	Gabapentin	Topiramate
Clinical profile							
Acute episodes							
Mania	++	++	++	+	(+)	(++)	++
Dysphoric mania	++	(++)	++	+	?	(+)	++
Family history negative	+	++	++	?	?	?	?
Depression		+	±	+	(++)	(+)	( )
Prophylaxis							
Mania	++	++	++	++	(+)	+	(+)
Depression	++	++	++	++	(++)	++	(±)
Rapid cycling	++	+	++	+++	(++)	(++)	+
Continuous cycling	±	++	(++)	(++)	?	?	+
Seizures							
Generalized, complex partial	0	++	++	±	++	++	++
Absence	0	–	++	?	++	–	–
Paroxysmal pain syndromes	0	++	+	–	?	(+)	?
Migraine	±	±	++	+	?	(+)	?
Side-effect profiles							
White blood count	↑↑*	↓↓	(↓)	–	–	–	–
Diabetes insipidus	↑↓*	→↓	–	–	–	–	–
Thyroid hormones, T₃, T₄	↑↓↑*	→↓	→	–	?	(↑)?	?
Thyroid stimulating hormone	↑↑*	–	?	–	?	–	?
Serum calcium	↑	→(↑)	?	?	?	?	–
Weight gain	↑↑	(↑)	↑↑[a]	–	–	←	–
Tremor	↑↑	–	↑↑	–	←	←	–
Memory disturbances	(↑)	(↑)	(↑)	↓	(↑)	←	↓
Diarrhoea, gastrointestinal distress	↑↑	(↑)	←	(↓)	–	(↑)	←
Teratogenesis	(↑)	←↑	←↑	–	–	–	?
Psoriasis	↑	–	–	–	–	–	–

Pruritic rash	—	—	↑↑	(↑)ᵃ	(↑)	(↑)	—
Alopecia	(↑)	—	—	↑	—	—	—
Agranulocytosis, aplastic anaemia	—	—	←	(↑)	—	—	—
Thrombocytopenia	—	—	(↑)	—	—	—	(↑)?
Hepatitis	—	—	←	←	—	←	←
Hyponatraemia, water intoxication	—	—	←	—	—	—	←
Dizziness, ataxia, diplopia	—	—	↑↑	(↑)	—	←	←
Hypercortisolaemia, escape from dexamethasone suppression	—	—	—	?	—	—	—

Clinical Efficacy: 0 = none, ± = equivocal, + = effective, ++ = very effective, ( ) = very weak data, ? = unknown, − − = exacerbation
Side Effects: ↑ = increase, ↓ = decrease, ( ) = inconsistent or rare, − = absent, − − = worse
*Li = Effect of lithium predominates over that of carbamazepine when used in combination
ᵃ = about 3 months after onset of VPA; prevent alopecia with zinc and selenium?

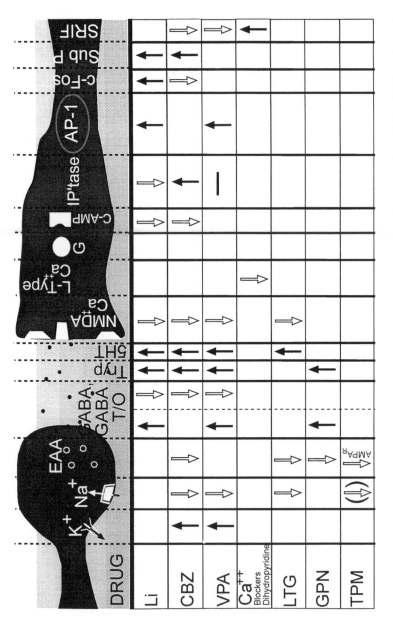

Figure 12.7 Mechanisms of mood stabilization; Li = lithium; CBZ = carbamazepine; VPA = verapamil; LTG = lamotrigine; GPN = gabapentin; TPM = topiramate; k = potassium; Na = sodium; EAA = excitatory amino acids; GABA = gamma-aminobutyric acids; T/O = turnover; Tryp = tryptophan; 5HT = serotonin; NMDA = N-methyl-D-aspartate; Ca = calcium; C-AMP = cyclic-adenosine monophosphate; IP'tase = inositol monophosphatase; AP-1 = activator protein –1; sub P = substance P; SRIF = somatostatin.

targets of therapeutics and new drug development are available for further systematic exploration. It also remains to be clarified whether the differences in mechanisms of action of these agents (Figure 12.7) will ultimately be attributable to a different range of clinical therapeutic effects, such that individual patients and subgroups can be more optimally treated with one type of drug compared with another. For example, to the extent that topiramate blocks the AMPA-glutamate receptor selectively, and this mechanism has been implicated in the maintenance of long-term potentiation (LTP) (Maren *et al.*, 1993), as opposed to the NMDA receptor which is crucial to its induction (Muller *et al.*, 1988), one could postulate that topiramate could play an important role in components of an illness such as post-traumatic stress disorder (PTSD) or sensitized neural substrates of recurrent affective disorder wherein hyperactivity of neural pathways has already been induced and is now being maintained by upregulated AMPA-receptor activity. This, and a variety of other formulations based on preclinical data, remain to be directly tested in the clinic.

However, this perspective highlights the potential importance not only of looking for similarities in the mechanism of action between lithium and valproate as elegantly dissected by Manji and associates (Manji *et al.*, 1996; Chen *et al.*, 1999), but also identifying and elaborating on possible differences as well. In addition, it is possible that multiple mechanisms of action targeted at the same inhibitory neurotransmitter system (for example, the GABAergic system) may be more effective in maximally potentiating this system than a single agent alone (see Figure 12.6). This has also proven to be the case for inhibition of overexcitation in glutamatergic (or cholinergic) pathways and would have additional rationales for complex pharmacotherapy (Post *et al.*, 1996b, 1998b). To the extent that one also separately targeted pathological versus adaptive mechanisms for inhibition and enhancement, respectively, the door is open for even more complex pharmacotherapeutic regimens.

Even prior to clarifying these issues, much clinical trials work remains to better define the use of currently available putative mood stabilizers for their optimal efficacy in bipolar disorder and how this might differ as a function of illness subtypes, stage of illness development, and other clinical and neurobiological predictors of response. Definition of some of these issues will require new methodological and clinical research design approaches to the illness as well as a new mandate better to fund and study this potentially life-threatening medical illness.

References

Ahrens, B., Muller-Oerlinghausen, B., Schou, M., *et al.* (1995). Excess cardiovascular and suicide mortality of affective disorders may be reduced by lithium prophylaxis. *J. Affect. Dis.*, **33**, 67–75.

Attal, N., Brasseur, L., Parker, F., *et al.* (1998). Effects of gabapentin on the different components of peripheral and central neuropathic pain syndromes: a pilot study. *Eur. Neurol.*, **40**, 191–200.

Avissar, S., Nechamkin, Y., Roitman, G., *et al.* (1997). Reduced G protein functions and immunoreactive levels in mononuclear leukocytes of patients with depression. *Am. J. Psychiatry*, **154**, 211–217.

Avissar, S. and Schreiber, G. (1992a). Interaction of antibipolar and antidepressant treatments with receptor-coupled G proteins. *Pharmacopsychiatry*, **25**, 44–50.

Avissar, S. and Schreiber, G. (1992b). Ziskind-Somerfeld Research Award. The involvement of guanine nucleotide binding proteins in the pathogenesis and treatment of affective disorders. *Biol. Psychiatry*, **31**, 435–459.

Avissar, S., Schreiber, G., Aulakh, C.S., *et al.* (1990). Carbamazepine and electroconvulsive shock attenuate β-adrenoceptor and muscarinic cholinoceptor coupling to G proteins in rat cortex. *Eur. J. Pharmacol.*, **189**, 99–103.

Backonja, M., Beydoun, A., Edwards, K.R., *et al.* (1998). Gabapentin for the symptomatic treatment of painful neuropathy in patients with diabetes mellitus: a randomized controlled trial. *J. Am. Med. Assoc.*, **280**, 1831–1836.

Banki, C.M., Karmacsi, L., Bissette, G., *et al.* (1992). Cerebrospinal fluid neuropeptides in mood disorder and dementia. *J. Affect. Dis.*, **25**, 39–45.

Bebchuk, J.M., Arfken, C.L., Dolan-Manji, S., *et al.* (1999). A preliminary investigation of a protein kinase c inhibitor (tamoxifen) in the treatment of acute mania. *Arch. Gen. Psychiatry* (in press).

Belmaker, R.H. (1984). Adenylate cyclase and the search for new compounds with the clinical profile of lithium. *Pharmacopsychiatry*, **17**, 9–15.

Belmaker, R.H., Avissar, S. and Schreiber, G. (1991). Effect of lithium on human neurotransmitter receptor systems and G proteins. In: *Lithium and the cell: Pharmacology and Biochemistry*, (N.J. Birch, ed.), London, Academic Press, pp. 113–119.

Benjamin, J., Agam, G., Levine, J., *et al.* (1995a). Inositol treatment in psychiatry. *Psychopharmacol. Bull.*, **31**, 167–175.

Benjamin, J., Levine, J., Fux, M., *et al.* (1995b). Double-blind, placebo-controlled, crossover trial of inositol treatment for panic disorder. *Am. J. Psychiatry*, **152**, 1084–1086.

Bernasconi, R. (1982). The GABA hypothesis of affective illness: influence of clinically effective antimanic drugs on GABA turnover. In: *Basic Mechanisms in the Action of Lithium: Proceedings of a Symposium Held at Schloss Ringberg, Bavaria, F.R.G., October 4–6, 1981* (H.M. Emrich, J.B. Aldenhoff and H.D. Lux, ed.), Amsterdam, Excerpta Medica, pp. 183–192.

Bernasconi, R., Hauser, K., Martin, P., *et al.* (1984). Biochemical aspects of the mechanism of action of valproate. In: *Anticonvulsants in Affective Disorders*, (H.M. Emrich, T. Okuma and A.A. Muller, ed.), Amsterdam, Excerpta Medica, pp. 14–32.

Berridge, M.J. (1989). The Albert Lasker Medical Awards. Inositol trisphosphate, calcium, lithium, and cell signaling. *J. Am. Med. Assoc.*, **262**, 1834–1841.

Brandt, L., Saveland, H., Ljunggren, B., *et al.* (1988). Control of epilepsy partialis continuans with intravenous nimodipine. Report of two cases. *J. Neurosurg.*, **69**, 949–950.

Calabrese, J.R., Rapport, D.J., Shelton, M.D., *et al.* (1998). Clinical studies on the use of lamotrigine in bipolar disorder. *Neuropsychobiology*, **38**, 185–191.

Calabrese, J.R., Bowden, C.L., Sachs, G.S., *et al.*, (1999). A double-blind placebo-controlled study of lamotrigine monotherapy in outpatients with bipolar I depression. Lamictal 602 study group. *J. Clin. Psychiatry*, **60**, 79–88.

Chen, R.W., and Chuang, D.M. (1999). Long term lithium treatment suppresses p53 and Bax expression but increases Bcl-2 expression. A prominent role in neuroprotection against excitotoxicity. *J. Biol. Chem.*, **274**, 6039–6042.

Chen, G., Zeng, W.Z., Yuan, P.X., *et al.*, (1999). The mood-stabilizing agents lithium and valproate robustly increase the levels of the neuroprotective protein 6cl-2 in the CNS. *J. Neurochem.* **72**, 879–882.

Colin, S.F., Chang, H.-C., Mollner, S., *et al.* (1991). Chronic lithium regulates the expression of adenylate cyclase and Gi-protein alpha subunit in rat cerebral cortex. *Proc. Natl. Acad. Sci. USA*, **88**, 10634–10637.

Coppen, A., Prange, A.J., Jr., Whybrow, P.C., et al. (1972). Abnormalities of indoleamines in affective disorders. Arch. Gen. Psychiatry, 26, 474–478.

Coyle, J.T. (1996). The glutamatergic dysfunction hypothesis for schizophrenia. Harv. Rev. Psychiatry, 3, 241–253.

Crundwell, J.K. (1994). Lithium and its potential benefit in reducing increased mortality rates due to suicide. Lithium, 5, 193–204.

Curzon, G. (1988). Serotonergic mechanisms of depression. Clin. Neuropharmacol., 11, S11–S20.

Czyrak, A., Mogilnicka, E. and Maj, J. (1989). Dihydropyridine calcium channel antagonists as antidepressant drugs in mice and rats. Neuropharmacology, 28, 229–233.

Dailey, J.W., Reith, M.E., Steidley, K.R., et al. (1998). Carbamazepine-induced release of serotonin from rat hippocampus in vitro. Epilepsia, 39, 1054–1063.

Dailey, J.W., Reith, M.E., Yan, Q.S., et al. (1997). Anticonvulsant doses of carbamazepine increase hippocampal extracellular serotonin in genetically epilepsy-prone rats: dose response relationships. Neurosci. Lett., 227, 13–16.

Dailey, J.W., Yan, Q.S., Adams-Curtis, L.E., et al. (1996). Neurochemical correlates of anti-epileptic drugs in the genetically epilepsy-prone rat (GEPR). Life Sci., 58, 259–266.

Dalby, N.O. and Nielsen, E.B. (1997). Comparison of the preclinical anticonvulsant profiles of tiagabine, lamotrigine, gabapentin and vigabatrin. Epilepsy Res., 28, 63–72.

de Falco, F.A., Bartiromo, U., Majello, L., et al. (1992). Calcium antogonist nimodipine in intractable epilepsy. Epilepsia, 33, 343–345.

de Jonge, M., Freidl, A. and de Vry, J. (1993). CNS Pharmacology of Nimodipine: Antidepressants effects, drug discrimination and Ca2+ Imaging. In: Drugs in Development, Vol. 2: Ca2+ Antagonists in the CNS (A. Scriabine, R.A. Janis and D.J. Triggle, eds), Branford, Neva Press, pp. 165–174.

Dixon, J.F. and Hokin, L.E. (1997). The antibipolar drug valproate mimics lithium in stimulating glutamate release and inositol 1,4,5-trisphosphate accumulation in brain cortex slices but not accumulation of inositol monophosphates and bisphosphates. Proc. Natl. Acad. Sci. USA, 94, 4757–4760.

Dixon, J.F., Los, G.V. and Hokin, L.E. (1994). Lithium stimulates glutamate 'release' and inositol 1,4,5-trisphosphate accumulation via activation of the N-methyl-D-aspartate receptor in monkey and mouse cerebral cortex slices. Proc. Natl. Acad. Sci. USA, 91, 8358–8362.

Dubovsky, S.L., Franks, R.D. and Allen, S. (1987). Verapamil: a new antimanic drug with potential interactions with lithium. J. Clin. Psychiatry, 48, 371–372.

Dubovsky, S.L., Franks, R.D., Lifschitz, M., et al. (1982). Effectiveness of verapamil in the treatment of a manic patient. Am. J. Psychiatry, 139, 502–504.

Dubovsky, S.L., Murphy, J., Thomas, M., et al. (1992). Abnormal intracellular calcium ion concentration in platelets and lymphocytes of bipolar patients. Am. J. Psychiatry, 149, 118–120.

Dubovsky, S.L., Thomas, M., Hijazi, A., et al. (1994). Intracellular calcium signaling in peripheral cells of patients with bipolar affective disorder. Eur. Arch. Psychiatry Clin. Neurosci., 243, 229–234.

Duman, R.S. (1998). Novel therapeutic approaches beyond the serotonin receptor. Biol. Psychiatry, 44, 324–335.

Duman, R.S., Heninger, G.R. and Nestler, E.J. (1997). A molecular and cellular theory of depression. Arch. Gen. Psychiatry, 54, 597–606.

Ehlers, C.L., Henriksen, S.J., Wang, M., et al. (1983). Corticotropin releasing factor produces increases in brain excitability and convulsive seizures in rats. Brain Res., 278, 332–336.

Fleischhacker, W.W., Hinterhuber, H., Bauer, H., et al. (1992). A multicenter double-blind study of three different doses of the new cAMP-phosphodiesterase inhibitor rolipram in patients with major depressive disorder. Neuropsychobiology, 26, 59–64.

Freedman, D.D. and Waters, D.D. (1987). 'Second generation' dihydropyridine calcium antagonists. Greater vascular selectivity and some unique applications. Drugs, 34, 578–598.

Friedman, E. and Wang, H.Y. (1996). Receptor-mediated activation of G proteins is increased in postmortem brains of bipolar affective disorder subjects. J. Neurochem., 67, 1145–1152.

Frye, M.A., Ketter, T.A., Osuch, E.A., *et al.* (1998). Gabapentin and lamotrigine monotherapy in mood disorder: an update (Abstract). *Syllabus and Proceedings Summary of the 151st Annual Meeting of the American Psychiatric Association*, Abstract No. 77D, 150.

Frye, M.A., Pazzaglia, P.J., Luckenbaugh, D., *et al.* (1997). Baseline CSF somatostatin predictive of nimodipine treatment response (Abstract). *Biol. Psychiatry*, **41**, 33S.

Geoffroy, M., Mogilnicka, E., Nielsen, M. and Rafaelsen, O.J. (1988). Effect of nifedipine on the shuttlebox escape deficit induced by inescapable shock in the rat. *Eur. J. Pharmacol.*, **154**, 277–283.

Gershon, S., Levine, J., Chengappa, R., *et al.* (1998). Controlled trial of inositol in treatment resistant depression (Abstract). *Abstracts of the XXIst CINP Congress*, Abstract STH1605.

Gold, P.W., Licinio, J., Wong, M.L., *et al.* (1995). Corticotropin releasing hormone in the pathophysiology of melancholic and atypical depression and in the mechanism of action of antidepressant drugs. *Ann. NY Acad. Sci.*, **771**, 716–729.

Hong, J.S., Tilson, H.A. and Yoshikawa, K. (1983). Effects of lithium and haloperidol administration on the rat brain levels of substance P. *J. Pharmacol. Exp. Ther.*, **224**, 590–593.

Hough, C.J., Irwin, R.P., Gao, X.-M., *et al.* (1996). Carbamazepine inhibition of N-Methyl-D-aspartate-evoked calcium influx in rat cerebellar granule cells. *J. Pharmacol. Exp. Ther.*, **276**, 143–149.

Jones, R.S., Mondadori, C. and Olpe, H.R. (1985). Neuronal sensitivity to substance P is increased after repeated treatment with tranylcypromine, carbamazepine or oxaprotaline, but decreased after repeated electroconvulsive shock. *Neuropharmacology*, **24**, 627–633.

Klein, E., Belmaker, R.H., Newman, M., *et al.* (1985). A comparison of lithium effects on human brain and rat brain noradrenaline-sensitive adenylate cyclase. *Acta Pharmacol. Toxicol. (Copenh.)*, **56** (Suppl. 1), 15–20.

Knapp, S. and Mandell, A.J. (1973). Short- and long-term lithium administration: effects on the brain's serotonergic biosynthetic systems. *Science*, **180**, 645–647.

Kramer, M.S., Cutler, N., Feighner, J., *et al.* (1998). Distinct mechanism for antidepressant activity by blockade of central substance P receptors. *Science*, **281**, 1640–1645.

Larkin, J.G., McKee, P.J., Blacklaw, J., Thompson, G.G., Morgan, I.C. and Brodie, M.J. (1991) Nimodipine in refractory epilepsy: a placebo-controlled, add-on study. *Epilepsy Res* **9**, 71–77.

Le Douarin, C., Oblin, A., Fage, D., *et al.* (1983). Influence of lithium on biochemical manifestations of striatal dopamine target cell supersensitivity induced by prolonged haloperidol treatment. *Eur. J. Pharmacol.*, **93**, 55–62.

Lesch, K.P., Aulakh, C.S., Tolliver, T.J., *et al.* (1991). Differential effects of long-term lithium and carbamazepine administration on Gs alpha and Gi alpha protein in rat brain. *Eur. J. Pharmacol.*, **207**, 355–359.

Levine, J. (1997). Controlled trials of inositol in psychiatry. *Eur. Neuropsychopharmacol.*, **7**, 147–155.

Levine, J., Barak, Y., Gonzalves, M., *et al.* (1995). Double-blind, controlled trial of inositol treatment of depression. *Am. J. Psychiatry*, **152**, 792–794.

Li, P.P., Tam, Y.K., Young, L.T., *et al.* (1991). Lithium decreases Gs, Gi-1 and Gi-2 alpha-subunit mRNA levels in rat cortex. *Eur. J. Pharmacol.*, **206**, 165–166.

Lloyd, K.G., Thuret, E.W. and Pilc, A. (1986). GABA and the mechanism of action of antidepressant drugs. In: *GABA and Mood Disorders: Experimental and Clinical Research* (G. Bartholini, K.G. Lloyd and P.L. Morselli, eds), LERS monograph series, **4**, New York, Raven Press, pp. 33–42.

Loosen, P.T. (1988). TRH: behavioral and endocrine effects in man. *Prog Neuropsychopharmacol. Biol. Psychiatry*, **12** (Suppl.), S87–117.

Macdonald, R.L. and Kelly, K.M. (1995). Antiepileptic drug mechanisms of action. *Epilepsia*, **36** (Suppl. 2), S2–12.

Maes, M., Calabrese, J., Jayathilake, K., *et al.* (1997). Effects of subchronic treatment with valproate on L-5-HTP-induced cortisol responses in mania: evidence for increased central serotonergic neurotransmission. *Psychiatry Res.*, **71**, 67–76.

Maitre, L., Baltzer, V. and Mondadori, C. (1984). Psychopharmacological and behavioural effects of anti-epileptic drugs in animals. In: *Anticonvulsants in Affective Disorders* (H.M. Emrich, T. Okuma and A.A. Muller, eds), Amsterdam, Excerpta Medica, pp. 3–13.

Manji, H., Bebchuk, J.M., Arfken, C.L., *et al.* (1998). Modulation of brain phosphoinositide signaling by lithium: Relationship to therapeutic response in manic-depressive illness (Abstract). *Abstracts of the XXIst CINP Congress*, Abstract STH1602.

Manji, H.K., Chen, G., Hsiao, J.K., Risby, E.D., *et al.* (1996). Regulation of signal transduction pathways by mood-stabilizing agents: implications for the delayed onset of therapeutic efficacy. *J. Clin. Psychiatry*, **57** (Suppl. 13), 34–46.

Manji, H.K., Potter, W.Z. and Lenox, R.H. (1995). Signal transduction pathways. Molecular targets for lithium's actions. *Arch. Gen. Psychiatry*, **52**, 531–543.

Manna, V. (1991). Bipolar affective disorders and role of intraneuronal calcium. Therapeutic effects of the treatment with lithium salts and/or calcium antagonist in patients with rapid polar inversion. *Minerva Med.*, **82**, 757–763.

Marangell, L.B., George, M.S., Callahan, A.M. *et al.* (1997). Effects of intrathecal protirelin (thyrotropin-releasing hormone) in refractory depressed patients. *Arch. Gen. Psychiatry*, **54**, 214–222.

Maren, S., Tocco, G., Standley, S., Baudry, M., *et al.* (1993). Postsynaptic factors in the expression of long-term potentiation (LTP): increased glutamate receptor binding following LTP induction in vivo. *Proc. Natl. Acad. Sci. USA*, **90**, 9654–9658.

Martin, P., Laurent, S., Massol, J., Childs, M. and Puech, A.J. (1989). Effects of dihydropyridine drugs on reversal by imipramine of helpless behavior in rats. *Eur. J. Pharmacol.*, **162**, 185–188.

Meltzer, H.L. (1990). Mode of action of lithium in affective disorders. An influence on intracellular calcium functions. *Pharmacol. Toxicol.*, **66**, 84–99.

Merren, M.D. (1998). Gabapentin for treatment of pain and tremor: a large case series. *South. Med. J.*, **91**, 739–744.

Meyer, F.B., Tally, P.W., Anderson, R.E., *et al.* (1986). Inhibition of electrically induced seizures by a dihydropyridine calcium channel blocker. *Brain Res.*, **384**, 180–183.

Minthon, L., Edvinsson, L. and Gustafson, L. (1997). Somatostatin and neuropeptide Y in cerebrospinal fluid: correlations with severity of disease and clinical signs in Alzheimer's disease and frontotemporal dementia. *Dement. Geriatr. Cogn. Disord.*, **8**, 232–239.

Mitchell, P.B., Manji, H.K., Chen, G., *et al.* (1997). High levels of Gs alpha in platelets of euthymic patients with bipolar affective disorder. *Am. J. Psychiatry*, **154**, 218–223.

Mitsushio, H., Takashima, M., Mataga, N., *et al.* (1988). Effects of chronic treatment with trihexyphenidyl and carbamazepine alone or in combination with haloperidol on substance P content in rat brain: a possible implication of substance P in affective disorders. *J. Pharmacol. Exp. Ther.*, **245**, 982–989.

Mogilnicka, E., Czyrak, A. and Maj, J. (1987). Dihydropyridine calcium channel antagonists reduce immobility in the mouse behavioral despair test; antidepressants facilitate nifedipine action. *Eur. J. Pharmacol.*, **138**, 413–416.

Mogilnicka, E., Czyrak, A. and Maj, J. (1988). BAY K 8644 enhances immobility in the mouse behavioral despair test, an effect blocked by nifedipine. *Eur. J. Pharmacol.*, **151**, 307–311.

Molchan, S.E., Hill, J.L., Martinez, R.A., *et al.* (1993). CSF somatostatin in Alzheimer's disease and major depression: relationship to hypothalamic-pituitary-adrenal axis and clinical measures. *Psychoneuroendocrinology*, **18**, 509–519.

Motohashi, N. (1992). GABA receptor alterations after chronic lithium administration. Comparison with carbamazepine and sodium valproate. *Prog. Neuropsychopharmacol. Biol. Psychiatry*, **16**, 571–579.

Motohashi, N., Ikawa, K. and Kariya, T. (1989). GABA$_B$ receptors are up-regulated by chronic treatment with lithium or carbamazepine. GABA hypothesis of affective disorders. *Eur. J. Pharmacol.*, **166**, 95–99.

Muller, D., Joly, M. and Lynch, G. (1988). Contributions of quisqualate and NMDA receptors to the induction and expression of LTP. *Science*, **242**, 1694–1697.

Nibuya, M., Nestler, E.J. and Duman, R.S. (1996). Chronic antidepressant administration increases the expression of cAMP response element binding protein (CREB) in rat hippocampus. *J. Neurosci.*, **16**, 2365–2372.

Nonaka, S. and Chuang, D.M. (1998). Neuroprotective effects of chronic lithium on focal cerebral ischemia in rats. *Neuroreport.*, **9**, 2081–2084.

Nonaka, S., Hough, C.J. and Chuang, D.M. (1998a). Chronic lithium treatment robustly protects neurons in the central nervous system against excitotoxicity by inhibiting N-methyl-D-aspartate receptor-mediated calcium influx. *Proc. Natl. Acad. Sci. USA*, **95**, 2642–2647.

Nonaka, S., Katsube, N. and Chuang, D.M. (1998b). Lithium protects rat cerebellar granule cells against apoptosis induced by anticonvulsants, phenytoin and carbamazepine. *J. Pharmacol. Exp. Ther.*, **286**, 539–547.

Nowak, G., Trullas, R., Layer, R.T., Skolnick, P. *et al.* (1993a). Adaptive changes in the N-methyl-D-aspartate receptor complex after chronic treatment with imipramine and l-amino-cyclopropanecarboxylic acid. *J. Pharmacol. Exp. Ther.*, **265**, 1380–1386.

Nowak, G., Paul, I.A., Popik, P., *et al.* (1993b). Ca2 + antagonists effect an antidepressant-like adaptation of the NMDA receptor complex. *Eur. J. Pharmacol.*, **247**, 101–102.

Okamoto, Y., Kagaya, A., Motohashi, N., *et al.* (1995). Inhibitory effects of lithium ion on intracellular Ca2 + mobilization in the rat hippocampal slices. *Neurochem. Int.*, **26**, 233–238.

Paczynski, R.P., Meyer, F.B. and Anderson, R.E. (1990). Effects of the dihydropyridine Ca2 + channel antagonist nimodipine on kainic acid-induced limbic seizures. *Epilepsy Res.*, **6**, 33–38.

Pande, A.C., Davidson, J.R., Jefferson, J.W. *et al.* (1999). Treatment of social phobia with gabapentin: a placebo-controlled study. *J. Clin. Psychopharmacol.*, **19**, 341–348.

Pani, L., Kuzmin, A., Diana, M., *et al.* (1990). Calcium receptor antagonists modify cocaine effects in the central nervous system differently. *Eur. J. Pharmacol.*, **190**, 217–221.

Paul, I.A., Nowak, G., Layer, R.T., *et al.* (1994). Adaptation of the N-methyl-D-aspartate receptor complex following chronic antidepressant treatments. *J. Pharmacol. Exp. Ther.*, **269**, 95–102.

Pazzaglia, P.J., George, M.S., Post, R.M., *et al.* (1995). Nimodipine increases CSF somatostatin in affectively ill patients. *Neuropsychopharmacology*, **13**, 75–83.

Pazzaglia, P.J., Post, R.M., Ketter, T.A., *et al.* (1998). Nimodipine monotherapy and carbamazepine augmentation in patients with refractory recurrent affective illness. *J. Clin. Psychopharmacol.*, **18**, 404–413.

Pazzaglia, P.J., Post, R.M., Ketter, T.A., *et al.* (1993). Preliminary controlled trial of nimodipine in ultra-rapid cycling affective dysregulation. *Psychiatry Res.*, **49**, 257–272.

Pollack, M.H., Matthews, J. and Scott, E.L. (1998). Gabapentin as a potential treatment for anxiety disorders (letter). *Am. J. Psychiatry*, **155**, 992–993.

Post, R.M. (1999). Calcium channel inhibitors. In: *Comprehensive Textbook of Psychiatry*, 7th edn: (B.J. Sadock, ed.), Baltimore Williams & Wilkins, (in press).

Post, R.M., Ballenger, J.C., Uhde, T.W., *et al.* (1982). Effect of carbamazepine on cyclic nucleotides in CSF of patients with affective illness. *Biol. Psychiatry*, **17**, 1037–1045.

Post, R.M. and Chuang, D.-M. (1991). Mechanism of action of lithium: Comparison and contrast with carbamazepine. In: *Lithium and the Cell: Pharmacology and Biochemistry* (N.J. Birch, ed.), London, Academic Press, pp. 199–241.

Post, R.M., Frye, M.A., Denicoff, K.H., *et al.* (1998a). Beyond lithium in the treatment of bipolar illness. *Neuropsychopharmacology*, **19**, 206–219.

Post, R.M., Frye, M.A., Leverich, G.S., *et al.* (1998b). The role of complex combination therapy in the treatment of refractory bipolar illness. *CNS Spectrums*, **3**, 66–86.

Post, R.M., Ketter, T.A., Denicoff, K., *et al.* (1996a). The place of anticonvulsant therapy in bipolar illness. *Psychopharmacology (Berl.)*, **128**, 115–129.

Post, R.M., Ketter, T.A., Jaffe, R.T., *et al.* (1991). Lack of beneficial effects of l-baclofen in affective disorder. *Int. Clin. Psychopharmacol.*, **6**, 197–207.

Post, R.M., Ketter, T.A., Pazzaglia, P.J., *et al.* (1996b). Rational polypharmacy in the bipolar affective disorders. *Epilepsy Res. Suppl.*, **11**, 153–180.

Post, R.M., Pazzaglia, P.J., Ketter, T.A., *et al.* (1999). Carbamazepine and nimodipine in affective illness: Efficacy, mechanisms of action, and interactions. In: *Book IV: Pharmacotherapy of Mood and Cognition* (S. Montgomery and U. Halbreich, eds), Washington, DC, American Psychiatric Press, (in press).

Post, R.M., Rubinow, D.R., Uhde, T.W., *et al.* (1985). Effects of carbamazepine on noradrenergic mechanisms in affectively ill patients. *Psychopharmacology (Berl.)*, **87**, 59–63.

Post, R.M. and Weiss, S.R. (1992). Ziskind-Somerfeld Research Award 1992. Endogenous biochemical abnormalities in affective illness: therapeutic versus pathogenic. *Biol. Psychiatry*, **32**, 469–484.

Post, R.M. and Weiss, S.R. (1998). Sensitization and kindling phenomena in mood, anxiety, and obsessive-compulsive disorders: the role of serotonergic mechanisms in illness progression. *Biol. Psychiatry*, **44**, 193–206.

Post, R.M., Weiss, S.R.B., Chuang, D.-M., *et al.* (1994). Mechanisms of action of carbamazepine in seizure and affective disorders. In: *Anticonvulsants in Mood Disorders* (R.T. Jaffe and J.R. Calabrese, eds), New York, Marcel Dekker, Inc., pp. 43–92.

Post, R.M., Weiss, S.R.B. and Chuang, D.-M. (1992). Mechanisms of action of anticonvulsants in affective disorders: comparisons with lithium. *J. Clin. Psychopharmacol.*, **12**, 23S–35S.

Post, R.M., Weiss, S.R.B., Clark, M., *et al.* (1999b). Lithium, carbamazepine, and valproate in affective illness: biochemical and neurobiological mechanisms. In: *Mechanisms of Action of Antibipolar Treatments* (H. Manji, ed.), Washington, DC, American Psychiatric Press, (in press).

Post, R.M., Weiss, S.R.B., Li, H., *et al.* (1998). Neural plasticity and emotional memory. *Development and Psychopathology*, **10**, 829–855.

Prange, A.J., Loosen, P.T. and Nemeroff, C.B. (1979). Peptides: application to research in nervous and mental disorders. In: *New Frontiers of Psychotropic Drug Research* (S. Fielding, ed.), New York, Futura Publishing Co., pp. 117–189.

Risch, S.C., Janowsky, D.S., Parker, D., *et al.* (1984). Neuroendocrine abnormalities in affective disorders: possible cholinergic mechanisms. In: *Neurobiology of Mood Disorders* (R.M. Post and J. C. Ballenger, eds), Baltimore, Williams & Wilkins, pp. 664–672.

Rosenfeld, W.E. (1997). Topiramate: a review of preclinical, pharmacokinetic, and clinical data. *Clin. Ther.*, **19**, 1294–1308.

Rossetti, Z.L., Pani, L., Kuzmin, A., *et al.* (1990). Dihydropyridine calcium antagonists prevent cocaine-, but not amphetamine-, induced dopamine release and motor activity in rats. *Acta Physiol. Hung.*, **75** (Supp.), 249–250.

Roy, A. (1993). Neuropeptides in relation to suicidal behavior in depression. *Neuropsychobiology*, **28**, 184–186.

Rubinow, D.R., Davis, C.L. and Post, R.M. (1992). Somatostatin in neuropsychiatric disorders. In: *Basic and Clinical Aspects of Neuroscience Vol. 4* (C. Weil, E.E. Muller and M.O. Thorner, eds), Berlin/Heidelberg, Springer-Verlag, pp. 29–42.

Rubinow, D.R., Gold, P.W., Post, R.M., *et al.* (1985). CSF somatostatin in affective illness and normal volunteers. *Prog. Neuropsychopharmacol. Biol. Psychiatry*, **9**, 393–400.

Schreiber, G., Avissar, S., Danon, A., *et al.* (1991). Hyperfunctional G proteins in mononuclear leukocytes of patients with mania. *Biol. Psychiatry*, **29**, 273–280.

Sherman, W.R., Munsell, L.Y., Gish, B.G., *et al.* (1985). Effects of systemically administered lithium on phosphoinositide metabolism in rat brain, kidney, and testis. *J. Neurochem.*, **44**, 798–807.

Siuciak, J.A., Lewis, D.R., Wiegand, S.J., *et al.* (1997). Antidepressant-like effect of brain-derived neurotrophic factor (BDNF). *Pharmacol. Biochem. Behav.*, **56**, 131–137.

Smith, M.A., Makino, S., Altemus, M., *et al.* (1995). Stress and antidepressants differentially regulate neurotrophin 3 mRNA expression in the locus coeruleus. *Proc. Natl. Acad. Sci. USA*, **92**, 8788–8792.

Snead, O.C. (1995). Basic mechanisms of generalized absence seizures. *Ann. Neurol.*, **37**, 146–157.

Sourkes, T.L. (1977). Biochemistry of mental depression. *Can. Psychiatr. Assoc. J.*, **22**, 467–481.

Souza, F.G., Mander, A.J. and Goodwin, G.M. (1990). The efficacy of lithium in prophylaxis of unipolar depression. Evidence from its discontinuation. *Br. J. Psychiatry*, **157**, 718–722.

Taylor, C.P., Gee, N.S., Su, T.Z., *et al.* (1998). A summary of mechanistic hypotheses of gabapentin pharmacology. *Epilepsy Res.*, **29**, 233–249.

Tolle, T.R., Castro-Lopes, J.M., Schadrack, J., *et al.* (1995). Anticonvulsants suppress c-Fos protein expression in spinal cord neurons following noxious thermal stimulation. *Exp. Neurol.*, **132**, 271–278.

Tondo, L., Baldessarini, R.J., Hennen, J., *et al.* (1998). Lithium treatment and risk of suicidal behavior in bipolar disorder patients. *J. Clin. Psychiatry*, **59**, 405–414.

Vadnal, R. and Parthasarathy, R. (1995). Myo-inositol monophosphatase: diverse effects of lithium, carbamazepine, and valproate. *Neuropsychopharmacology*, **12**, 277–285.

Vezzani, A., Wu, H.Q., Stasi, M.A., *et al.* (1988). Effect of various calcium channel blockers on three different models of limbic seizures in rats. *Neuropharmacology*, **27**, 451–458.

Waldmeier, P.C., Baumann, P.A., Wicki, P., *et al.* (1995). Similar potency of carbamazepine, oxcarbazepine, and lamotrigine in inhibiting the release of glutamate and other neurotransmitters. *Neurology*, **45**, 1907–1913.

Wang, S.J., Huang, C.C., Hsu, K.S., *et al.* (1996). Inhibition of N-type calcium currents by lamotrigine in rat amygdalar neurones. *NeuroReport.*, **7**, 3037–3040.

Wang, S.J., Tsai, J.J. and Gean, P.W. (1998). Lamotrigine inhibits depolarization-evoked Ca++ influx in dissociated amygdala neurons. *Synapse*, **29**, 355–362.

Weiss, S.R.B., Nierenberg, J., Lewis, R., *et al.* (1992). Corticotropin-releasing hormone: Potentiation of cocaine-kindled seizures and lethality. *Epilepsia*, **33**, 248–254.

White, H.S. (1997). Clinical significance of animal seizure models and mechanism of action studies of potential antiepileptic drugs. *Epilepsia*, **38** (Suppl. 1), S9–17.

Wurpel, J.N. and Iyer, S.N. (1994). Calcium channel blockers verapamil and nimodipine inhibit kindling in adult and immature rats. *Epilepsia*, **35**, 443–449.

Young, L.T., Li, P.P., Kish, S.J., *et al.* (1993). Cerebral cortex Gsα protein levels and forskolin-stimulated cyclic AMP formation are increased in bipolar affective disorder. *J. Neurochem.*, **61**, 890–898.

Young, L.T., Li, P.P., Kish, S.J., *et al.* (1991). Postmortem cerebral cortex Gs alpha-subunit levels are elevated in bipolar affective disorder. *Brain Res.*, **553**, 323–326.

13

Lithium: clinical use in mania and prophylaxis of affective disorders

John Cookson and Gary Sachs

Key points

- Lithium remains a first-line treatment for mania.
- Acute lithium toxicity can cause permanent neurological damage.
- Most patients with mania require antipsychotic drugs.
- Lithium remains a first-line treatment for the prophylaxis of bipolar disorder.
- Abrupt discontinuation of lithium can trigger mania in up to 50% of cases.
- Lithium is not usually successful as monotherapy.
- Careful selection and monitoring of patients is important when using lithium.

Introduction

Bipolar mood disorder, still widely referred to as manic depressive illness, is a common psychiatric condition which is often complicated by loss of employment, marital discord, substance abuse, suicide and violence. Lithium is the most widely accepted treatment for bipolar illness. The limitations of lithium therapy are increasingly apparent. Early claims for its efficacy as monotherapy seem unduly optimistic. Lithium remains a first-line treatment for mania, especially in the USA, although European clinicians would generally use it in combination with, or as adjunct to, other drugs. Decisions about treatment have grown complex in the light of new research and with the advent of new treatments, particularly anticonvulsants.

Cade's (1949) report of lithium's antimanic effects began the psychopharmacological era in psychiatry, and the prophylactic efficacy of lithium in bipolar disorder was established by 1968. The history of the use of lithium in medicine has been described comprehensively by Neil Johnson (1984). The pivotal studies, which were the basis for our use of lithium, were carried out more than 25 years ago. Some psychiatrists came to regard lithium as a specific treatment for bipolar illness. In the USA FDA approval for lithium was granted in 1970. By then, lithium therapy was widely regarded as the treatment of choice for bipolar mood disorder in the USA and was used extensively in Europe.

This development had a major impact on the treatment of bipolar disorder in the USA. When Baldessarini (1970) compared the frequency of affective illness to schizophrenia in patients discharged from hospital before and after the introduction of lithium, a reciprocal pattern was noted, with increasingly frequent diagnosis of bipolar illness and decreasing frequency of schizophrenia. Stoll *et al.* (1993) confirmed this finding in the discharge diagnoses of six psychiatric hospitals from the early 1970s. In the UK, the situation was different; there, affective illness was often diagnosed in patients whom US colleagues regarded as having schizophrenia. This resulted from differences in definition, with a broader concept of schizophrenia in the USA, as shown by the US-UK diagnostic project (Cooper *et al.*, 1972). Subsequently the general acceptance of criteria-based diagnostic systems, particularly DSM-III in 1982, introduced greater diagnostic reliability; however, the definition of bipolar mood disorder was broadened to include patients with mood-incongruent psychotic features, who would previously have been regarded as having schizoaffective disorder or schizophrenia. Thus the availability of lithium and the wider use of standard diagnostic systems have led patients to receive a diagnosis of bipolar disorder who might previously have been diagnosed with schizophrenia, at least in the USA. Many of the randomized-controlled trials of lithium were carried out before this shift in the diagnosis of bipolar disorder. This may help to reconcile the oft-quoted expectation that lithium is effective for all but 20–40% of bipolar patients with recent studies which suggest that lithium is far less effective.

Over the past 25 years there have been two further discoveries which necessitate a reappraisal of the place of lithium in treatment (Cookson, 1997) – the occurrence of permanent neurological sequelae as a result of acute lithium toxicity (Schou, 1984), and the recognition that mania may occur as a result of abrupt discontinuation of lithium (Mander and Loudon, 1988). The mode(s) of action of lithium have been considered in Chapter 12.

Placebo-controlled studies of the use of lithium
Mania

Following Cade's description of the anti-manic effects of lithium, there were four placebo-controlled studies of lithium in mania that used a crossover design. These were conducted in Denmark by Schou *et al.* (1954) and later in double-blind designs in England by Maggs (1963) and in the USA by Goodwin *et al.* (1969) and Stokes *et al.* (1971). In a total of 116 patients on lithium, there was an overall response rate of 78%, much greater than the placebo response rate (40% in one study).

Bowden *et al.* (1994) compared valproate (as Divalproex) to lithium or placebo in a 3-week parallel-group, double-blind study of 179 patients, half of whom had been unresponsive to lithium previously. The proportion of patients showing 50% improvement was greater for valproate (48%) and lithium (49%) than for placebo (25%). Few patients had a return to normal functioning within 3 weeks. Thus, in routine practice for acute mania, both lithium and valproate are useful as adjuncts to antipsychotic drugs, rather than as monotherapy. Lithium has a 'lag' in its effect, taking a few days to begin, and 2–3 weeks to approach its full effect on mania – sometimes taking longer. This limits lithium as a treatment for acute mania and makes monotherapy risky for all but the mildest cases. Subsequent analyses indicate that patients with mixed affective states may benefit more from valproate than from lithium.

Usually, clinicians must initiate other types of treatment for acute mania. Commonly, when a rapid response is required, treatment is initiated with antipsychotic medication. Some data suggest that anticonvulsants may also have a more rapid onset of antimanic action than lithium. Some open reports suggest rapid improvement (within 3 days) in a proportion of patients in response to valproate when treatment is initiated at doses of 20–30 mg/kg (Keck et al., 1993; McElroy et al., 1993).

Acute bipolar depression

The earliest assessments of lithium as an antidepressant were negative (Cade, 1949; Noack and Trautner, 1951). However there is compelling evidence from systematic reviews and meta-analysis of randomized clinical trials (RCTs) that lithium is superior to placebo for bipolar depression (Souza and Goodwin, 1991; Zornberg and Pope, 1993). Zornberg and Pope (1993) noted that lithium was superior in eight out of nine comparisons. Among these, Goodwin et al. (1969) obtained particularly good results with improvement in 10 of 13 bipolar depressed patients during lithium treatment. Seven of those 10 were considered to be unequivocal responders because their depression recurred during the placebo treatment phase. Several authors emphasize the relative slowness of improvement, for instance imipramine responders improved within the first week of treatment while lithium responders needed 2–3 weeks of treatment to begin to demonstrate response (Worrall et al., 1979). Factors limiting the generalizability of these research studies to routine clinical practice include the exclusion of patients with rapid-cycling, psychotic depression, or treatment-resistant depression (those having failed two or more previous somatic treatment trials).

The claim that lithium possesses acute antidepressant activity requires qualification. In the sole available direct comparison with more than four subjects of lithium against a standard antidepressant, imipramine was found to be superior (Fieve et al., 1968). Despite this finding, the use of lithium as an initial treatment for bipolar depression is reasonable. Himmelhoch (1994) notes that at low doses, lithium monotherapy is frequently effective in bipolar depression. In our clinical research programme, within 3 weeks of initiating lithium monotherapy, one-third of previously unmedicated bipolar depressed patients met criteria for recovery (Sachs, unpublished data).

Many clinicians use standard antidepressants in combination with lithium for patients with bipolar depression. The only study addressing this issue gives a confusing result. A double-blind RCT of bipolar depressed patients compared adjunctive treatment with imipramine, paroxetine or placebo. All patients were on lithium and had serum levels above 0.5 mmol/l at the time of enrollment (Pitts et al.; 1997). Overall no advantage was found for combining lithium with either antidepressant. However, in patients with serum lithium levels below 0.8 mmol/l, there was a significant advantage for paroxetine over placebo. This suggests an advantage for standard antidepressants in the treatment of those patients who cannot tolerate or do not respond to lithium at serum levels above 0.8 mmol/l.

Increasing lithium dose should not be viewed as a potent intervention, and patients should not be required to endure the adverse effects associated with maximal lithium levels. For most breakthrough depressions, it is reasonable to offer a trial of antidepressant medication while maintaining a serum lithium level in the therapeutic range. The antidepressant effect of lithium may be greatest for bipolar patients who become depressed while unmedicated.

Prophylaxis of bipolar disorder

Interpretation of the 10 large, double-blind comparative trials of lithium versus placebo in the prophylaxis of bipolar patients requires attention to details of study design. In some cases, this tends to produce results that overestimate the benefit of lithium for routine clinical practice. Two studies used double-blind discontinuation, with patients already on lithium being assigned randomly either to continue on lithium or to switch to placebo. In the study by Baastrup et al. (1970), 55% of patients who switched to placebo and none of those who continued on lithium relapsed within 5 months. About half of the relapses were manias, and half were depression. However, this design is severely undermined by the occurrence of lithium withdrawal mania (see below). One study used a crossover design that also involved a lithium withdrawal phase (Cundall et al., 1972). The required prospective design was used by Coppen et al. (1971) in the UK, by Prien et al. (1973) in the USA and in five other smaller studies. Overall in 204 patients on lithium prospectively, about 35% relapsed in the study period (which varied from 4 months to 3 years), compared to about 80% of 221 patients on placebo (see Goodwin and Jamison, 1990).

In these studies, the efficacy of lithium was more apparent for manic than for depressive relapses. However, retrospective mirror-image studies suggested that the efficacy in preventing depression might be as great as that in preventing mania (Poole et al., 1978; Holinger and Wolpert, 1979). Lithium improves both the severity and frequency of episodes. Usually it also stabilizes the mood between major episodes. Kukopoulos and Reginaldi (1973) argue that the reduction in depression is secondary to the prevention of mania, which would otherwise be followed by a post-manic depressive phase. Complaints about depressive recurrences on lithium are common, however, and patients are considered more likely to report dysphoria than to complain about their hypomanic symptoms. Keller et al. (1992) found that symptoms of mood elevation led to mania twice as often as subsyndromal depressive symptoms led to full depression.

The prophylaxis of unipolar depression

The broader concept of unipolar depression and the relatively short follow-up periods limit the prospective studies of lithium in the prophylaxis of unipolar depression. Some trials fail to distinguish between preventing the re-emergence of the index episode (a 'relapse' within the first 6 months) and true prophylaxis (against 'recurrence' after 6 months). Two of the above prospective trials included unipolar depressives. They found no difference in the efficacy of lithium compared to that in bipolar patients (Coppen et al.,

1971; Prien *et al.*, 1973). Prien *et al.* (1984) found imipramine superior to lithium in the prophylaxis of the most severe depressive episodes and of equal efficacy for moderately severe depression. A comprehensive meta-analysis left no reason to doubt the efficacy of lithium in the prophylaxis of unipolar depressive illness; alternative treatment with antidepressant monoamine reuptake inhibitors (MARIs) may be safer in overdose, or better tolerated, but their greater efficacy is arguable (Souza and Goodwin, 1991). It is possible that some individuals may benefit particularly from lithium prophylaxis.

Predicting response to lithium

Patients with typical bipolar disorder and complete recovery between episodes are more likely to benefit from lithium prophylaxis (Grof *et al.*, 1993). A family history of bipolar disorder is strongly associated with prophylactic efficacy. Neurological signs predict a poor response to lithium (Himmelhoch *et al.*, 1980). Patients whose first episode was manic rather than depressive do better on lithium (Prien *et al.*, 1984; Faedda *et al.*, 1991). A good response to lithium in acute mania or depression may predict prophylactic efficacy. Manic patients who respond tend to be classical manics rather than mixed or schizoaffective (Himmelhoch *et al.*, 1976; Goodnick and Meltzer, 1984; Swann *et al.*, 1986). Elated-grandiose manics showed a better response than destructive-paranoid manics in one study (Murphy and Beigel, 1974) but not in another (Swann *et al.*, 1986). Dysphoric manics were less likely to improve (Post *et al.*, 1989). Patients with a rapid-cycling phase of illness are often less responsive to lithium (Dunner and Fieve, 1974; Dilsaver *et al.*, 1993). Other factors militating against prophylactic efficacy are poor adherence to treatment, drug abuse, and a larger number of previous episodes. In the prophylaxis of unipolar depressive disorder, a good response to lithium is predicted by a family history of mania or response to lithium, stable premorbid personality, low neuroticism and good interepisode functioning (Coppen and Abou-Saleh, 1983).

Lithium: side effects

Lithium, even at therapeutic doses, has actions on many bodily systems. These are important, as some require intervention. They also contribute to non-compliance. The majority of patients on lithium experience at least one side effect, depending on the dosage used (Vestergaard *et al.*, 1980). All patients should be informed about side effects and signs of toxicity.

Thyroid

Lithium tends to reduce thyroid function. The most sensitive laboratory index, increased TSH, occurs in 23% of patients (Transbol *et al.*, 1978). Thyroid enlargement (goitre) develops in about 5% of patients (Myers *et al.*, 1985), and clinical hypothyroidism occurs in 5–10% of patients depending upon the dose and duration of treatment (Yassa *et al.*, 1988). Patients with pre-existing thyroid antibodies or a family history of thyroid disease are at greater risk of developing hypothyroidism (Lazarus *et al.*, 1981), and lithium treatment can increase antibody levels (Calabrese *et al.*, 1985; Myers *et al.*, 1985). The development of hypothyroidism is often signalled by weight gain and lethargy and should be distinguished from depression. Treatment with l-thyroxine is usually straightforward. The occurrence of thyrotoxicosis during lithium treatment has also been described, and there may be a rebound exacerbation when lithium is discontinued.

Kidney

Polyuria and excessive thirst with polydipsia are noted by about one-third of patients on lithium. The condition is usually reversible but, after long-term treatment, it may become irreversible (Bucht *et al.*, 1980). Giving lithium once daily, as opposed to divided doses, was associated with lower daily urine volumes in some studies, although others found no difference (Bowen *et al.*, 1991). For patients in whom a reduction in dose is not appropriate in order to avoid polyuria, the loop diuretic frusemide or amiloride with or without potassium supplements may be helpful. In 1977, Hestbech *et al.* reported histological changes in patients on lithium including glomerular damage, interstitial fibrosis and tubular atrophy (focal interstitial nephropaphy). However, similar findings were later made in bipolar subjects who had received no lithium treatment.

Further work has shown that during long-term treatment with lithium, monitored at therapeutic doses, no deterioration occurs in the glomerular filtration rate in the vast majority of patients. However, occasional cases of chronic renal failure have been reported and attributed by nephrologists to lithium, even in patients whose lithium levels have been monitored carefully. Some regard this to be a rare idiosyncratic reaction to lithium (Waller and Edwards, 1989), but it is not clear that this rate exceeds that expected for idiopathic renal failure in the general population. Episodes of lithium toxicity may produce renal damage with reduced glomerular filtration rates (Johnson, 1984). Claims that renal impairment is more likely to be found in patients after more than 20 years on lithium await replication.

Central nervous system

A fine tremor of the hands, similar to that found in those with anxiety occurs in about 25% of patients. Tricyclic antidepressants and selective serotonin reuptake inhibitors (SSRIs) can worsen the tremor. Beta-blockers such as propanolol (starting at 10 mg bid) reduce the tremor and are probably best taken intermittently. Lithium can increase extrapyramidal (parkinsonian) side effects in patients on antipsychotic drugs (Tyrer *et al.*, 1980) and can itself produce cogwheel rigidity in a small minority of patients (Asnis *et al.*, 1979). In contrast to antipsychotic-induced parkinsonism, this does not improve with anticholinergic drugs. Cerebellar tremor and incoordination are signs of toxicity, as are more severe forms of fine tremor and parkinsonism.

Mental and cognitive effects

There is some objective evidence of an effect of therapeutic levels of lithium upon memory, but not all studies show this. Patients interviewed about possible side effects frequently affirm memory problems. The use of ECT for patients on lithium has been associated with acute organic brain syndrome or prolonged confusional states, but a retrospective case-control study did not find a higher frequency of adverse effects of ECT in patients on lithium (Jha *et al.*, 1996). Schou (1979), who interviewed 24 successful artists and professionals taking lithium, explored the possible effect of lithium upon creativity. Although six wished to discontinue lithium believing it diminished their creativity, the majority considered that their long-term productivity and creativity were higher under lithium treatment despite missing some hypomanic swings.

In therapeutic doses, lithium does not impair psychomotor coordination. It is not a bar to driving private motor vehicles, although a diagnosis of manic-depressive illness excludes patients from driving certain public service vehicles in the UK and the USA. After an admission for mania, the patient may not drive for 6–12 months according to the UK Driver and Vehicle Licensing Agency.

Cardiovascular effects

Lithium can produce benign reversible T-wave flattening or inversion, a pattern similar to that with hypokalaemia. Cardiac dysrhythmias are rare with therapeutic doses especially in younger patients, but sinus node arrhythmias have been described (sick sinus syndrome) (Mitchell and MacKenzie, 1982). Higher rates of arrhythmia should be expected when lithium is used in combination with carbamazepine than with either drug alone (Steckler, 1994). Caution should be exercised when using lithium with the elderly and patients with cardiac failure. The mortality rate among patients on lithium is similar to that of manic depressives before lithium was introduced (Norton and Whalley, 1984). Nilsson (1998) reported that lithium treatment ameliorated the excessive cardiovascular mortality formerly found in untreated bipolar patients.

Skin

Lithium can produce or exacerbate acne and psoriasis. Tetracyclines should be used with caution because of their possible interaction with lithium, but retinoids can be used. Hair loss and altered texture may also occur in about 6% of patients on lithium, and there may be golden discoloration of the distal nail plates.

Parathyroid, bones and teeth

Lithium produces mild increases in parathyroid hormone level and serum calcium. Stancer and Forbath (1989) reported clinical hyperparathyroidism in patients on lithium. No long-term effects on bone have been found in animals or humans (Birch *et al.*, 1982). It is unknown whether this applies to the growing bones of children. There is no evidence of a direct effect of lithium upon the teeth, but lithium's side effects of dry mouth or increased consumption of sweet drinks can lead to cavities.

Metabolic effects and weight gain

About 25% of patients gain more than 4.5 kg (10 lb) in weight. The mechanism is unknown. Although increased consumption of sweet drinks is cited, an increase in food intake and altered metabolism are also possible. Lithium produces subtle alterations in glucose and insulin metabolism and may occasionally worsen control of diabetes. Fluid retention and oedema may occur. Lithium may antagonize aldosterone and increase angiotensin levels (Stewart et al., 1988). In a study over 1 year, more patients reported weight gain as a side effect on valproate (21%) and lithium (13%) than on placebo (7%) (Bowden et al., 1999).

Gastrointestinal

About one-third of patients experience mild abdominal discomfort, especially at higher dosages. Loose motions sometimes occur during the first few weeks of treatment, especially with higher doses. By using divided doses, these side effects can usually be avoided. Sometimes a slow release preparation is tolerated better, but occasionally these irritate the lower bowel. Severe or persistent diarrhoea suggests toxicity.

Sexual function

Impairment of sexual drive, arousal and ejaculation has been attributed to lithium but this is rare (Blay et al., 1982). The LH response to LHRH is potentated by lithium treatment, similarly to the potentiation of the TSH response to TRH.

Neuromuscular junction

Lithium reduces acetylcholine release and impairs neuromuscular transmission. Normally the safety factor in neuromuscular transmission is sufficient to overcome these effects. Lithium potentiates neuromuscular blocking agents, including succinyl choline, and exacerbates myasthenia gravis.

Respiratory effects

Lithium can produce respiratory depression in patients with chronic obstructive airway disease, especially at toxic blood levels (Lawler and Cove-Smith, 1986). Lower therapeutic levels reduce the reactivity of bronchial smooth muscle and may benefit some patients with asthma (Knox et al., 1992).

Blood and bone marrow

Lithium produces a benign reversible leucocytosis probably by an effect on marrow growth factors.

Contraindications

There are no absolute contraindications to lithium treatment but caution is required in people with renal failure, heart failure, recent myocardial infarction, electrolyte imbalance, the elderly and in patients who are unreliable in taking medication. In the USA lithium is generally withheld prior to electroconvulsive therapy to reduce the risk of arrhythmia. The ECT Handbook (Kellner et al., 1997) advises stopping lithium 36–48 hours before ECT and holding it until after the final ECT treatment, to avoid delirium or prolonged seizures. Many clinicians withhold solely the dose of lithium immediately preceding an ECT session, and some simply continue routine lithium dosing.

Pregnancy

Initial concern about the risk of teratogenicity was based largely on the frequency of abnormalities reported to the Lithium Information Centre in Wisconsin. These voluntary reports included particularly high rates of Ebstein's anomaly and suggested fetal exposure to lithium, especially in the first trimester, carried substantially greater risk of other malformations as well. Recent cohort studies suggest the risk of major congenital abnormalities may be 4–12%, compared to 2–4% in women taking other drugs not known to be teratogenic (Kallen and Tandberg, 1983; Jacobson et al., 1992; Cohen et al., 1994). As Cohen and Rosenbaum's (1998) and Llewellyn et al.'s (1998) reviews note, first trimester exposure to lithium is associated with an increased relative risk of Ebstein's anomaly which is 10–20 times that of the general population. However, the absolute risk of 0.05–0.1% is low. Screening tests, including high-resolution ultrasound and echocardiography examination of the fetus at 16–18 weeks' gestation, are advisable in women exposed to lithium in early pregnancy.

Perinatal toxicity is reported in neonates delivered from mothers taking lithium. Hypotonicity and cyanosis characterize this 'floppy baby syndrome'. A naturalistic study (Cohen et al., 1995), however, found no evidence of neonatal toxicity in the newborns of bipolar women treated with lithium at the time of labour and delivery. A 5-year follow-up of children with second and third trimester exposure to lithium born without congenital malformations found no significant behavioural toxicity (Schou, 1976). Lithium is secreted in breast milk and serum lithium levels in nursing infants are reported to be 10–50% of the mothers' serum level (Weinstein and Goldfield, 1973). It remains unclear what effect this low lithium intake might have on well-hydrated, breast-feeding infants. Women accepting this risk and wishing to breast feed should be counselled to provide supplemental fluids and discontinue breast feeding under circumstances of increased fluid loss or decreased intake. A switch from lithium to an anticonvulsant medication for prophylaxis during pregnancy is not recommended. The risks of teratogenicity associated with valproate and carbamazepine are higher than with lithium, and a lithium-responsive patient may not be protected by these anticonvulsants.

Even the remote possibility of teratogenicity or developmental effects upon the child causes understandable concern among those planning to conceive. Pregnancy in bipolar patients may be managed acceptably without psychotropic drugs. This risk is likely lowest in women with only one prior episode (Cohen and Rosenbaum, 1998). Women choosing to discontinue lithium should be encouraged to taper medication gradually (over several weeks or months) and only after an euthymic period of 1 year or longer. If alternative medication is needed when pregnancy is planned, antipsychotics or antidepressants are probably the safest. There is a risk of transient, extrapyramidal side effects in the neonate if antipsychotics are continued. These issues are considered further in Chapter 19.

Lithium toxicity – clinical features

Lithium toxicity is indicated by the development of three groups of symptoms – gastrointestinal, motor – especially cerebellar, and cerebral (see Table 13.1). Nausea and diarrhoea progress to vomiting and incontinence. Marked fine tremor progresses to a coarse (cerebellar or parkinsonian) tremor, giddiness, cerebellar ataxia, and slurred speech, and to gross incoordination with choreiform movements and muscular twitching (myoclonus), upper motor neuron signs (spasticity and extensor plantar reflexes), EEG abnormalities and seizures. In mild toxicity there is impairment of concentration, but this deteriorates into drowsiness and disorientation. In more severe toxicity, there is marked apathy and impaired consciousness leading to coma. A Creutzfeldt-Jakob like syndrome with characteristic EEG changes, myoclonus and cognitive deterioration has been described in patients on lithium and was, in these cases, reversible (Smith and Kocen, 1988).

Table 13.1 Symptoms of lithium toxicity

	Gastrointestinal	Motor	Cerebral
Mild	Nausea Diarrhoea	Severe fine tremor	Poor concentration
Moderate	Vomiting	Coarse tremor Cerebellar ataxia Slurred speech	Drowsiness Disorientation
Severe	Vomiting Incontinence	Choreiform/parkinsonian movement General muscle twitching (myoclonus) Spasticity and cerebellar dysfunction EEG abnormalities and seizures	Apathy Coma

Diagnosis of toxicity

Lithium toxicity should be assumed in patients on lithium who have vomiting, severe nausea, cerebellar signs or disorientation. Lithium treatment should be stopped immediately, and serum lithium, urea and electrolyte levels should be measured. However, the severity of toxicity bears little relationship to serum lithium levels (Hansen and Amdisen, 1978), and neurotoxicity can occur with serum levels in the usual therapeutic range (West and Meltzer, 1979). Many of the features of toxicity may reflect high intracellular, rather than extracellular, levels. Diagnosis should be based upon clinical judgement and not upon the blood level. Lithium should only be restarted (at an adjusted dose) when the patient's condition has improved or an alternative cause of the symptoms has been found.

Treatment of lithium toxicity

Often, cessation of lithium and provision of adequate salt and fluids, including saline infusions, will suffice to reduce toxicity. In patients with high serum levels (greater than 3 mmol/l) or coma, haemodialysis can speed the removal of lithium and reduce the risk of permanent neurological damage (Johnson, 1984).

Outcome of lithium toxicity

Patients who survive episodes of lithium toxicity will often make a full recovery. However, a proportion has persistent renal or neurological damage with cerebellar symptoms, spasticity and cognitive impairment. This outcome is more likely if patients are continued on lithium while showing signs of toxicity or during intercurrent physical illnesses (Schou, 1984). Patients with persistent neurological damage had also shown more advanced signs of toxicity (Hansen and Amdisen, 1978). The signs of toxicity develop gradually over several days during continued lithium treatment and, in some cases, continue to develop for days after treatment is stopped. Serum lithium levels can also continue to rise after treatment is stopped, probably through release of lithium from intracellular stores (Sellers *et al.*, 1982).

Factors predisposing to lithium toxicity

Conditions of salt depletion (diarrhoea, vomiting, excessive sweating during fever or in hot climates) can lead to lithium retention. Drugs which reduce the renal excretion of lithium include thiazide diuretics (but not frusemide or amiloride), certain non-steroidal anti-inflammatory drugs (ibuprofen, indomethacin, piroxicam, naproxen, and phenylbutazone, but not aspirin, paracetamol or sulindac), certain antibiotics (erythromycin, metronidazole and probably tetracyclines) and calcium antagonists. These drugs should be avoided if possible. If they must be used, the dose of lithium should be reduced and blood levels monitored. In patients with serious intercurrent illnesses, especially infections, lithium should be stopped or reduced in dose and carefully monitored until the patient's condition is stable.

Gastroenteritis is particularly liable to lead to toxicity. In the elderly, renal function is decreased. Lower doses are required, and toxicity can develop more readily (Stone, 1989).

Practical aspects of lithium treatment

A physical examination and tests of the blood and urine should, if possible, precede drug treatment. If not, they should take place soon after the patient is sedated in order to elucidate any intercurrent physical illness, especially infection, and any causes of secondary mania (e.g. drugs). Determination of baseline renal, hepatic and thyroid function would also be helpful.

Selection of patients

The Guidelines of the American Psychiatric Association (1997) recommend lithium as a first-line treatment for acute mania. Antipsychotics and benzo-diazepines are recommended only as 'adjuncts' for the control of agitation and behavioural disturbance and to sedate the patient until the effect of the 'mood-stabilizer' develops. The Statement of the Carolina Consensus Panel appears to corroborate this opinion (Francis et al., 1998). In Europe, psychiatrists view this advice with scepticism. There, antipsychotics are widely regarded in Europe as first-line treatment for acute mania; lithium is added for patients who are known to have responded to it in the past or as an adjunct for those who remain manic after 2 weeks of adequate doses of an antipsychotic. This difference in approach may be more theoretical than real; in reputable centres in both the USA and Europe, surveys show that the majority of manic patients are discharged from hospital still taking antipsychotic medication and remain on it after 6 months (Licht et al., 1994; McElroy et al., 1996).

Maintenance treatment with lithium should be considered after a second major episode of bipolar disorder or third episode of unipolar disorder, especially if the interval between episodes has been less than 5 years. The interval between the first and second episodes tends to be longer than between subsequent episodes. Maintenance treatment should therefore only be used after a first episode if the dangers of a subsequent episode are thought to justify it – for instance, if the episode was severe and disruptive, had a relatively sudden onset and was not precipitated by external factors, if the person's job is very sensitive, or if there is a suicide risk. Some experts recommend lithium therapy after a first manic episode when the patient has a strong family history of bipolar disorder. It has been suggested that patients who have already experienced more than two mood episodes are less likely than others to benefit from lithium prophylaxis (Gelenberg et al., 1989). However, this needs further research, as cases exist in which patients improve after multiple mood episodes. For instance, Robert Lowell's bipolar illness improved on lithium although he had experienced more than 20 episodes when commenced on it (Jamison, 1994).

Lithium blood levels, therapeutic range and monitoring

The narrow gap or overlap between therapeutic and toxic blood levels of lithium necessitates careful monitoring of lithium levels, usually based on samples taken 12 hours after the last dose. The pharmacokinetics of lithium involve rapid and almost complete absorption from the gastrointestinal tract, with a peak blood level at 2–4 hours after an oral dose, followed by distribution in body fluids and slow penetration of the intracellular space and brain. The eventual concentration in cerebrospinal fluid is about 40–50% of that in plasma. Elimination is largely by the kidney, and the plasma half-life varies from 7 to 20 hours in physically healthy individuals. It is longer in the elderly or physically unwell. Thornhill and Field (1982) found it to range from 15 to 55 hours in euthymic, psychiatric patients. Thus on a regular dose, steady state blood levels would be reached after a period of between 2 and 9 days.

Preparations of lithium are available which differ substantially in time to peak serum level and Cmax than others, but the serum level 12 hours after a dose is about the same. For instance, the peak levels of controlled release lithium preparations are about 25–40% lower and are delayed by about 3 hours compared to immediate release lithium (Shelley and Silverstone, 1986; Kirkwood *et al.*, 1994). While equal doses of different preparations produce nearly equal serum lithium levels at 12 hours, the area under the curve is about 10% greater for controlled release preparations. There may be differences in tolerability, and controlled release forms may produce slightly higher levels in the brain than the immediate release forms.

Recent studies have indicated that blood levels lower than those formerly used are sufficient in prophylaxis (Coppen *et al.*, 1983). Thus, efficacy was preserved until levels were below 0.6 mmol/l. For some patients, lower levels than this would suffice, although Gelenberg *et al.* (1989) found that a group with levels of 0.8–1.0 mmol/l had a better outcome than a group with levels of 0.4–0.6 mmol/l. In the elderly, a level of 0.5 mmol/l is recommended (Hardy *et al.*, 1987). Recommendations vary about monitoring lithium, renal and thyroid function tests, but even in the most stable patient, these tests should be performed at least once a year. During less stable phases, lithium levels should be done more frequently.

Antidepressants and lithium

Lithium does not induce mania and reduces the risk of affective switch during treatment with standard antidepressant agents (Quitkin *et al.*, 1981). In cases where depression occurs despite adequate lithium maintenance – breakthrough depression – some experts suggest that raising lithium levels will optimize antidepressant efficacy (Jann *et al.*, 1982; Price *et al.*, 1984). However, cases have been described who were refractory to high therapeutic lithium levels (Himmelhoch, 1994). Also, low doses and low serum levels of lithium (450–600 mg and 0.35 mmol/l–0.65 mmol/l) can be more effective in treating anergically depressed bipolar patients than higher doses (Himmelhoch *et al.*, 1980; Himmelhoch, 1987).

In patients with bipolar I disorder, the course of antidepressant MARI treatment should be gradually discontinued as the depression improves, to reduce the risk of triggering a manic episode and to avoid the induction of rapid-cycling (Wehr and Goodwin, 1979). Kane *et al.* (1982) found lithium more effective than imipramine or placebo in preventing depressive recurrences in bipolar II patients. The combination of lithium and a MARI may be more effective in preventing depression than either drug alone (Shapiro *et al.*, 1989). There is evidence that SSRIs such as paroxetine are less likely to trigger mania than tricyclic antidepressants (TCAs) (Montgomery and Roberts, 1994). However, some bipolar individuals are readily switched into mania by SSRIs.

Lithium–antipsychotic combinations

Combinations of high levels of lithium with high doses of antipsychotics, including haloperidol have been associated with severe neurological symptoms, hyperthermia, impaired consciousness and irreversible brain damage (Cohen and Cohen, 1974; Loudon and Waring, 1976). The conditions resemble both lithium toxicity and neuroleptic malignant syndrome. Antipsychotic drugs can increase intracellular lithium levels suggesting a possible mechanism for this interaction (Von Knorring, 1990). Subsequent studies have demonstrated the safety of combining haloperidol (up to 30 mg/day) with lithium at levels of up to 1 mmol/l (see Johnson *et al.*, 1990). When combining lithium with antipsychotics, blood levels should generally be maintained below 1 mmol/l. Staff should be advised to observe and report the development of neurological symptoms, and lithium should be temporarily discontinued if such symptoms develop. The combination of antipsychotics and lithium can also lead to troublesome somnambulism, which would require a dose reduction (Charney *et al.*, 1979).

Rapid-cycling and mixed episodes

Treatment of bipolar patients with mixed episodes or rapid-cycling is challenging. Such patients have high rates of chronicity (Keller *et al.*, 1986), substance abuse, self-destructive behaviour, and other comorbid neuropsychiatric illness. Unfortunately, these more pernicious subtypes account for between 30% and 60% of bipolar patients in some US studies; the proportion may be lower in European experience. Antidepressant drugs, especially TCAs, can produce rapid cycling and should be discontinued if cycling occurs (Wehr *et al.*, 1988).

Patients with mixed episodes and/or rapid-cycling are usually less responsive to lithium than typical bipolar patients (Dilsaver *et al.*, 1993; Murphy and Beigel, 1974; Himmelhoch *et al.*, 1976; Himmelhoch and Garfinkel, 1986; Swann *et al.*, 1986; Secunda *et al.*, 1985, 1986, 1987). Compiling these reports, 36% of patients with mixed mania and 75% of patients with pure episodes responded well to lithium (McElroy *et al.*, 1992). Methodological limitations included lack of control groups and varying treatment periods ranging from 24 days to 5 years. Those rapid-cycling patients who have never been exposed to antidepressants may respond well to lithium (Kukopulos *et al.*, 1980).

Patients with rapid-cycling or mixed episodes may respond more favourably to the anticonvulsants carbamazepine or valproate than to lithium (Post *et al.*, 1987; Hayes, 1989; McFarland *et al.*, 1990; Calabrese *et al.*, 1992; Clothier *et al.*, 1992; Freeman *et al.*, 1992). In the double-blind study of Bowden *et al.* (1994) the response to valproate was at least as good for mixed episodes as for pure mania. Anticonvulsants can be useful as first-line treatment, but many patients with mixed episodes or rapid-cycling will benefit from combination treatment. Polypharmacy is often required and can be carried out safely with careful monitoring. Practice in the USA seems more inclined towards polypharmacy than in Europe, where a more purist approach still prevails.

Withdrawal of lithium

Symptoms of anxiety, irritability and emotional lability can follow sudden discontinuation of lithium (King and Hullin, 1983). In a double-blind, placebo-controlled, cross-over study, sudden cessation of lithium in bipolar patients led to the development of mania within 2–3 weeks in 50% (7/14) of the patients (Mander and Loudon, 1988).

A review of all published studies suggests that half the bipolar patients who discontinued lithium had a mood episode within 5 months, usually of mania (Suppes *et al.*, 1991). In a naturalistic study, discontinuation over more than 2 weeks was associated with fewer recurrences than was abrupt discontinuation (Baldessarini *et al.*, 1996). Discontinuation of lithium should therefore be gradual. Case reports suggest that discontinuation of lithium can not only cause recurrent affective episodes but also induce episodes that are unresponsive to the reintroduction of lithium (Post, 1990). Recent longitudinal experience reported by Coryell *et al.* (1998) and Tondo *et al.* (1998) does not reveal decreased response when lithium is reintroduced for treatment of subsequent episodes. Also, there are as yet no prospective studies that support this hypothesis. Bowden *et al.* (1999) found that upon entry to a double-blind maintenance study, relapse rates in lithium-treated subjects randomized to either valproate or placebo were no higher than relapse rate for those randomized to continue lithium for maintenance treatment. The possible occurrence of lithium withdrawal mania should be part of the information given to patients when started on lithium. It has been estimated that to balance the risk of mania from abrupt discontinuation, a first episode manic patient would need to continue on lithium for a minimum of 2 years (Goodwin, 1994).

There are no clear guidelines for deciding when to advise patients to stop lithium. If they have relapses in spite of good adherence to treatment and satisfactory blood levels or if they have remained well on lithium for 3–4 years, the benefits and risks of continuing lithium should be reviewed. Patients whose mood has been stable are less likely to relapse when stopping lithium than those who have continued to show mild mood swings ('metastable'). Lithium may be reduced at the rate of one-quarter to one-eighth of the original dose every 2 months to minimize the risk of precipitating with-drawal mania. Further studies are needed to clarify this.

Natural outcome on lithium

Dickson and Kendell (1986) reported a three-fold increase in admissions for mania in Edinburgh during the period 1970–1981 when the use of lithium increased. This highlights the difficulty of delivering an effective treatment to a community. A large proportion of patients at risk does not seek treat-ment, and many that seek help do adhere poorly to lithium. In addition, there is the risk of withdrawal mania for those who stop treatment too abruptly – for instance, when patients feel no need for medication during a mild upswing of mood. A naturalistic follow-up in the USA found no difference in outcome over 18 months between bipolar patients discharged on or off lithium (Harrow et al., 1990). However, these patients were not randomly assigned. Gillberg et al. (1993) found a particularly poor social outcome in adolescents with bipolar disorder whose treatment usually included trials of lithium. None were able to maintain employment, and all were on public assistance by the age of 30.

Under circumstances where steps are taken to encourage and check adherence, relapse rates and affective morbidity as low as those in controlled trials can be achieved for patients in naturalistic studies while on lithium (McCreadie and Morrison, 1985; Coppen and Abou-Saleh, 1988). This is part of the rationale for specialist lithium or affective disorder clinics. Some clinics provide immediate measurement of blood lithium levels by use of lithium sensitive electrodes rather than the usual flame photometer method. A case record study of 827 manic-depressive or schizoaffective patients treated with lithium for more than 6 months showed that mortality was reduced to that of the general population (Müller-Oerlinghausen et al., 1992). A similar finding was reported by Coppen et al. (1991). However Vestergaard and Aagaard (1991) found a higher mortality over 5 years in 133 lithium-treated affective disorder patients than in the general population (Relative Risk 4.35). Of 22 deaths in this study, nine were suicide.

Adherence to treatment

In the UK the use of lithium is only about 0.8 per 1000 population, even in centres with active lithium clinics (McCreadie and Morrison, 1985); about half the patients who commenced on lithium discontinued it within 1 year, but a quarter remained on it for over 10 years. The patients who are less likely to adhere to treatment with lithium tend to be younger, male, and have had fewer previous episodes of illness. The reasons they give for stopping are: drug side effects, missing periods of elation, feeling well and in no need of treatment, feeling depressed or less productive, or not wanting to depend on medication. The side effects most often given as reasons for non-adherence are excessive thirst and polyuria, tremor, mem-ory impairment, and weight gain. A 5-year follow-up conducted in Naples of all patients commenced on lithium, showed only 23% continuing on it without recurrence for 5 years. Another 29% had continued lithium and suffered a recurrence but had a reduction in the amount of hospitalization by more than 50% compared to the pretreatment period. Only 39% of patients were managed for 5 years on lithium alone. Most of those who stopped lithium did so on their own initiative; the most common reasons given were: perceived ineffectiveness (37%), side effects (28%), no need for the medication (18%), found it inconvenient (12%), or felt a loss of drive (5%) (Maj et al., 1998).

In order to increase adherence (or the modern equivalent 'concordance'), the doctor should take side effects seriously, keep lithium levels as low as possible, educate the patients and their families about their illness and the use of lithium, and discuss adherence with the patient. For non-adherent patients, the regular contact provided by counselling or psychotherapy (e.g. cognitive-behavioural therapy) can be useful and has been shown to improve compliance and affective morbidity (Glick et al., 1985). It may be helpful to plot a 'life chart' with the patient.

Alternatives to lithium in prophylaxis

Even in favourable clinical trials, lithium prophylaxis was unsuccessful in over 30% of patients. More recent studies put the average failure rate much higher and alternative treatments are clearly needed (Prien and Gelenberg, 1989; Post, 1990). Many patients require a combination of mood stabilizers. The combination of lithium with an antipsychotic is common, but lithium may also be combined with carbamazepine. These combinations increase the risk of lithium neurotoxicity. The combination of lithium and valproate is probably the safest and often efficacious (Freeman and Stoll, 1998). These issues are considered further in Chapters 14, 15 and 16.

Conclusion

The discovery of lithium as a treatment for mania by Cade in 1949 can be regarded as the beginning of the modern era of effective drug treatments in psychiatry (Shorter, 1997). However, experience over the past 25 years indicates that lithium is far short of an ideal treatment even when administered expertly to 'concordant' patients. There is a striking difference between the results of early controlled trials and the outcome on lithium in open clinical practice. Some even doubt the validity of the clinical trials (Moncrieff, 1997). Lithium, the smallest metal cation, is a relatively crude treatment, substituting in many biological processes for the physiological cations sodium, potassium, calcium and magnesium. It has numerous side effects. The fact that it remains in widespread use testifies to the strength of evidence arising both from controlled trials and from extensive clinical experience. It is likely to remain in use until equally or more effective treatments with fewer side effects become available. The literature does now permit a more sophisticated view of the usefulness of lithium in bipolar illness. In most cases, patients will benefit from adjunctive therapies together with lithium, but in a substantial number, lithium is of little benefit. Alternative rather than adjunctive treatments would be appropriate.

How long should patients be treated with lithium before this is declared ineffective? The literature lacks a consensus definition of lithium non-responders. Schou (1968) suggests that lithium prophylaxis becomes more effective after the first year. It is unlikely, however, that a patient is benefiting from lithium treatment if his or her rate of cycling is unchanged after 2 years. At that time, a gradual discontinuation (no more than 300–600 mg per month) can be undertaken with continued monitoring. It is often difficult to assess the relationship between treatment and outcome simply by reviewing medical records. Mood charting provides a superior means of assessing the outcome of treatment and making this easily accessible to other doctors. With some encouragement most bipolar outpatients can chart their mood on a daily basis, as can some inpatients. Monthly mood charting by the clinician requires only a few seconds and aids greatly in assessing the outcome of treatment. Samples of a simple mood chart are shown in Figure 13.1.

Acknowledgement

We are grateful to Ms Marnie Sambur for her assistance in preparing this manuscript.

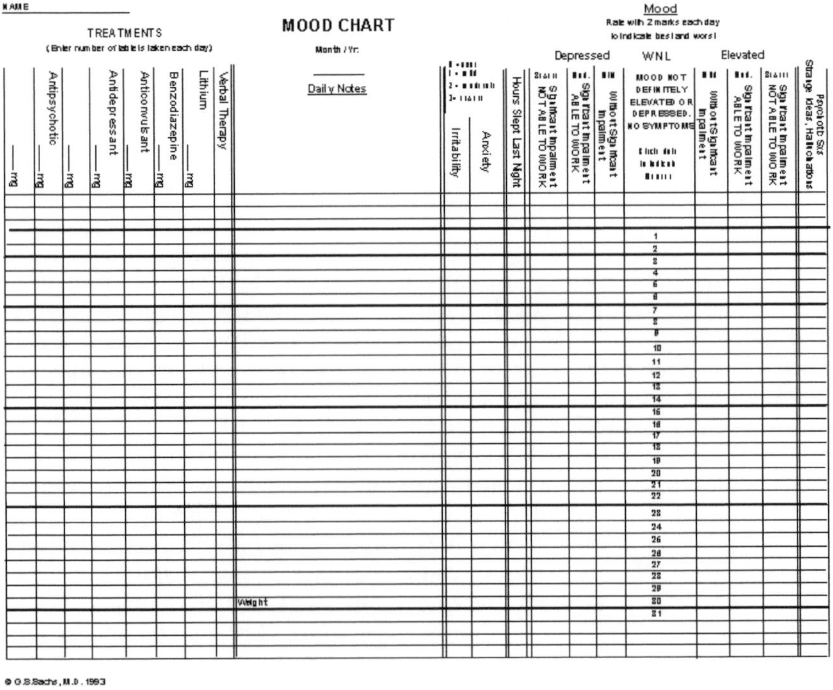

Figure 13.1 A simple mood chart

References

American Psychiatric Association (1997). Expert consensus guidelines are released for treatment of bipolar disorder. *Am. Fam. Phys.* **55**, 1447–1449.

Asnis, G.M., Asnis, D., Dunner, D.L., *et al.* (1979). Cogwheel rigidity during chronic lithium therapy. *Am. J. Psychiatry*, **136**, 1225–1226.

Baastrup, P.C., Poulsen, J.C., Schou, M., *et al.* (1970). Prophylactic lithium: Double-blind discontinuation in manic-depressive and recurrent-depressive disorder. *Lancet*, **2**, 326–330.

Baldessarini, R.J. (1970). Frequency of diagnoses of schizophrenia versus affective disorders from 1944 to 1968. *Am. J. Psychiatry*, **127**, 757–763.

Baldessarini, R.J., Tondo, L., Faedda, G.L., *et al.* (1996). Effects of the rate of discontinuing lithium maintenance treatment in bipolar disorders. *J. Clin. Psychiatry*, **57**, 441–448.

Birch, N.J., Horsman, A. and Hullin, R.P. (1982). Lithium, bone and body weight studies in long-term lithium-treated patients and in the rat. *Neuropsychobiology*, **8**, 86–92.

Blay, S.L., Toledo Ferraz, M.P. and Calil, H.M. (1982). Lithium-induced male sexual impairment: two case reports. *J. Clin. Psychiatry*, **43**, 497–498.

Bowden, C.L., Lecrubier, Y., Bauer, M., *et al.* (1999). Maintenance therapies and management of rapid cycling bipolar disorder. *J. Affect. Dis.* (in press).

Bowden, C.L., Brugger, A.M., Swann, A.C., *et al.* (1994). Efficacy of Divalproex vs. lithium and placebo in the treatment of mania. *J. Am. Med. Assoc.*, **271**, 918–924.

Bowen, R.C., Grof, P. and Grof, E. (1991). Less frequent lithium administration and lower urine volume. *Am. J. Psychiatry*, **148**, 189–192.

Bucht, G., Wahlin, A., Wentzel, T., *et al.* (1980). Renal function and morphology in long-term lithium and combined lithium–neuroleptic treatment. *Acta Med. Scand.*, **208**, 381–385.

Cade, J.F.J. (1949). Lithium salts in the treatment of psychotic excitement. *Med. J. Aust.*, **36**, 349–352.

Calabrese, J.R., Gulledge, A.D., Hahn, K., *et al.* (1985). Autoimmune thyroiditis in manic-depressive patients treated with lithium. *Am. J. Psychiatry*, **142**, 1318–1321.

Calabrese, J.R., Markovitz, P.J., Kimmel, S.E., *et al.* (1992). Spectrum of efficiency of valproate in 78 rapid-cycling bipolar patients. *J. Clin. Psychopharmacol.*, **12**, 53S–56S.

Charney, D.S., Kales, A., Soldatos, C., *et al.* (1979). Somnambulistic-like episode, secondary to contained lithium-neuroleptic treatment. *Brit. J. Psychiatry*, **135**, 418–424.

Clothier, J., Swann, A.C. and Freeman, T. (1992). Dysphoric mania. *J. Clin. Psychopharmacol.*, **12**, 13S–16S.

Cohen, L.S., Friedman, J.M., Jefferson, J.W., *et al.* (1994). A reevaluation of risk of in utero exposure to lithium. *J. Am. Med. Assoc*, **271**, 146–150.

Cohen, L.S., Sichel, D.A., Robertson, L.M., *et al.* (1995). Postpartum prophylaxis for women with bipolar disorder. *Am. J. Psychiatry*, **152**, 1641–1645.

Cohen, L.S. and Rosenbaum, J.F. (1998). Psychotropic drug use during pregnancy: weighing the risks. *J. Clin. Psychiatry*, **59** (Suppl. 2), 18–28.

Cohen, W.J. and Cohen, N.H. (1974). Lithium carbonate, haloperidol, and irreversible brain damage. *J. Am. Med. Assoc.*, **230**, 1283–1287.

Cookson, J.C. (1997). Lithium: balancing risks and benefits. *Brit. J. Psychiatry*, **171**, 120–124.

Cooper, J.E., Kendell, R.E., Gurland, B.J., *et al.* (1972). *Psychiatric Diagnosis in New York and London: A Comparative Study of Mental Hospital Admissions.* Maudsley Monograph No. 20. London, Oxford University Press.

Coppen, A. and Abou-Saleh, M.T. (1983). Lithium in prophylaxis of unipolar depression: a review. *J. Roy. Soc. Med.*, **76**, 297–301.

Coppen, A. and Abou-Saleh M.T. (1988). Lithium therapy: from clinical trials to practical management. *Acta Psychiatrica Scand.*, **78**, 754–762.

Coppen, A., Noguera, R., Bailey, J., *et al.* (1971). Prophylactic lithium in affective disorders: Controlled trial. *Lancet*, **2**, 275–279.

Coppen, A., Abou-Saleh, M.T., Milln, P., *et al.* (1983). Decreasing lithium dosage reduces morbidity and side effects during prophylaxis. *J. Affect. Dis.*, **5**, 353–362.

Coppen, A., Standish-Barry, H., Bailey, J., *et al.* (1991). Does lithium reduce the mortality of recurrent mood disorders? *J. Affect. Dis.*, **23**, 1–7.

Coryell, W., Solomon, D., Leon, A.C., *et al.* (1998). Lithium discontinuation and subsequent effectiveness. *Am. J. Psychiatry*, **155**, 895–898.

Cundall, R.L., Brooks, P.W., Murray, L.G. (1972). A controlled evaluation of lithium prophylaxis in affective disorders. *Psychol. Med.*, **2**, 308–311.

Dickson, W.E. and Kendell, R.E. (1986). Does maintenance lithium therapy prevent recurrences of mania under ordinary clinical conditions? *Psychol. Med.*, **16**, 521–530.

Dilsaver, S.C., Swann, A.C., Shoaib, A.M., *et al.* (1993). The manic syndrome: factors which may predict a patient's response to lithium, carbamazepine and valproate. *J. Psychiatric Neurosci.*, **18**, 61–66.

Dunner, D.L. and Fieve, R.R. (1974). Clinical factors in lithium prophylaxis failure. *Arch. Gen. Psychiatry*, **30**: 229–233.

Faedda, G.L., Baldessarini, R.J., Tohen, M., *et al.* (1991). Episode sequence in bipolar disorder and response to lithium treatment. *Am. J. Psychiatry*, **148**, 1237–1239.

Fieve, R.R., Platman, S.R., and Plutchick, R.R. (1968). The use of lithium in affective disorders I: Acute endogenous depression. *Am. J. Psychiatry*, **125**, 487–491.

Francis, A.J., Kahn, D.A., Carpenter, D., *et al.* (1998). The expert consensus guidelines for treating depression in bipolar disorder. *J. Clin. Psychiatry*, **59** (Suppl. 4), 73–79.

Freeman, T.W., Clothier, J.L., Pazzaglia, P., *et al.* (1992). A double-blind comparison of valproate and lithium in the treatment of acute mania. *Am. J. Psychiatry*, **149**, 108–111.

Freeman, M.P. and Stoll, A.L. (1998). Mood stabilizer combinations: a review of safety and efficacy. *Am. J. Psychiatry*, **155**, 12–21.

Gelenberg, A.J., Kane, J.M., Keller, M.B., *et al.* (1989). Comparison of standard and low serum levels of lithium for maintenance treatment of bipolar disorder. *New Eng. J. Med.*, **321**, 1489–1493.

Gillberg, I.C., Hellgren, L., Gillberg, C. (1993). Psychotic disorders diagnosed in adolescence: outcome at age 30 years. *J. Childh. Psychol. Psychiatry*, **34**, 1173–1185.

Glick, I.D., Clarkin, J.F., Spencer, J.H., *et al.* (1985). A controlled evaluation of inpatient family intervention: Preliminary results of the six-month follow-up. *Arch. Gen. Psychiatry*, **42**, 882–886.

Goodnick, P.J. and Meltzer, H.Y. (1984). Treatment of schizoaffective disorders. *Schizophrenia Bull.*, **10**, 30–48.

Goodwin, F.K. and Jamison, K.R. (1990). *Manic-Depressive Illness*. Oxford, Oxford University Press.

Goodwin, F.K., Murphy, D.C. and Bunney, W.F. (1969). Lithium carbonate treatment in depression and mania: a longitudinal double-blind study. *Arch. Gen. Psychiatry.*, **21**, 486–496.

Goodwin, G.M. (1994). Recurrence of mania after lithium withdrawal. Implications for the use of lithium in the treatment of bipolar affective disorder. *Brit. J. Psychiatry* **164**, 149–152.

Grof, P., Alda, M., Grof, E., *et al.* (1993). The challenge of predicting response to stabilising lithium treatment. *Brit. J. Psychiatry*, **163** (Suppl. 21), 16–19.

Hansen, H.E. and Amdisen, A. (1978). Lithium intoxication (Report of 23 cases and a review of 100 cases from the literature). *Q. J. Med.*, **47**, 123–144.

Hardy, B.G., Shulman, K.I., Mackenzie, S.E., *et al.* (1987). Pharmacokinetics of lithium in the elderly. *J. Clin. Psychopharmacol.*, **7**, 153–158.

Harrow, M., Goldberg, J.F., Grossman, L.S., *et al.* (1990). Outcome in manic disorder: a naturalistic follow-up study. *Arch. Gen. Psychiatry*, **47**, 665–671.

Hayes, S.G. (1989). Long-term use of valproate in psychiatric disorders. *J. Clin. Psychiatry*, **50** (Suppl.), 35–39.

Hestbech, J., Hansen, H.E., Amdisen, A. *et al.* (1977). Chronic real lesions following long-term treatment with lithium. *Kidney Int.*, **12**, 205–213.

Himmelhoch, J.M. (1987). Lest treatment abet suicide. *J. Clin. Psychiatry*, **48** (Suppl.), 44–54.

Himmelhoch, J.M. (1994). On the failure to recognize lithium failure. *Psychiatric Annl.*, **24**, 241–250.

Himmelhoch, J.M., Mulla, D., Neil, J.F., *et al*. (1976). Incidence and significance of mixed affective states in a bipolar population. *Arch. Gen. Psychiatry*, **33**, 1062–1066.

Himmelhoch, J.M., Neil, J.F., May, S.J., *et al*. (1980). Age, dementia, dyskinesias, and lithium response. *Am. J. Psychiatry*, **137**, 941–945.

Himmelhoch, J.M. and Garfinkel, M.E. (1986). Sources of lithium resistance in mixed mania. *Psychopharmacol. Bull.*, **22**, 613–620.

Holinger, P.C. and Wolpert, E. A. (1979). A ten-year follow-up of lithium use. *Irish Med. J.*, **156**, 99–104.

Jacobson, S.J., Jones, K., Johnson, K., *et al*. (1992). Prospective multi-centre study of pregnancy outcome after lithium exposure during first trimester. *Lancet*, **339**, 530–533.

Jamison, K.R. (1994). *Touched with Fire: Manic-Depressive Illness and the Artistic Temperament*. Simon and Shuster, New York.

Jann, M.W., Bitar, A. H. and Rao, A. (1982). Lithium prophylaxis of tricyclic-antidepressant-induced mania in bipolar patients. *Am. J. Psychiatry*, **139**, 683–684.

Jha, A.K., Stein, G.S. and Fenwick, P. (1996). Negative interaction between lithium and electroconvulsion therapy. A case-controlled study. *Br J. Psychiatry*, **168**, 241–243.

Johnson, D.A.W., Lowe, M.R. and Batchelor, D.H. (1990). Combined lithium-neuroleptic therapy for manic-depressive illness. *Hum. Psychopharmacol.*, **5** (Suppl), 262–297.

Johnson, G. (1984). Lithium. *Med. J. Aust.*, **141**, 595–601.

Johnson, F.N. (1984). *The History of Lithium Therapy*. London, MacMillan.

Kallen, B. and Tandberg, A. (1983). Lithium and pregnancy: a cohort study on manic-depressive women. *Acta Psychiatrica Scand.*, **68**, 134–139.

Kane, J.M., Quitkin, F.M., Rifkin, A. (1982). Lithium carbonate and imipramine in the prophylaxis of unipolar and bipolar II illness. *Arch. Gen. Psychiatry*, **39**, 1065–1069.

Keck, P.E., McElroy, S.L., Tugrul, K.C., *et al*. (1993). Valproate oral loading in the treatment of acute mania. *J. Clin. Psychiatry*, **54**, 305–308.

Keller, M.B., Lavori, P.W., Coryell, W., *et al*. (1986). Differential outcome of pure manic, mixed/cycling, and pure depressive episodes in patients with bipolar illness. *J. Am. Med. Assoc.*, **255**, 3138–3142.

Keller, M.A., Lavori, P.W., Kane, J.M., *et al*. (1992). Subsyndromal symptoms in bipolar disorder. A comparison of standard and low serum levels of lithium. *Arch. Gen. Psychiatry*, **49**, 31–376.

Kellner, C.H., Pritchett, J.T., Beale, M.D., *et al*. (1997). *Handbook of ECT*. Washington, American Psychiatric Press.

King, J.R. and Hullin, R.P. (1983). Withdrawal symptoms from lithium: four case reports and a questionnaire study. *Brit. J. Psychiatry*, **143**, 30–35.

Kirkwood, C.K., Wilson, S.K., Hayes, P.E., *et al*. (1994). Single-dose bioavailability of two extended-release lithium carbonate products. *Am. J. Hosp. Pharmacol.*, **51**, 486–489.

Knox, A.J., Higgins, B.G., Hall, I.P., *et al*. (1992). Effect of oral lithium on bronchial reactivity in asthma. *Clin. Sci.*, **82**, 407–412.

Kramlinger, K.G. and Post, R.M. (1996). Ultra-rapid and ultradian cycling in bipolar affective illness. *B. J. Psychiatry*, **168**, 314–323.

Kukopulos, A. and Reginaldi, D. (1973). Does lithium prevent depressions by suppressing mania? *Int. Pharmacopsychiatry*, **8**, 152–158.

Kukopulos, A., Reginaldi, D., Laddoma, P., *et al*. (1980). Course of the manic-depressive cycle and changes caused by treatment. *Pharmakopsychiatric Neuropsychopharmacol.*, **13**, 156–167.

Lawler, P.G. and Cove-Smith, J.R. (1986). Acute respiratory failure following lithium intoxication. *Anaesthesia*, **41**, 623–627.

Lazarus, J.H., John, R., Bennie, E.H., *et al*. (1981). Lithium therapy and thyroid function: a long-term study. *Psychol. Med.*, **11**, 85–92.

Licht, R.W., Gouliaev, G., Vestergaard, P., *et al*., (1994). Treatment of manic episodes in Scandinavia; the use of neuroleptic drugs in a clinical routine setting. *J. Affective Disorders*, **32**, 179–185.

Llewellyn, A., Stowe, Z.N. and Strader, J.R. (1998). The use of lithium and management of women with bipolar disorder during pregnancy and lactation. *J. Clin. psychiatry*, **59** (Suppl. 6), 57–64.

Loudon, J.B. and Waring, H. (1976). Toxic reactions to lithium and haloperidol. *Lancet*, **2**, 1088.

Maggs, R. (1963). Treatment of manic illness with lithium carbonate. *B. J. Psychiatry*, **109**, 56–65.

Maj, M., Pirozzi, R., Magliano, L., *et al.* (1998). Long-term outcome of lithium prophylaxis in bipolar disorder: a 5-year prospective study of 402 patients at a lithium clinic. *Am. J. Psychiatry*, **155**, 30–35.

Mander, A.J. and Loudon, J.B. (1988). Rapid recurrence of mania following abrupt discontinuation of lithium. *Lancet*, ii, 15–17.

McCreadie, R.G. and Morrison, D.P. (1985). The impact of lithium in South-West Scotland. *Br. J. Psychiatry*, **146**, 70–74.

McElroy, S.L., Keck, P.E., Pope, H.G., *et al.* (1992). Clinical and research implications of the diagnosis of dysphoric or mixed mania or hypomania. *Am. J. Psychiatry*, **149**, 1633–1644.

McElroy, S.L., Keck, P.E., Tugrul, K.C., *et al.* (1993). Valproate as a loading treatment in acute mania. *Neuropsychobiology*, **27**, 146–149.

McElroy, S.L., Keck, P.E. and Strakowshi, S.M. (1996). Mania, psychosis and antipsychotics. *J. Clin. Psychiatry*, **57** (Suppl. 3), 14–26.

McFarland, B.H., Miller, M.R. and Straumfjord, A.A. (1990). Valproate use in the older manic patient. *J. Clin. Psychiatry*, **51**, 479–481.

Mitchell, J.E. and MacKenzie, T.B. (1982). Cardiac effects of lithium therapy in man: a review. *J. Clin. Psychiatry*, **43**, 47–51.

Moncrieff, J. (1977). Lithium: evidence reconsidered. *Br. J. Psychiatry*, **171**, 113–119.

Montgomery, S.A. and Roberts, A. (1994). SSRIs: well-tolerated treatment for depression. *Hum. Psychopharmacol.*, **9**, S7–S10.

Müller-Oerlinghausen, B., Ahren, B., Grof, E., *et al.* (1992). The effects of long-term lithium treatment on the mortality of patients with manic-depressive and schizo-affective illness. *Acta Psychiatrica Scand.*, **86**, 218–222.

Murphy, D.L. and Beigel, A. (1974). Depression, elation, and lithium carbonate responses in manic patient sub-groups. *Arch. Gen. Psychiatry*, **31**, 643–648.

Myers, D.H., Carter, R.A., Burns, B.H., *et al.* (1985). A prospective study of the effects of lithium on thyroid function and on the prevalence of thyroid antibodies. *Psychol. Med.*, **15**, 55–61.

Nilsson, A. (1998). Does lithium reduce suicide rates in recurrent mood disorders. Presented at the XXIst CINP Congress, Glasgow 1998.

Noack, C.H. and Trautner, E.M. (1951). The lithium treatment of maniacal psychosis. *Med. J. Aust.*, **2**, 219–222.

Norton, B. and Whalley, L.J. (1984). Mortality of a lithium-treated population. *Br. J. Psychiatry*, **145**, 277–282.

Pitts, C.D., Young, M.L., Oakes, R., *et al.* (1997) Comparative safety of paroxetine versus imipramine in the treatment of bipolar depression. Presented at the American Psychiatric Association annual meeting, San Diego.

Poole, A.J., James, H.D. and Hughes, W. C. (1978). Treatment experience in the lithium clinic at St Thomas' Hospital. *J. Roy. Soc. Med.*, **71**, 890–894.

Post, R.M. (1990). Prophylaxis of bipolar disorders. *Int. Rev. Psychiatry*, **2**, 227–320.

Post, R.M., Uhde, T.W., Roy-Byrne, P.P., *et al.* (1987). Correlates of antimanic responses to carbamazepine. *Psychiatry Res.*, **21**, 71–83.

Post, R.M., Rubinow, D.R., Uhde, T.W., *et al.* (1989). Dysphoric mania: Clinical and biological correlates. *Arch. Gen. Psychiatry*, **46**, 353–358.

Price, L.H., Charney, D.S. and Heninger, G.R. (1984). Manic symptoms following addition of lithium to antidepressant treatment. *J. Clin. Psychopharmacol.*, **4**, 361–362.

Prien, R.F., Caffey, E.M. Jr and Klett, C.J. (1973). Prophylactic efficacy of lithium carbonate in manic-depressive illness. *Arch. Gen. Psychiatry*, **28**, 337–341.

Prien, R.F., Kupfer, D.J., Mansky, P.A., *et al.* (1984). Drug therapy in the prevention of recurrences in unipolar and bipolar affective disorder: report of the NIMH Collaborative Study Group comparing lithium carbonate, imipramine, and a lithium carbonate-imipramine combination. *Arch. Gen. Psychiatry*, **41**, 1096–1104.

Prien, R.F. and Gelenberg, A.J. (1989). Alternatives to lithium for preventive treatment of bipolar disorder. *Am. J. Psychiatry*, **146**, 840–848.

Quitkin, F.M., Kane, J., Rifkin, A., *et al.* (1981). Prophylactic lithium carbonate with and without imipramine for bipolar I patients: A double-blind study. *Arch. Gen. Psychiatry*, **38**, 902–907.

Schou, M. (1968). Lithium in psychiatric therapy and prophylaxis. *J. Psychiatric Res.*, **6**, 67–95.

Schou, M. (1976). What happened later to the lithium babies: a follow-up study of children born without malformations. *Acta Psychiatricia Scand.*, **54**, 193–197.

Schou, M. (1979). Artistic productivity and lithium prophylaxis in manic-depressive illness. *Br. J. Psychiatry*, **135**, 97–103.

Schou, M. (1984). Long-lasting neurological sequelae after lithium intoxication. *Acta Psychiatrica Scand.*, **70**, 594–602.

Schou, M., Juel-Nielson, N., Stromgren, E., *et al.* (1954). The treatment of manic psychoses by administration of lithium salts. *J. Neurol. Neurosurg. Psychiatry*, **17**, 250–260.

Secunda, S.K., Katz, M.M., Swann, A., *et al.* (1985). Mania: diagnosis, state measurement and prediction of treatment response. *J. Affect. Dis.*, **8**, 113–121.

Secunda, S.K., Cross, C.K., Koslow, S., *et al.* (1986). Biochemistry and suicidal behavior in depressed patients. *Biol. Psychiatry*, **21**, 756–767.

Secunda, S.K., Swann, A., Katz, M.M., *et al.* (1987). Diagnosis and treatment of mixed mania. *Am. J. Psychiatry*, **144**, 96–98.

Sellers, J., Tyrer, P., Whiteley, A., *et al.* (1982). Neurotoxic effects of lithium with delayed rise in serum lithium levels. *Br. J. Psychiatry*, **140**, 623–625.

Shapiro, D.R., Quitkin, F.M. and Fleiss, J.L. (1989). Response to maintenance therapy in bipolar illness. Effect of index episode. *Arch. Gen. Psychiatry*, **46**, 401–405.

Shelley, R.K. and Silverstone, T. (1986). Single dose pharmacokinetics of 5 formulations of lithium: a controlled comparison in healthy subjects. *Int. Clin. Psychopharmacol.*, **1**, 324–331.

Shorter, E. (1997). *A History of Psychiatry: from the Asylum to the Age of Prozac.* New York: John Wiley & Sons.

Smith, S.J.M. and Kocen, R.S. (1988). A Creutzfeldt-Jakob like syndrome due to lithium toxicity. *J. Neurol. Neurosurg. Psychiatry*, **158**, 120–123.

Souza, F.G.M. and Goodwin, G.M. (1991). Lithium treatment and prophylaxis in unipolar depression: a meta-analysis. *Br. J. Psychiatry*, **158**, 666–675.

Squillace, K., Post, R.M., Savard, R., *et al.* (1984). Life charting of the longitudinal course of recurrent affective illness. In: *Neurobiology of Mood Disorders* (R.M. Post and J.C. Ballenger, eds), Baltimore, Williams & Wilkins, pp. 38–59.

Stancer, H.C. and Forbath, N. (1989). Hyperparathyroidism, hypothyroidism, and impaired renal function after 10 to 20 years of lithium treatment. *Arch. Int. Med.*, **149**, 1042–1045.

Steckler, T.L. (1994). Lithium- and carbamazepine-associated sinus node dysfunction: nine-year experience in a psychiatric hospital. *J. Clin. Psychopharmacol.*, **14**, 336–339.

Stewart, P.M., Atherden, S.M., Stewart, S.E., *et al.* (1988). Lithium carbonate – a competitive aldosterone antagonist? *Br. J. Psychiatry*, **153**, 205–207.

Stokes, P.E., Shamoian, C.A., Stoll, P.M., *et al.* (1971). Efficacy of lithium as acute treatment of manic-depressive illness. *Lancet*, **1**, 1319–1325.

Stoll, A.L., Tohen, M., Baldessarini, R.J., *et al.* (1993). Shifts in diagnostic frequencies of schizophrenia and major affective disorders at six North American Psychiatric hospitals, 1972–1988. *Am. J. Psychiatry*, **150**, 1668–1673.

Stone, K. (1989). Mania in the elderly. *Br. J. Psychiatry*, **155**, 220–224.

Suppes, T., Baldessarini, R., Faedda, G.L., *et al.* (1991). Risk of recurrence following disconti-nuation of lithium treatment in bipolar disorder. *Arch. Gen. Psychiatry*, **48**, 1082–1088.

Swann, A.C., Secunda, S.K., Katz, M.M., *et al.* (1986). Lithium treatment of mania: clinical characteristics, specificity of symptom change, and outcome. *Psychiatry Res.*, **18**, 127–141.

Thisted, E. and Ebbesen, F. (1993). Malformations, withdrawal manifestations and hypogly-caemia after exposure to vaproate in utero. *Arch. Dis. Childh.*, **69**, 288–291.

Thornhill, D.P. and Field, S.P. (1982). Distribution of lithium elimination in a selected population of psychiatric patients. *Eur. J. Clin. Pharmacol.*, **21**, 351–354.

Tondo, L., Baldessarini, R.J., Hennen, J., *et al.* (1998). Lithium maintenance treatment of depression and mania in bipolar I and bipolar II disorders. *Am. J. Psychiatry*, **155**, 638–646.

Transbol, I, Christiansen, C. and Baastrup, P.C. (1978). Endocrine effects of lithium: I. Hypothyroidism, its prevalence in long-term treated patients. *Acta Endocrinol.*, **87**, 759–767.

Tyrer, P., Alexander, M.S., Regan, A., *et al.* (1980). An extrapyramindal syndrome after lithium therapy. *Brit. J. Psychiatry*, **136**, 191–194.

Vestergaard, P., Amdisen, A. and Schou, M. (1980). Clinically significant side effects of lithium treatment. A survey of 237 patients in long-term treatment. *Acta Psychiatrica Scand.*, **62**, 193–200.

Vestergaard, P. and Aagaard, J. (1991). Five-year mortality in lithium-treated manic-depressive patients. *J. Affect. Dis.*, **21**, 33–38.

Von Knorring, L. (1990). Possible mechanisms for the presumed interaction between lithium and neuroleptics. *Hum. Psychopharmacol.*, **5**, 287–292.

Waller, D.G. and Edwards, J.G. (1989). Lithium and the kidney: an update. *Psychol. Med.*, **19**, 825–831.

Wehr, T.A. and Goodwin, F.K. (1979). Rapid cycling in manic-depressives induced by tricyclic antidepressants. *Arch. Gen. Psychiatry*, **36**, 555–559.

Wehr, R.A., Sack, D.A., Rosenthal, N.E., *et al.* (1988). Rapid cycling affective disorder: contributing factors and treatment responses in 51 patients. *Am. J. Psychiatry*, **145**, 179–184.

Weinstein, M.R. and Goldfield, M.D. (1973). Lithium carbonate in obstetrics: guidelines for clinical use. *Am. J. Obstet. Gynecol.*, **116**, 15–22.

West, A.P. and Meltzer, H.Y. (1979). Paradoxical lithium neurotoxicity: a report of five cases and a hypothesis about risk for neurotoxicity. *Am. J. Psychiatry*, **136**, 963–966.

Wood, A.J. and Goodwin, G.M. (1987). A review of the biochemical and neuropharmacological actions of lithium. *Psychol., Med.*, **17**, 579–600.

Worrall, E.P., Moody, J.P., Peet, M., *et al.* (1979). Controlled studies of the acute antidepressant effects of lithium. *Brit. J. Psychiatry*, **135**, 255–262.

Yassa, R., Saunders, A., Nastase, C., *et al.* (1988). Lithium induced thyroid disorders: a prevalence study. *J. Clin. Psychiatry*, **49**, 14–16.

Zornberg, G.L. and Pope, H.G. (1993). Treatment of depression in bipolar disorder: new directions for research. *J. Clin. Psychopharmacol.*, **13**, 397–408.

14

Carbamazepine and valproate: use in mood disorders

Charles Bowden and Bruno Müller-Oerlinghausen

Key points

- Valproate and carbamazepine have extensive research based evidence of benefit for bipolar disorder treatment.
- Valproate acts somewhat more rapidly than lithium or carbamazepine in acute mania.
- Carbamazepine and valproate are probably more effective than lithium for bipolar disorder secondary to neurological conditions and some other atypical forms.
- Antisuicidal action has been shown for lithium, not however for carbamazepine or valproate long-term treatment.
- Carbamazepine has risk of allergic skin reaction, and requires gradual dosage escalation. It is contraindicated during pregnancy.
- Valproate can cause gastrointestinal irritability and weight gain. It is contraindicated during pregnancy.
- These two drugs provide important therapeutic options for bipolar disorder, and have contributed to increased study of other drugs first studied as antiepileptic agents.

Introduction

Valproate and carbamazepine represent the first two, and most extensively studied of a group of medications initially approved as anti-epileptic compounds that have been shown to have antimanic and, probably, mood stabilizing properties. Although each drug is reviewed separately in this chapter, several factors common to these two drugs warrant discussion. The interest in these drugs sprang from recognition that lithium was of particular benefit in a subgroup of patients with affective disorders and that its specific adverse effect profile constrained its utility (Stokes *et al.*, 1971). The first published study of valproate in bipolar disorder appeared prior to regulatory approval of lithium for acute mania.

Whereas early open reports of valproate and carbamazepine were consistently positive in bipolar disorder, particularly for treatment of acute mania, recent research has differed for the two compounds, with more randomized placebo-controlled studies of valproate. Recognition of the utility of both drugs in the case of bipolar disorder has contributed to increased research interest in the disorder on two fronts. Pharmaceutical companies have become keenly interested in the potential of other drugs initially studied as treatments for epilepsy. There is also increased interest in factors associated with response or non-response to a treatment, in part stemming from evidence that the predictors may differ across drugs.

History

Lithium is considered the first rank drug for episode-preventive treatment of bipolar patients in the USA as well as in Europe. Nevertheless, lithium is not efficacious in all patients and its effectiveness can be markedly lowered by selecting the wrong patients (e.g. with atypical psychopathology), by non-compliance, or by troubling side effects (Grof et al., 1993; Grof, 1998). Among alternatives, several anticonvulsants at present possess the greatest therapeutic benefits. Most likely diphenylhydantoin was the first anticonvulsant tried – with little success in endogenous psychoses (Kalinowsky and Putnam, 1943). The benefit for manic episodes of valproate, which chemically is dipropylacetic acid, was first described by French investigators (Lambert et al., 1966, 1975) and was confirmed over the next two decades by a consistently positive series of both open trial and randomized, prospective, placebo-controlled studies (Pope et al., 1991; Emrich and Wolf, 1992; Bowden et al., 1994). Independently of Lambert, Japanese researchers reported some years later on the antimanic effects of carbamazepine (CBZ) (Takezaki and Hanaoka, 1971). Acute and prophylactic effects of CBZ in patients with affective disorders were observed in a large number of patients by Okuma et al. (1973, 1979) who also reported that CBZ had a more pronounced preventive effect on manic than on depressive episodes. The replication of these preliminary findings in a small, crossover placebo-controlled study, by Ballenger and Post (1980), on the acute antimanic effect stimulated further clinical studies of CBZ in bipolar spectrum disorders. In 1983 Post et al. reported some prophylactic benefits of CBZ in bipolar patients, although more recent studies suggest lesser effectiveness for prophylaxis when used as monotherapy (Post et al., 1983; Dardennes et al., 1995; Denicoff et al., 1997; Greil et al., 1997a). Oxcarbazepine, the keto-derivative of carbamazepine and valproate was also shown to be effective as an antimanic agent (Emrich et al., 1984; Cabrera et al., 1986).

Carbamazepine

Indications

Open studies suggest that CBZ possesses episode-preventive efficacy in recurrent affective disorders, preferentially bipolar patients. Based on double-blind comparator studies comprising 284 patients, equal prophylactic efficacy of CBZ and lithium was claimed by several authors (Placidi et al., 1986; Simhandl and Denk, 1994). However, these studies had several methodological limitations such as small samples, inclusion of lithium non-responders or rapid cyclers, short observation periods, and analyses limited to study completers. A meta-analysis of four such studies (Dardennes et al., 1995) concluded that equipotency of CBZ and lithium was not supported and that efficacy of CBZ appeared to be less than that of lithium. Other authors have also questioned the long-term efficacy of CBZ (Murphy et al., 1989). However, several authors found carbamazepine superior to lithium in rapid cyclers (Emrich, 1990). The largest prospective, randomized, open trial comparing the prophylactic efficacy of CBZ and lithium as monotherapy has recently been completed. Over a 2.5-year period, lithium was superior to CBZ in 171 bipolar patients (DSM-IV). The statistical significance differed according to the selected outcome criteria (Greil et al., 1997a). The relative efficacy of lithium was greatest in the subgroup of 67 'classical' patients, i.e. bipolar I without mood-incongruent delusions and without comorbidity (Greil et al., 1998). For the 'non-classical' group a trend in favour of CBZ was found. Secondary data also suggested that rapid-cycling, mixed states, or mood incongruent delusions predict a somewhat better response to CBZ than to lithium. Among the 90 schizoaffective patients (ICD-9), outcome with CBZ was better than with lithium in those with more schizophrenia-like or depressive disorders, but not in patients fulfilling DSM-III-R criteria of bipolar disorder. Lithium and CBZ were generally equivalent in the maintenance treatment of more broadly defined schizoaffective disorders (Greil et al., 1997b). Preliminary findings from a recently completed randomized, double-blind, 1-year study in 168 bipolar patients suggest 'non-inferiority' of CBZ compared to lithium within a 15% confidence interval (Berky et al., 1998). Premature discontinuation due to severe adverse drug reactions, especially dermatological, are more than twice as common in the CBZ-treated groups (Greil et al., 1997a; Berky et al., 1998). In the aggregate these studies provide some evidence that CBZ is more beneficial than lithium in patients with non-classical bipolar disorder, mixed states, or rapid-cycling. The data suggest lesser efficacy for CBZ than lithium in classical bipolar patients.

Carbamazepine has also been used successfully as an adjunct to antipsychotic medication in schizophrenic patients, although it markedly reduces the plasma level of haloperidol and other neuroleptics (Dose et al., 1987; Goff and Baldessarini, 1993). Carbamazepine may be tried in patients with agitated or aggressive behaviour including those with dementia (Barratt, 1993; Tariot et al., 1998).

In the MAP-study, six suicidal acts occurred in the CBZ-group, whereas none occurred in the lithium group (Thies-Flechtner et al., 1996). This effectiveness of lithium in reducing suicidal behaviour is in accord with most other reports (Tondo et al., 1997; Schou, 1998). We therefore suggest that in an apparent lithium non-responder who has a history of suicide attempts and for whom a trial of CBZ seems indicated, lithium should not be discontinued, but that CBZ should be added to lithium in order to maintain an antisuicidal effect (Nilsson and Axelsson, 1990; Müller-Oerlinghausen et al., 1992; Müller-Oerlinghausen et al., 1996).

Several open case reports, and retrospective studies suggest that lithium/CBZ combination therapy is often effective for patients not responding to monotherapy with either lithium or CBZ. With one exception (Fritze et al., 1994), the findings suggest a superior effect of the combination as compared to monotherapy (Nolen, 1983; Ballenger, 1988; Di Costanzo and Schifano, 1991; Peselow et al., 1994).

Adverse effects

Initially, gastrointestinal effects, headache, dizziness or visual disturbances are observed. Such adverse effects are dose-dependent. Elderly patients may develop cardiac arrhythmia, or confusional states. Allergic skin reactions occur frequently and amount to around 10% of the total of observed side effects in carbamazepine-treated subjects. Severe complications such as Steven-Johnson-syndrome or Lyell-syndrome were reported occasionally (Tennis and Stern, 1997). Mild leukopenia or thrombocytopenia as well as increases of liver transaminases can be observed. The risk of severe neural tube defects if used during the first trimester of pregnancy is 0.5–1.0% (Lindhout and Omtzigt, 1992).

Dosing, monitoring, and interactions

For maintenance treatment the dose of CBZ should be titrated only slowly, i.e. within 2–4 weeks, to the required serum level in order to avoid initial neuromuscular side effects and unnecessary drop outs. A CBZ serum level, assessed 12 hours after intake of last tablet, should be aimed at achieving a serum level of 6–10 µg/ml. This will usually be achieved by administering a daily dose of 600–1200 mg/day (in 3–4 fractions). In view of the short half-life, shortened additionally under prolonged treatment by the auto enzyme inducing effect of CBZ, sustained release preparations should be preferred for long-term medication. When switching patients from lithium to CBZ it is advisable not to stop lithium abruptly, but to taper its serum level down and dose up CBZ at the same time in an overlapping mode. The accepted ranges of serum levels for both compounds (lithium 0.6–0.8 mmol/l; CBZ 6–10 µg/ml) can usually be maintained when combining them, although in some susceptible patients (see below) neurotoxic symptoms may require reduced serum levels. Necessary controls include blood cell counts, including platelet counts, and liver as well as coagulation function tests (weekly during the first month, later on at monthly intervals). Medication should be discontinued in case of dermatological reactions, leukopenia, thrombocytopenia (< 50 000/ mm³), or γ-GT values beyond 80 µ/l. Carbamazepine induction of hepatic enzyme 3A4 results in subtherapeutic activities of drugs solely or principally metabolized by this oxidative enzyme isoform (e.g. alprazolam, bupropion, oral contraceptives, nefazodone, fluvoxamine) (Spina et al., 1996).

Valproate

Valproate has been established as significantly superior to placebo in alleviation of acute manic episodes in two random, double-blind studies in which no neuroleptics were allowed and only limited, brief use of benzodiazepine was permitted (Pope et al., 1991; Bowden et al., 1994). Both studies were conducted in patients whose illnesses were sufficiently severe to require hospitalization. The study by Bowden et al. included a lithium comparator group and is the largest placebo-controlled study of lithium in acute mania. In the aggregate, lithium and divalproex were similarly effective. Onset of response was somewhat earlier among those treated with divalproex and

Table 14.1 Dosing, controls, precautions for carbamazepine and valproate (modified according to Emrich and Dietrich, 1997)

	Carbamazepine (CBZ)	Valproate
Daily dose (mg/day)	600–1200	500–3000
Plasma level (μg/ml)	6–10	45–110
Initial dose (mg)	200	250 tid to 30 mg/kg
Increase of single dose (mg)	100–200 every 1–3 days	200–500 every 1–3 days
Contraindications	Atrioventricular block, pregnancy (first trimester), preceding bone marrow disorder	Hepatic dysfunction, pregnancy (first trimester)
Lab controls	Blood cell and platelet counts, liver and coagulation tests	As for CBZ; plus amylase activity
Withdrawal in case of	Allergic reactions, marked leukopenia, or thrombopenia, γ-GT > 80 U/l	GI symptoms, nausea, vomiting of unknown aetiology

magnitude of improvement on some key disturbed behaviour (e.g., reduced need for sleep) was greater with divalproex than lithium (Bowden, 1996). Serum levels above 45 μg (315 nmol/ml) were associated with greater likelihoods of improvement in both studies (Bowden et al., 1996).

Open reports of valproate in the prophylaxis of bipolar disorder indicate reduction in both the frequency and intensity of episodes, with suggestion of greater benefit on manic symptomatology (Puzynski and Klosiewicz, 1984; Klosiewicz, 1985; Calabrese et al., 1992). No placebo-controlled trials have been published. A 1-year maintenance trial of divalproex compared to placebo and lithium has been completed and is in preparation for publication (Bowden et al., 1997).

Predictors of response

Two studies have shown that divalproex was more effective than lithium in patients with mixed manic episodes (Freeman et al., 1992; Bowden, 1995; Swann et al., 1997). Further analysis of the study by Bowden et al. indicated that presence of two or more purely depressive symptoms distinguished patients with poor response to lithium, and suggest that such criteria may be more useful than the DSM-IV criteria for mixed mania (Swann et al., 1997). Acutely manic rapid-cycling patients responded as well as did non-rapid-cycling patients (Bowden et al., 1994). Whereas an increased lifetime number of episodes was associated with non-response to lithium, the response to divalproex remained superior to placebo independent of number of episodes of mania or depression. Response to divalproex and lithium was equivalent and superior to placebo among patients with eight or fewer lifetime episodes (Swann et al., 1999). An open, non-comparative study also reported high rates of response of rapid-cycling patients (Calabrese and Delucchi, 1990). Approximately half of the patients received concurrent lithium.

Open reports indicate that valproate is also effective in patients with hypomanic states and cyclothymic disorders (Lambert, 1984; Jocobsen, 1993). Numerous reports of valproate's effectiveness in a range of conditions which display some but not all of the DSM-IV criteria for bipolar disorder have been published. In general, those reports suggest that impulsive aggressive behaviour, especially if episodically occurring, regardless of episode duration, may benefit (Sival et al., 1994; Puryear et al., 1995; Bowden, 1998).

Valproate is effective in reduction of frequency of migraine headaches (Silberstein et al., 1993; Jensen et al., 1994), which is highly associated with bipolar disorder (Breslau et al., 1994). It is approved by the FDA for this use in the USA. Small case series suggest that panic attacks and bulimia, also comorbidly occurring with bipolar disorder, may benefit from valproate (Lum et al., 1990; Primeau et al., 1990).

Adverse effects

Tolerability and adverse effect experiences derived from the longer, more extensive use of valproate and carbamazepine in the treatment of epilepsy are generally relevant to their use in bipolar disorder. Valproate is well tolerated, both acutely and chronically, with low rates of cognitive and sensory impairment. Adverse events more common with divalproex than with placebo were nausea and reduced platelet count (Bowden et al., 1994). The reduction of platelet count and white blood count is positively correlated with serum level of valproate; therefore reduction in dosage may ameliorate such lowering. The gastrointestinal irritant effect of valproate is lower with the divalproex form of valproate than with sodium valproate (Wilder et al., 1983). Valproate may cause hair loss, probably secondary to chelation of trace metals such as selenium and zinc. Separation of valproate dosing from meals or vitamin use by several hours may eliminate the problem, as may supplementing with a multiple vitamin containing selenium and zinc. Valproate can elevate hepatic enzyme activity and has been associated with hepatic failure. Hepatic failure secondary to valproate use has been reported in persons under the age of 2 years, but not in persons older than 2 years of age. Cautious use of valproate is indicated in the presence of active level hepatic disease. In recent placebo-controlled acute and 1-year maintenance trials hepatic enzyme levels did not increase with valproate treatment, despite consistently high serum levels of around 85 µg/ml (595 nmol/ml). Valproate (as well as carbamazepine) is associated with an increased risk of neural tube defects (1–2%) if used during the first trimester of pregnancy, and its use is therefore discouraged for this period (Lindhout and Omtzigt, 1992). Valproate is present in much reduced concentration in breast-fed infants; therefore, it might be safely taken by a mother breast-feeding her child.

Dosing

For treatment of mania, valproate is started at 250 mg tid. If GI tolerability is satisfactory, as is usually the case with the divalproex formulation, dosing can be started at 20–30 mg/kg/day, which will yield a generally therapeutic serum level of 45 µg/315 mm or greater within 2 days. This results in significant improvement within 3 days, which is probably a bit faster than improvement within 5–7 days observed without a loading dose approach. Dosage can be adjusted based on day 3–5 serum levels to achieve a serum level between 45 and 110 µg/ml. There is no linear relationship with response within that range, but patients with less than satisfactory responses at the lower end of the range can usually tolerate well an increase to the higher end of the range. Characteristic adverse events become more prevalent above 100 µg/ml. Case series suggest that patients with comorbid neurological disorder may require somewhat higher levels, whereas patients with hypomania somewhat lower levels (Sovner, 1989; Jacobsen, 1993). Valproate levels are only moderately affected by drugs that inhibit hepatic oxidative enzymes. However, free valproate levels are transiently increased by the many psychotropic drugs that bind substantially to plasma proteins, or even by a fatty meal.

Maintenance dosing

Maintenance therapy dosing for valproate is empirically rather than experimentally based. Most studies have continued serum levels similar to those established during treatment for acute mania. Empirically, it is our practice to maintain serum levels at the same levels as needed for acute episodes, but to lower dosage if any serious or functionally impairing side effects develop. We do this because full tolerability is a primary goal for lifelong prophylaxis. If the lowered dose does not retain full prophylactic efficacy, we add another drug, most often lithium, an atypical antipsychotic, or lamotrigine rather than force a poorly tolerated dosage of either valproate or carbamazepine.

Maintenance therapy guidelines for carbamazepine are similar to acute treatment guidelines. Patients who get beyond the dosage adjustment phase of carbamazepine treatment generally have fewer neuromuscular adverse effects than they experienced acutely, which is the converse of the poorer long-term tolerability often associated with lithium therapy.

Future role

In the USA, divalproex will continue to gain broader use, both for mania and maintenance treatment, generally as the first choice drug. Its compatibility with other drugs will result in extensive combined drug therapy. Most use will be as single daily dosing. Use will broaden diagnostically to include some patients with episodic, impulsive irritability and aggressive behaviours, largely independent of syndromal diagnosis.

In Europe, use of valproate will continue to be as a second choice drug unless regulatory approval of divalproex or other forms of valproate with good gastrointestinal tolerability occur. Less long-term use of valproate will occur than in the USA. Niche use will continue in both the USA and Europe for patients with comorbid panic episodes and migraine (see Table 14.2).

Both in the USA and Europe, carbamazepine will continue to be used as a second choice drug, usually in combination with other mood stabilizers. Expanded use will be limited by its 3A4 enzyme inducing properties, propensity to cause serious vascular rash, and its non-patented status.

Table 14.2 Differences in valproate and carbamazepine use in USA and Europe

USA	Europe
Divalproex approved for mania	Valproate not approved for bipolar disorder
Divalproex used more often than lithium	Valproate little used
Carbamazepine unapproved	Carbamazepine approved in some countries
Carbamazepine used as second line	Carbamazpine used as second line
Extensive use in lithium refractory subtypes	Use in atypical forms, categorized differently than in USA, also use in lithium refractory patients
Vigorous prophylaxis from first episode	Varying practices regarding eligibility for prophylactic therapy

References

Ballenger, J.C. (1988). The clinical use of carbamazepine in affective disorders. *J. Clin. Psychiatry*, **49**, 13–19.

Ballenger, J.C. and Post, R.M. (1980). Carbamazepine in manic-depressive illness: a new treatment. *Am. J. Psychiatry*, **137**, 782–790.

Barratt, E.S. (1993). The use of anticonvulsants in aggression and violence. *Psychopharmacol. Bull.*, **29**, 75–81.

Berky, M., Wolf, C. and Kovács, G. (1998). Carbamazepine versus lithium in bipolar affective disorders. *Eur. Arch. Psychiatry Clin. Neurosci.*, **248**, S119.

Bowden, C.L. (1995). Predictors of response to divalproex and lithium. *J. Clin. Psychiatry*, **56**, 25–30.

Bowden, C.L. (1996). Role of newer medications for bipolar disorder. *J. Clin. Psychopharmacol.* **16** (Suppl. 1), 48S–55S.

Bowden, C.L. (1998). Anticonvulsants in bipolar elderly. In *Geriatric Psychopharmacology* (J.C. Nelson, ed.), New York, Marcel Dekker, Inc., pp. 285–300.

Bowden, C.L., Brugger, A.M., Swann, A.C., *et al.* (1994). Efficacy of divalproex vs lithium and placebo in the treatment of mania. *J. Am. Med. Assoc.*, **271**, 918–924.

Bowden, C.L., Janicak, P.G., Orsulak, P., *et al.* (1996). Relation of serum valproate concentration to response in mania. *Am. J. Psychiatry*, **153**, 765–770.

Bowden, C.L., Swann, A.C., Calabrese, J.R., *et al.* (1997). Maintenance clinical trials in bipolar disorder: design implications of the divalproex-lithium-placebo study. *Psychopharmacol. Bull.*, **33**, 693–699.

Breslau, N., Merikangas, K. and Bowden, C.L. (1994) Comorbidity of migraine and major affective disorders. *Neurology*, **44** (Suppl. 7), S17–S22.

Cabrera, J.F., Muhlbauer, H.D., Schley, J., *et al.* (1986). Long-term randomized clinical trial on oxcarbazepine vs. lithium in bipolar and schizoaffective disorders: preliminary results. *Pharmacopsychiatry*, **19**, 282–283.

Calabrese, J.R. and Delucchi, G.A. (1990). Spectrum of efficacy of valproate in 55 patients with rapid-cycling bipolar disorder. *Am. J. Psychiatry*, **147**, 431–434.

Calabrese, J.R., Markovitz, P.J., Kimmel, S.E., *et al.* (1992). Spectrum of efficacy of valproate in 78 rapid-cycling bipolar patients. *J. Clin. Psychopharmacol.*, **12**, 53S–56S.

Dardennes, R., Even, C., Bange, F., *et al.* (1995). Comparison of carbamazepine and lithium in the prophylaxis of bipolar disorders. A meta-analysis. *Br. J Psychiatry*, **166**, 378–381.

Denicoff, K.D., Smith-Jackson, E.E., Bryan, A.L., *et al.* (1997). Valproate prophylaxis in a prospective clinical trial of refractory bipolar disorder. *Am. J. Psychiatry*, **154**, 1456–1458.

Di Costanzo, E. and Schifano, F. (1991). Lithium alone or in combination with carbamazepine for the treatment of rapid-cycling bipolar affective disorder. *Acta Psychiatrica Scand.*, **83**, 456–459.

Dose, M., Apelt, S. and Emrich, H.M. (1987). Carbamazepine as adjunct of antipsychotic therapy. *Psychiatry Res.*, **22**, 303–310.

Emrich, H.M. (1990). Alternatives to lithium prophylaxis for affective and schizoaffective disorders. In: *Affective and Schizoaffective Disorders: Similarities and Differences* (A. Marneros and M. Tsuang, eds), Berlin, Heidelberg, New York, Tokyo, Springer, pp. 262–273.

Emrich, H.M. and Dietrich, D.E. (1997). Langzeitprophylaxe mit Antikonvulsia. In: *Die Lithiumtherapie Nutzen, Risiken, Alternativen*. 2nd Edition. (B. Müeller-Oerlinghausen, W. Griel, A. Berghöfer, eds), Springer-Verlag Berlin-Heidelberg-New York, pp. 484–500.

Emrich, H.M., Dose, M. and von Zerssen, D. (1984). Action of sodium-valproate and of oxcarbazepine in patients with affective disorders. In: *Anticonvulsants in Affective Disorders* (H.M. Emrich, T. Okuma and A.A. Müller, eds), Amsterdam, Excerpta Medica, pp. 45–55.

Amrich, H.M. and Wolf, R. (1992). Valproate treatment of mania. *Prog. Neuropsychopharmacol. Biol. Psychiatry*, **16**, 691–701.

Freeman, T.W., Clothier, J.L., Pazzaglia, P., *et al.* (1992). A double-blind comparison of valproate and lithium in the treatment of acute mania. *Am. J. Psychiatry*, **149**, 108–111.

Fritze, J., Beneke, M., Lanczik, M., *et al.* (1994). Carbamazepine as adjunct or alternative to lithium in the prophylaxis of recurrent affective disorders. *Pharmacopsychiatry*, **27**, 181–185.

Goff, D.C. and Baldessarini, R.J. (1993). Drug interactions with antipsychotic agents. *J. Clin. Psychopharmacol.*, **13**, 57–67.

Greil, W., Kleindienst, N., Erazo, N., *et al.* (1998). Differential response to lithium and carbazepine in the prophylaxis of bipolar disorder. *J. Clin. Psychopharmacol.*, **18**, 455–460.

Greil, W., Ludwig-Mayerhofer, W., Erazo, N., *et al.* (1997a). Lithium versus carbamazepine in the maintenance treatment of bipolar disorders – a randomised study. *J. Affect. Dis.*, **43**, 151–161.

Greil, W., Ludwig-Mayrhofer, W., Erazo, N., *et al.* (1997b). Lithium vs. carbamazepine in the maintenance treatment of schizoaffective disorder: a randomised study. *Eur. Arch. Psychiatry Clin. Neurosci*, **247**, 42–50.

Grof, P. (1998). Has the effectiveness of lithium changed? Impact of the variety of lithium's effects. *Neuropsychopharmacology*, **19**, 183–188.

Grof, P., Alda, M., Grof, E., *et al.* (1993). The challenge of predicting response to stabilizing lithium treatment. The importance of patient selection (Review). *Br. J. Psychiatry*, **163(S)**, 16–19.

Jacobsen, F.M. (1993) Low dose valproate: a new treatment for cyclothymia, mild rapid cycling disorders, and premenstrual syndrome. *J. Clin. Psychiatry*, **54**, 229–234.

Jensen, R., Brinck, T. and Olesen, J. (1994). Sodium valproate has a prophylactic effect in migraine without aura. A triple-blind, placebo-controlled crossover study. *Neurology*, **44**, 647–651.

Kalinowsky, L.B. and Putnam, T.J. (1943). Attempts at treatment of schizophrenia and other nonepileptic psychoses with dilantin. *Arch. Neurol. Psychiatry*, **49**, 414–420.

Klosiewicz, L. (1985). Preventive effect of valproic acid amide in affective diseases. *Psychiatria Polska*, **19**, 23–29.

Lambert, P.A. (1984). Acute and prophylactic therapies of patients with affective disorders using valpromide (dipropylacetamide). In *Anticonvulsants in Affective Disorders* (H.M. Emrich, T. Okuma and A.A. Muller, eds), Amsterdam, Excerpta Medica, pp. 33–44.

Lambert, P.A., Carraz, G., Borselli, S., *et al.* (1975). Le dipropyl-acetamide dans le traitement de la psychose maniaco-depressive. *L'Encephale*, **1**, 31.

Lambert, P.A., Cavaz, G., Borselli, S., *et al.* (1966). Action neuropsychotrope d'un nouvel anti-epileplique: Le Depamide. *Ann. Med. Psychol.*, **1**, 707–710.

Lindhout, D. and Omtzigt, J.G.C. (1992). Pregnancy and the risk of teratogenicity. *Epilepsia*, **33** (Suppl.), S41–S48.

Lum, M., Fontaine, R., Elie, R., *et al.* (1990). Divalproex sodium's antipanic effect in panic disorder: a placebo-controlled study. *Biol. Psychiatry*, **27**, 164A–165A.

Murphy, D.J., Gannon, M.A. and McGennis, A. (1989). Carbamazepine in bipolar affective disorder. *Lancet*, **2**, 1151–1152.

Müller-Oerlinghausen, B., Mueser-Causemann, B. and Volk, J. (1992). Suicides and parasuicides in a high-risk patient group on and off lithium long-term medication. *J. Affect. Dis.*, **25**, 261–270.

Müller-Oerlinghausen, B., Wolf, T., Ahrens, B., *et al.* (1996). Mortality of patients who dropped out from regular lithium prophylaxis: a collaborative study by the International Group for the Study of Lithium-Treated Patients. *Acta Psychiatrica Scand.*, **94**, 344–347.

Nilsson, A. and Axelsson, R. (1990). Lithium discontinuers. I. Clinical characteristics and outcome. *Acta Psychiatrica Scand.*, **82**, 433–438.

Nolen, W.A. (1983). Carbamazepine, a possible adjunct or alternative to lithium in bipolar disorder. *Acta Psychiatrica Scand.*, **67**, 218–225.

Okuma, T., Inanaga, K., Otsuki, S., *et al.* (1979). Comparison of the antimanic efficacy of carbamazepine and chlorpromazine: a double-blind controlled study. *Psychopharmacology*, **66**, 211–217.

Okuma, T., Kishimoto, A., Inoue, K., *et al.* (1973). Anti-manic and prophylactic effects of carbamazepine (Tegretol) on manic depressive psychosis: a preliminary report. *Folia Psychiatr. Neurol. JPN*, **27**, 283–297.

Peselow, E.D., Fieve, R.R., Difiglia, C., *et al.* (1994). Lithium prophylaxis of bipolar illness: the value of combination treatment. *Br. J. Psychiatry*, **164**, 208–214.

Placidi, G.F., Lenzi, A., Lazzerini, F., *et al.* (1986). The comparative efficacy and safety of carbamazepine versus lithium: a randomized, double-blind, 3-year trial in 83 patients. *J. Clin. Psychiatry*, **47**, 490–494.

Pope, H.G., Jr, McElroy, S.L., Keck, P.E., Jr. *et al.* (1991). Valproate in the treatment of acute mania: a placebo-controlled study. *Arch. Gen. Psychiatry*, **48**, 62–68.

Post, R.M., Uhde, T.W., Ballenger, J., *et al.* (1983). Prophylactic efficacy of carbamazepine in manic-depressive illness. *Am. J. Psychiatry*, **140**, 1602–1604.

Primeau, F., Fontaine, R. and Beauclair, L. (1990). Valproic acid and panic disorder. *Can. J. Psychiatry*, **35**, 248–250.

Puryear, L.J., Kunik, M.E. and Workman, R., Jr (1995). Tolerability of divalproex sodium in elderly psychiatric patients with mixed diagnoses. *J. Geriatric Psychiatry Neurol.*, **8**, 234–237.

Puzynski, S. and Klosiewicz, L. (1984). Valproic acid amide as a prophylactic agent in affective and schizoaffective disorders. *Psychopharm. Bull.*, **20**, 151–159.

Schou, M. (1998). The effect of prophylactic lithium treatment on mortality and suicidal behavior: a review for clinicians. *J. Affect. Dis.*, **50**, 253–259.

Silberstein, S.D., Saper, J.R. and Mathew, N.T. (1993). The safety and efficacy of divalproex sodium in the prophylaxis of migraine headache: a multicenter double-blind, placebo-controlled trial. *Headache*, **33**, 264–265.

Simhandl, C. and Denk, E. (1994). Carbamazepin in der Rezidivprophylaxe unipolarer und bipolarer affektiver Erkankungen. In: *Ziele und Ergebnisse der Medikamentösen Prophylaxe Affektiver Psychosen* (B. Müller-Oerlinghausen and A. Berghöfer, eds), New York, Thieme, Stuttgart, pp. 121–126.

Sival, R.C., Haffmans, P.M., van Gent, P.P., *et al.* (1994). The effects of sodium valproate on disturbed behavior in dementia. *J. Am. Geriartr. Soc.*, **42**, 906–907.

Sovner, R. (1989). The use of valproate in the treatment of mentally retarded persons with typical and atypical bipolar disorders. *J. Clin. Psychiatry*, **50**, 40–43.

Spina, E., Pisani, F. and Perucca, E. (1996). Clinically significant pharmacokinetic drug interactions with carbamazepine – an update. *Clin. Pharmacokinet.*, **31**, 198–214.

Stokes, P.E., Shamoian, C.A., Stoll, P.M., *et al.* (1971). Efficacy of lithium as acute treatment of manic-depressive illness. *Lancet*, **1**, 1319–1325.

Swann, A.C., Bowden, C.L., Calabrese, J.R., *et al.* (1999). Mania: illness course and acute response to lithium, divalproex, or placebo. *Am. J. Psychiatry*, **156**, 1264–1266.

Swann, A.C., Bowden, C.L., Morris, D., *et al.* (1997). Depression during mania: treatment response to lithium or divalproex. *Arch. Gen. Psychiatry*, **54**, 37–42.

Takezaki, H. and Hanaoka, M. (1971). The use of carbamazepine (Tegretol) in the control of manic depressive psychosis and other manic, depressive states (Abstract). *Seishin Shikeigaku Zasshi – Psychiatri, Neurol. Jpn.* **13**, 173–183.

Tariot, P.N., Erb, R., Podgorski, C.A., *et al.* (1998). Efficacy and tolerability of carbamazepine for agitation and aggression in dementia. *Am. J. Psychiatry*, **155**, 54–61.

Tennis, P. and Ster, R.S. (1997). Risk of serious cutaneous disorders after initiation of use of phenytoin, carbamazepine, or sodium valproate: a record linkage study. *Neurology*, **49**, 542–546.

Thies-Flechtner, K., Müller-Oerlinghausen, B., Seibert, W., *et al.* (1996). Effect of prophylactic treatment on suicide risk in patients with major affective disorders: data from a randomized prospective trial. *Pharmacopsychiatry*, **29**, 103–107.

Tondo, L., Jamison, K.R. and Baldessarini, R.J. (1997). Effect of lithium maintenance on suicidal behavior in major mood disorders. In: *The Neurobiology of Suicide. From the Bench to the Clinic* (D.M. Stoff and J.J. Mann, eds), New York, Annals of the New York Academy of Sciences, pp. 339–351.

Wilder, B.J., Karas, B.J., Penry, J.K., *et al.* (1983). Gastrointestinal tolerance of divalproex sodium. *Neurology*, **33**, 808–811.

15

Lamotrigine, gabapentin and the new anticonvulsants: efficacy in mood disorders

Nicol Ferrier and Joseph Calabrese

Key points

- Lamotrigine exhibits a broad spectrum of efficacy for depressed, manic, and mixed patterns of bipolar disorder.
- Serious dermatological side effects of lamotrigine occur in approximately 0.3% of patients.
- Gabapentin may be effective in bipolar disorder, especially for rapid-cycling.
- Topiramate is showing preliminary evidence of efficacy for treatment-refractory mania.

Introduction

Recent research has highlighted that a significant number of patients with bipolar affective disorder (BPAD) have a poor outcome (Cole *et al.*, 1993). The most commonly cited reason for poor outcome has become the development of rapid- or ultra-rapid-cycling, but mixed states, prolonged depression, and severe mania are also associated with poor outcome. The number of patients with poor outcome is unclear as detailed epidemiological studies have not been done. It has been estimated that approximately one-third of BPAD patients do not respond fully to lithium (Prien and Gelenberg, 1989; Post, 1990). It is also known that a significant number of patients discontinue lithium because of side effects (Post, 1990) which, in itself, may cause further problems because of the phenomenon of lithium-induced discontinuation effects.

Alternatives and supplements to lithium in the treatment of bipolar affective disorders, particularly with poor outcome, has recently been reviewed by Dubovsky and Buzan (1997). A range of studies performed over the past decade have shown that some of the anticonvulsants are effective in the acute and prophylactic treatment of patients with bipolar disorder including those inadequately responsive to or intolerant of lithium (Calabrese *et al.*, 1995). There is now good evidence for both carbamazepine and sodium valproate's efficacy in acute mania. In addition, there is also some evidence of efficacy in the acute treatment of depression, as well as the prevention of relapse and recurrence for both phases of the illness. A number of retrospective studies have suggested that patients with poor or predicted poor outcome are likely to respond better to anticonvulsants than lithium (McElroy *et al.*, 1992; American Psychiatric Association, 1994). Indeed, carbamazepine and valproate are considered by many authorities to be the first line of mood stabilizing agents along with lithium in the treatment of bipolar disorder. Although it is presently unknown whether the mechanism(s) of action underlying the antiepileptic properties of these drugs are responsible for their mood stabilizing effects, it has been suggested that other anticonvulsants should be screened for mood stabilizing and mood improving properties.

This chapter reviews the thymoleptic properties of lamotrigine, gabapentin, and briefly, other new anticonvulsants (topiramate and tiagabine).

Lamotrigine

New drugs are needed that possess efficacy in the depressed phase of bipolar I disorder and, in particular, are able to do so without causing a switch into hypomania/mania or rapid-cycling. Early controlled data suggest that lamotrigine possesses this unique spectrum of efficacy. In 14 clinical reports involving 207 patients with bipolar disorder (66 with rapid-cycling), lamotrigine has been observed to possess moderate to marked efficacy in depression, hypomania, and mixed states, but the drug's efficacy in hospitalized mania remains unclear (Calabrese et al., 1988a). In the largest of these clinical reports, the spectrum of efficacy of lamotrigine was examined in a 48-week, open-label, prospective trial of lamotrigine in 75 patients with either bipolar I or II disorder (Calabrese et al., in press, a). Lamotrigine was used as add-on therapy ($n = 60$) or monotherapy ($n = 15$) in patients presenting in depressed, hypomanic, manic, or mixed states. Of the 40 depressed patients included in the analysis, 48% exhibited a marked response and 20% a moderate response as measured by reductions in the 17-item Hamilton Depression Scale (HAMD17) scores. Of the 31 presenting hypomanic, manic, or mixed, 81% displayed a marked response and 3% a moderate response on the Mania Rating Scale (MRS). The magnitude of overall observed improvement was substantial with the depressed patients exhibiting a 42% decrease in HAM-D scores from baseline to endpoint, and the patients presenting hypomanic/manic/mixed exhibiting a 74% decrease in MRS scores from baseline to endpoint. The most common drug-related adverse events included dizziness, tremor, somnolence, headache, nausea, and rash. Rash was the most common adverse event resulting in drug discontinuation (9% of patients). One patient developed a serious rash which required hospitalization. Lamotrigine appeared to exhibit a broad spectrum of efficacy in the management of the depressed, hypomanic, manic, and mixed phase of bipolar disorder.

The findings of these clinical reports have led to the development of a series of controlled trials. Two of these controlled trials have been completed and support the impression that lamotrigine has mood stabilizing properties. An initial controlled study was conducted to evaluate the efficacy and safety of two doses of lamotrigine compared with placebo in the treatment of a major depressive episode in patients with bipolar I disorder (Calabrese et al., 1999b). Outpatients with bipolar I disorder experiencing a major depressive episode ($n = 195$) received lamotrigine (50 or 200 mg/day) or placebo as monotherapy for 7 weeks. Psychiatric evaluations, including the HAMD17, the Montgomery-Asberg Depression Rating Scale (MADRS), the MRS, and the Clinical Global Impressions Scale for Severity (CGI-S) and Improvement (CGI-I), were completed weekly. Lamotrigine 200 mg/day demonstrated significant antidepressant efficacy on HAMD17, HAMD Item 1, MADRS, CGI-S, and CGI-I compared with placebo. Improvements were seen as early as week 3. Lamotrigine 50 mg/day also demonstrated efficacy compared with placebo on several measures. The proportion of patients exhibiting a marked response on CGI-I was 51%, 41% and 26% for lamotrigine 200 mg/day, lamotrigine 50 mg/day, and placebo groups, respectively. The rate of the development of hypomania/mania/mixed states on lamotrigine ($n = 129$) in this trial did not significantly differ from that on placebo ($n = 65$), 5.4% vs. 4.6%. Adverse events and other safety results were similar across treatment groups (including switch rates), except for the higher rate of headaches in the lamotrigine groups. The conclusion was that lamotrigine monotherapy was an effective and well-tolerated treatment for bipolar depression.

In a preliminary National Institute of Mental Health (NIMH) communication which compared the efficacy of gabapentin, lamotrigine, and placebo in a double-blind cross-over design, Frye and colleagues (1998) reported that lamotrigine, but not gabapentin, was superior to placebo in mixed cohort of patients with bipolar I and II disorder, as well as recurrent major depression.

Lamotrigine is an anticonvulsant drug of the phenyltriazine class which has been shown to be effective as add-on treatment and monotherapy for partial complex seizures (Schachter et al., 1995). The mechanism by which lamotrigine exerts its anticonvulsant effect is different from that of the other anticonvulsants. This drug interacts preferentially with the slow inactivated state of sodium channels to prolong neuronal inactivation. This effect is augmented by a use-dependent action in which further inhibition by the drug develops during rapid, repetitive stimulation. As a result, the release of excitatory amino acids such as glutamate, is reduced, which may also play a role in the anticonvulsant effects of the drug. The effects of lamotrigine on sodium channels probably accounts for its efficacy in partial and secondarily generalized seizures. However, it does not explain its efficacy in primary generalized seizures, as other drugs which block sodium channels are ineffective for this seizure type. In addition, lamotrigine has been observed to inhibit cortical and amygdaloid kindling which may be of theoretical interest (Post, 1992) in bipolar disorder (Leach et al., 1986; Xie, 1995; Gilman, 1995).

This compound is primarily metabolized through glucuronidation, but some minor metabolism through methylation and oxidation does occur. Lamotrigine is absorbed completely (bioavailability, 98%) and rapidly (peak concentrations, 2.5 hours), moderately protein bound (55%), and possesses a comparatively long half-life when dosed chronically (25 hours) (Table 15.1) (Leach et al., 1986; Messenheimer, 1995). Routine monitoring of chemistries, complete blood counts, blood pressure, and heart rate is not necessary. Body weight remains relatively stable with chronic lamotrigine use. In the management of epilepsy, there does not appear to be a correlation between blood level and efficacy. When lamotrigine is administered as monotherapy, or along with agents that do not induce or inhibit hepatic enzyme systems, it is dosed according to the following schedule: weeks 1–2: 25 mg daily; weeks 3–4: 25 mg twice daily; week 5: 50 mg twice daily, then an

Table 15.1 Pharmacokinetic profiles

	Bioavailability (%)	Peak absorption (h)	Elimination half-life (h)	Protein binding (%)	Therapeutic range (mg/day)
LTG	98	2.5	25	55	50–300
GBP	60	2–4	6	< 3	600–3600
TPM	81–95	2	21	15	100–400

LTG: lamotrigine, GBP: gabapentin, TPM: topiramate.

increase in the total daily dose by 50 mg increments every 7 days up to a maximum of 500 mg daily.

Although lamotrigine itself has no significant effect on the hepatic cyclo-oxygenase system or on the metabolism of other antiepileptic drugs, valproate inhibits the metabolism of lamotrigine by immediately and significantly competing for metabolism through glucuronidation. As a result of this, the mean half-life of lamotrigine is immediately increased to about 70 hours and steady state lamotrigine plasma concentrations are increased. Therefore, when lamotrigine is added to ongoing treatment with valproate, the initial dose of lamotrigine should be 25 mg every other day – half of the mono-therapy dose. When valproate is added to ongoing treatment with lamotri-gine, the daily dose of lamotrigine should be immediately decreased by approximately one-half. Carbamazepine induces the metabolism of lamotri-gine by gradually decreasing the mean half-life of lamotrigine to about 12 hours and reducing steady state lamotrigine plasma concentrations. Therefore, when lamotrigine is added to ongoing treatment with carbama-zepine, the initial dose of lamotrigine is 50 mg daily, double the monotherapy dose. When carbamazepine is added to ongoing treatment with lamotrigine, the dose of lamotrigine must be gradually doubled over 1–3 weeks.

The most common side effects associated with the use of lamotrigine in combination with other psychiatric drugs in bipolar disorder include dizzi-ness, tremor, somnolence, headache, nausea, and rash (Calabrese et al., 1999a). Rash is the most common adverse event resulting in drug disconti-nuation. The nature of the reported adverse events in bipolar disorder are consistent with those observed in patients with epilepsy. In open-label and placebo-controlled epilepsy clinical trials involving 3501 patients, rash has been observed to occur in 10% of lamotrigine and 5% of placebo patients. Rash led to drug discontinuation in 3.8% of lamotrigine patients (Physician's Desk Reference, 1997). The spectrum of lamotrigine-associated cutaneous reactions include simple morbilliform (measle-like) rash, hives, angioedema, Stevens-Johnson syndrome, toxic epidermal necrolysis, and hypersensitivity reaction syndrome. The rate of serious rash resulting in hospitalization and discontinuation of treatment is reported to be one in 300 and usually occurs within 2–8 weeks of initiation of treatment. The incidence of rash is higher in patients taking concomitant valproate, and higher if the recommended initial lamotrigine dose and titration schedules are exceeded. The prevalance of serious rash resulting in hospitalization is significantly higher (approximately one in 100) in children ($\leq$ 16 years of age) than in adults. The consensus of clinical opinion is that, unless an alternative aetiology can be clearly identified, the drug should be discontinued when patients present with rash of any kind regardless of severity, since the clinician is unable to predict which cutaneous reactions will become serious. Strict adherence to the recommended dose escalation schedule may diminish the likelihood of rash. Lamotrigine is a Category C teratogen which indicates that studies in women and animals are not available.

Lamotrigine treatment appears to be associated with a low incidence of the adverse events that are usually observed with the currently available mood stabilizers, such as memory deficits/listlessness, weight gain, and alopecia. On the other hand, there is one feature of this drug's pharmacological profile that deserves special attention. The drug must be titrated slowly to minimize the likelihood of rash and dosing must be adjusted for concurrent use of hepatic enzyme inducers or inhibitors.

Gabapentin

Gabapentin is an antiepileptic agent (a cyclohexane derivative of gamma-aminobutyric acid (GABA)) with an unknown mechanism of action. It is currently in clinical use as an add-on therapy in patients with partial seizures resistant to conventional therapies (US Gabapentin Study Group, 1993).

Gabapentin is not metabolized in humans. It is not protein bound, has no known pharmacokinetic interactions with valproic acid, carbamazepine, other anticonvulsants, or oral contraceptives and is renally excreted unchanged (see Table 15.1). Gabapentin has a high therapeutic index and a relatively benign side-effect profile. Side effects reported with gabapentin are transient and minor, the most common being somnolence, dizziness, ataxia, and fatigue (Dichter and Brodie, 1996). It is not associated with haematological or hepatic problems and does not require serum concentration monitoring. These properties make gabapentin an attractive medication choice for bipolar patients who are receiving several psychotropic medications, those with hepatic or haematological disturbance, and those in whom blood monitoring of levels is problematical. In addition to these pharmacokinetic and pharmacological advantages, there are theoretical reasons why gabapentin may be of interest in mood disorders. The mechanism(s) of action of anticonvulsants in bipolar disorder is not known and the mechanism of therapeutic action of gabapentin is unknown. Recently, it has been shown to bind to a subunit of a voltage-dependent calcium channel (Gee et al., 1996). Gabapentin has also been shown to increase the enzyme activity of glutamic acid decarboxylase in vitro (Taylor et al., 1992), GABA turnover in vivo (Loesher et al., 1991), and non-synaptic GABA response in vitro (Brown et al., 1996). Gabapentin reduces potassium-induced release of several monoamine neurotransmitters (noradrenaline, dopamine, serotonin) from brain tissue in vitro (Reimann, 1983). In human subjects, gabapentin has been shown to increase whole blood serotonin (Rao et al., 1988), lengthen sleep stages 3 and 4 without changes in REM sleep, and to produce subtle psychotropic effects (Saletu et al., 1986).

Mood effects of gabapentin in patients without mood disorder

Gabapentin is well-tolerated in epileptic patients and produces good effects on seizure control. There has been a variety of open studies of patients with epilepsy which have reported positive benefits of gabapentin on mood, cognition, and quality of life (Sussman, 1997). Dimond *et al.* (1996) reviewed five double-blind clinical trials (totalling 700 patients) of gabapentin as add-on therapy in patients with epilepsy. Forty-six per cent of gabapentin-treated patients reported improvements in general well-being as compared with 29% of the placebo-treated patients. Caution is required since this finding is based on a retrospective examination of data from trials in epilepsy where psychological effects were not the primary focus and validated mood ratings were not employed. It appears that gabapentin's beneficial effects on psychological function in add-on therapy trials differ from the usual reports of the negative influence of antiepileptic polytherapy on attention, concentration, drive, mood, and sociability (Ludgate *et al.*, 1985). It is noteworthy that some patients reported improvement in mood even in the absence of seizure control. Leach *et al.* (1997), in a small double-blind study of gabapentin, found an improvement in cognition which related to the improvement in seizure control with no improvement in mood compared with placebo. A few case reports have described the development of disinhibition or hypomanic symptoms in epileptic patients (Wolf *et al.*, 1996) and patients with learning disabilities (Short and Cooke, 1995; Tallian *et al.*, 1996).

A single case report (Regan and Gordon, 1997) reported that a patient with Alzheimer's disease with intense agitation settled well on gabapentin, decreasing the need for antipsychotic medication. The nature of this patient's mood state was not clear. Pande *et al.* (1998) in a placebo-controlled study of gabapentin in social phobia found a significant improvement using gabapentin (doses flexibly between 600 and 3600 mg/day) in those patients completing more than 2 weeks of treatment.

Gabapentin in affective disorders

Two case reports (Ryback and Ryback, 1995; Stanton *et al.*, 1997) described apparent benefits of gabapentin in patients with behavioural dyscontrol and refractory mania respectively. Six open studies of gabapentin in various phases of bipolar disorder have been reported. McElroy *et al.* (1997) and Erfurth *et al.* (1998) have reported efficacy in mania and hypomania when the drug was used as add-on therapy – results as sole therapy were less clear with the possibility of a rather delayed effect. Young *et al.* (1997) reported a modest but significant reduction in depression rating scales in depressed bipolar patients treated with gabapentin. Some patients exhibited an apparent marked response, some of whom were treated with gabapentin as monotherapy. Longer-term prophylactic benefits in bipolar disorder are suggested by three open studies where gabapentin has been used as add-on therapy (Ryback *et al.* (1997) ($n = 73$), Bennett *et al.* (1997) ($n = 5$), Schaffer and Schaffer (1997) ($n = 18$)). In general, good outcomes were obtained (using the patient as their own control) particularly in rapid-cycling and refractory patients with evidence of a prolonged effect and few, mostly mild, side effects. It should be noted that in all three studies, there was a very large variation in the dose administered. The data suggest that doses between 1500 and 2400 mg are efficacious in prophylaxis. Whether the dose required varies for different clinical situations and levels of severity is presently unknown.

A recent study compared the efficacy of gabapentin, lamotrigine, and placebo in a cross-over design (Frye *et al.*, 1998). Gabapentin was not superior to placebo in this double-blind study in a mixed cohort of patients with bipolar I and II disorder, as well as recurrent major depression, although the short time on each agent (6 weeks) may have induced a false-negative result. Recently a double-blind randomized placebo-controlled study of gabapentin as adjunctive treatment to lithium and/or valproate in refractory lymphoma failed to show any significant effects. The dose-range was flexible (900–3600 mg/day) and the placebo response large, factors which may have mitigated against a specific positive result. (Pande, 1999).

Despite the limitations of the data, it appears that gabapentin may have efficacy in bipolar affective disorder, particularly in rapid-cycling disorder at doses of between 1500 mg and 2400 mg, at which it is well-tolerated, although care is needed to monitor for side effects, particularly worsening of the psychiatric state.

Other anticonvulsants

Topiramate, a structurally novel carbohydrate compound with documented anticonvulsant efficacy and safety, has recently been shown to have preliminary evidence of efficacy in treatment-refractory mania (Calabrese *et al.*, 1998b). Topiramate is a sulphamate-substituted derivative of the naturally occurring monosaccharide D-fructose and possesses carbonic anhydrase inhibiting properties. (See Table 15.1 for its pharmacokinetic profile.) There are now a total of eight preliminary communications involving a total of 177 patients with bipolar disorder (Calabrese *et al.*, 1998b; McElroy *et al.*, 1998; Marcotte and Gullick, 1998; Hussain and Chaudry, 1999; Kusumakar *et al.*, 1999; Chengappa *et al.*, 1999; Prado-Lima *et al.*, 1999; Gordon and Price, 1999) which have presented preliminary evidence for some antimanic effects and mood stabilizing effects in some patients. Side effects in patients with bipolar disorder included paraesthesias, nausea, constipation, decreased appetite/weight loss, dizziness, tinnitus, and abnormal thinking. Recently, an early clinical report has begun to explore the use of tiagabine in acutely manic hospitalized patients, but preliminary results from this trial do not appear promising (Walden *et al.*, 1998).

References

American Psychiatric Association (1994). Work group on bipolar disorder. Practice guideline for treatment of patients with bipolar disorder. *Am. J. Psychiatry*, **151**, 1–36.

Bennett, J., Goldman, W.T. and Suppes, T. (1997). Gabapentin for bipolar and schizoaffective disorders (letter). *J. Clin. Psychopharmacol.*, **17**, 141–142.

Brown, J.P., Boden, P., Singh, L., *et al.* (1996). Mechanisms of action of gabapentin. *Rev. Contemp. Pharmacother.*, **7**, 203–214.

Calabrese, J.R., Bowden, C.B. and Woyshville, M.J. (1995). Lithium and anticonvulsants in the treatment of bipolar disorder. In *Psychopharmacology: The Fourth Generation of Progress*, (F.E. Bloom, D.J. Kupfer, eds), New York, Raven Press, pp. 1099–1111.

Calabrese, J.R., Rapport, D.J., Shelton, M.D., *et al.* (1998a). Clinical studies on the use of lamotrigine in bipolar disorder. *Neuropsychobiology*, **38**, 185–191.

Calabrese, J.R., Bowden, C.L., McElroy, S.L., *et al.* (1999a). Spectrum of activity of lamotrigine in treatment-refractory bipolar disorder. *Am. J. Psychiatry*, **156**, 1019–1023.

Calabrese, J.R., Bowden, C.L., Sachs, G.S., *et al.* (1999b). A double-blind placebo-controlled study of lamotrigine monotherapy in outpatients with bipolar I depression. *J. Clin. Psychiatry*, **60**, 79–88.

Calabrese, J.R., Shelton, M.D., Keck, P.E., *et al.* (1998b). Topiramate in severe treatment-refractory mania. *Annual Meeting of the American Psychiatric Association.* Abstract NR202, p. 121.

Chengappa, K.N.R., Rathore, D., Levine, J., *et al.* (1999). Use of topiramate for bipolar disorder. XI World Congress of Psychiatry, Hamburg, Germany. Poster 03–17, 116 abstract.

Cole, A.J., Scott, J., Ferrier, I.N., *et al.* (1993). Patterns of treatment resistance in bipolar affective disorder. *Acta Psychiat. Scand.*, **88**, 121–123.

Dichter, M.A. and Brodie, M.J. (1996). New antiepileptic drugs. *N. Engl. J. Med.*, **334**, 1583–1590.

Dimond, K.R., Pande, A.C., Lamoreaux, L., *et al.* (1996). Effect of gabapentin (Neurontin) on mood and well-being in patients with epilepsy. *Prog. Neuro-Psychopharmacol. Biol. Psych.*, **20**, 407–417.

Dubovsky, S.L. and Buzan, R.D. (1997). Novel alternatives and supplements to lithium and anticonvulsants for bipolar affective disorder. *J. Clin. Psychiatry*, **58**, 224–242.

Erfurth, A., Kammerer, C., Grunze, H., *et al.* (1998). An open label study of gabapentin in the treatment of acute mania. *J. Psychiat. Res.*, **32**, 261–264.

Frye, M.A., Ketter, T.A., Osuch, E.A., *et al.* (1998). Gabapentin and lamotrigine monotherapy in mood disorders. *Presented at the Annual Meeting of the American Psychiatric Association.* Abstract No. 77D, p. 150.

Gee, N.S., Brown, J.P., Dissanayake, V.U., *et al.* (1996). The novel anticonvulsant drug, gabapentin (Neurontin), binds to the alpha2delta subunit of a calcium channel. *J. Biol. Chem.*, **271**, 5768–5776.

Gilman, J.T. (1995). Lamotrigine: an antiepileptic agent for the treatment of partial seizures. *Ann. Pharmacother.*, **29**, 144–151.

Gordon, A. and Price, L.H. (1999). Mood stabilization and weight loss with topiramate. *Am. J. Psychiatry*, **156**, 968–969.

Hussain, M. and Chaudry, Z. (1999). Treatment of bipolar depression with topiramate. XI World Congress of Psychiatry, Hamburg, Germany. Free Communication, 41–5, 58, abstract.

Kusumakar, V., Yatham, L., Kutcher, S., O'Donovan, C. (1999). Use of topiramate in rapid cycling bipolar women. XI World Congress of Psychiatry, Hamburg, Germany. Poster 07–33, 122, abstract.

Leach, J.P., Girvan, J., Paul, A., *et al.* (1997). Gabapentin and cognition: a double-blind dose-ranging placebo-controlled study in refractory epilepsy. *J. Neurol. Neurosurg. Psychiatry*, **62**, 372–376.

Leach, M.J., Marden, C.M. and Miller, A.A. (1986). Pharmacological studies on lamotrigine, a novel potential antiepileptic drug: II. Neurochemical studies on the mechanism of action. *Epilepsia*, **27**, 490–497.

Loescher, W., Hanack, D. and Taylor, C.P. (1991). Gabapentin increases amino-oxyacetic acid-induced GABA accumulation in several regions of rat brain. *Neurosci. Lett.*, **128**, 150–154.

Ludgate, J., Keating, J., O'Dwyer, R., *et al.* (1985). An improvement in cognitive function following polypharmacy reduction in a group of epileptic patients. *Acta Neurolog. Scand.*, **71**, 448–452.

Marcotte, D. and Gullick, A. (1998). Use of topiramate, a new antiepileptic drug, as a mood stabilizer. *XXIst Collegium Internationale Neuro-Psychopharmacologicum*, Abstract No. 3033, p. 287.

McElroy, S.L., Kmetz, G.F. and Keck, P.E. (1998). A pilot trial of adjunctive topiramate in the treatment of bipolar disorder. *XXIst Collegium Internationale Neuro-Psychopharmacologicum.* Abstract No. 3006, p. 281.

McElroy, S.L., Keck, P.E., Pope, H.G., *et al.* (1992). Valproate in the treatment of bipolar disorder: literature review and clinical guidelines. *J. Clin. Psychopharm.*, **12**, 42S–51S.

McElroy, S.L., Saufullo, C.A., Keck, P.E., *et al.* (1997). A pilot trial of adjunctive gabapentin in the treatment of bipolar disorder. *Ann. Clin. Psychiatry*, **9**, 99–104.

Messenheimer, J.A. (1995). Lamotrigine. *Epilepsia*, **36** (Suppl. 2), S87–S94.

Pande, A.C. (1999). Combination treatment in bipolar disorder. *Bipolar Disorders*, **1**, Supp. 1, 17.

Pande, A.C., Davidson, J.R.T., Greist, J.H., *et al.* (1998). A placebo-controlled study of gabapentin in social phobia. *Am. Coll. Neuropsychopharmacol.* Abstracts. p. 141.

Physicians Desk Reference (1997). Prescribing Information For Lamictal (1997). Medical Economics Data Production Co., Montvale, N.J.

Post, R.M. (1990). Non-lithium treatment for bipolar disorder. *J. Clin. Psychiatry*, **51**, 9–16.

Post, R.M. (1992). Transduction of psychosocial stress into the neurobiology of recurrent affective disorder. *Am. J. Psychiatry*, **149**, 999–1010.

Prado-Lima, P.A.S. and Bacattchuk, J. (1999). Topiramate in treatment-refractory depression. XI World Congress of Psychiatry, Hamburg, Germany. Poster 15-3, 126, abstract.

Prien, R.F. and Gelenberg, A.J. (1989). Alternatives to lithium for preventative treatment of bipolar disorder. *Am. J. Psychiatry*, **146**, 840–848.

Rao, M.L., Clarenbach, P., Vahlensleck, M., *et al.* (1988). Gabapentin augments whole blood serotonin in healthy young men. *J. Neural. Transm.*, **73**, 129–134.

Regan, W.M. and Gordon, S.M. (1997). Gabapentin for behavioural agitation in Alzheimer's disease. *J. Clin. Psychopharmacol.*, **17**, 58–59.

Reimann, W. (1983). Inhibition by GABA, baclofen and gabapentin of dopamine release from rabbit caudate nucleus. Are there common or different sites of action? *Eur. J. Pharmacol.*, **94**, 341–344.

Ryback, R.S., Brodksy, L. and Manufasi, F. (1997). Gabapentin in bipolar disorder (letter). *J. Neuropsychiatry*, **9**, 301.

Ryback, R. and Ryback, L. (1995). Gabapentin for behavioral dyscontrol. *Am. J. Psychiatry*, **152**, 1399.

Saletu, B., Grunberger, J. and Unzmayer, L. (1986). Evaluation of encephalotropic and psychotropic properties of gabapentin in man by pharmaco-EEG and psychometry. *Int. J. Clin. Pharmacol. Ther. Toxicol.*, **24**, 362–373.

Schaffer, C. and Schaffer, L. (1997). Gabapentin in the treatment of bipolar disorder. *Am. J. Psychiatry*, **154**, 291–292.

Schachter, S.C., Leppik, E., Matsuo, F., *et al.* (1995). Lamotrigine: a six month, placebo-controlled, safety and tolerance study. *J. Epilepsy*, **8**, 201–209.

Short, C. and Cooke, L. (1995). Hypomania induced by gabapentin. *Br. J. Psychiatry*, **166**, 679–680.

Stanton, S.P., Keck, P.E. and McElroy, S.L. (1997). Treatment of acute mania with gabapentin. *Am. J. Psychiatry*, **154**, 287.

Sussman, N. (1997). Gabapentin and lamotrigine; alternative agents for the treatment of bipolar disorder. *Primary Psychiatry*, August, 25–42.

Tallian, K.B., Nahata, M.C., Lo, W., *et al.* (1996). Gabapentin associated with aggressive behavior in pediatric patients with seizures. *Epilepsia*, **37**, 501–502.

Taylor, C.P., Vartanian, M.G., Andruszkiewicz, R., *et al.* (1992). 3-Alkyl GABA and 3-alkyglutamic acid analogues: two new classes of anticonvulsant agents. *Epilepsy Res.*, **11**, 103–110.

US Gabapentin Study Group (1993). Gabapentin as add-on therapy in refractory epilepsy: a double-blind, placebo-controlled, parallel group study. *Neurology*, **43**, 2292–2298.

Walden, J., Erfuth, A., Amann, B., *et al.* (1998). An open trial of the antimanic efficacy of the GAT-1 inhibitor, tiagabine. *Presented at the First Annual European Meeting of the Stanley Foundation Bipolar Disorders Symposium*, London, England, 1998.

Wolf, S., Shimnar, S., Kang, H., *et al.* (1996). Gabapentin toxicity in children manifesting as behavioral changes. *Epilepsia*, **36**, 1203–1205.

Xie, X. (1995). Interaction of the antiepileptic drug lamotrigine with recombinant rat brain type IIA Na$^+$ channels and with native Na$^+$ channels in rat hippocampal neurones. *Arch. Eur. J. Physiol.*, **430**, 437–446.

Young, L.T., Robb, J.D., Patells-Siotis, I., *et al.* (1997). Acute treatment of bipolar depression with gabapentin. *Biol. Psychiatry*, **42**, 851–853.

16

Antipsychotic medications in the treatment of mood disorders

Paul Keck and Rasmus Licht

Key points

- Typical antipsychotic medications have been used as an initial treatment for acute mania, as an adjunctive treatment for acute mania or depression, and as an augmentation strategy for maintenance therapy in refractory mood disorders.
- There is emerging evidence of efficacy for clozapine, risperidone, and olanzapine in the treatment of mania.
- There is less evidence for the role of these agents in treating depressions.
- The heightened risk of tardive dyskinesia in patients with mood disorders who receive typical antipsychotics is a compelling justification for the replacement of typical by atypical agents when antipsychotics are indicated in the management of mood disorders

---

Psychosis in mood disorders

Psychosis occurs commonly during the manic, mixed, and depressive episodes of bipolar disorder (McElroy *et al.*, 1996; Tohen and Zarate, 1998). In their review of 26 studies examining the prevalence of psychotic features in mania, Goodwin and Jamison (1990) found that 47% of manic episodes were accompanied by grandiose delusions, 28% by persecutory delusions, 18% by auditory hallucinations, and 18% by schneiderian first-rank symptoms. A number of other studies have revealed that, although mood-congruent or grandiose delusions may represent the most common presentation of psychosis in mania, mood-incongruent and bizarre delusions, including schneiderian first-rank symptoms also occur during manic episodes (Carlson and Goodwin, 1973; Pope and Lipinsky, 1978; Tohen *et al.*, 1992). In addition to the high prevalence of delusions and hallucinations in mania, numerous studies have found rates of thought disorder in mania comparable to those in schizophrenia (Breakey and Goodell, 1972; Andreasen 1979; Simpson and Davis, 1985; Harrow *et al.*, 1982, 1986, 1992a,b; Goodwin and Jamison, 1990). Since no single psychotic symptom or constellation of symptoms have been shown to be pathognomic for any specific psychiatric disorder, and since every type of psychotic symptom has been reported to occur in mania, bipolar mania must always be considered in the differential diagnosis of any patient presenting with psychosis (Pope and Lipinsky, 1978; McElroy *et al.*, 1996).

The prevalence and presentation of psychosis in bipolar depression has been less well studied (Goodwin and Jamison, 1990). Pooled data from the available studies suggest that, although delusions, hallucinations and thought disorder frequently occur in bipolar depression, psychotic features overall are more common in mania than depression (Goodwin and Jamison, 1990).

Similarly, data regarding the prevalence of psychotic depression among patients with major depressive disorder are sparse. However, the available data from clinical populations suggest that psychotic depression is common, accounting for approximately 25% of depressed patients (Coryell et al., 1984; Rothschild, 1996). Furthermore, there appear to be sufficient and important clinical differences between psychotic and non-psychotic major depression to consider them as distinct depressive syndromes (Schatzberg and Rothschild, 1992). These differences include greater episode severity (Frances et al., 1981; Coryell et al., 1984, 1985; Lykouras et al., 1986; Parker et al., 1991), duration (Coryell et al., 1996), and short-term disability (Coryell et al., 1987) associated with psychotic depression.

In this chapter, we review the role of standard and atpyical antipsychotic medications in the treatment of patients with bipolar disorder and major depressive disorder with psychotic features (delusional or psychotic depression). In particular, we address similarities and differences in pharmacological treatment approaches between the USA and Europe.

Standard antipsychotics in the treatment of mood disorders

Prior to the availability of mood-stabilizing agents (e.g. lithium, valproate, carbamazepine), standard antipsychotic medications represented the treatment of choice for acute mania and were also often used as maintenance treatment (Licht, 1998). Despite the increasing availability of mood-stabilizing agents devoid of the adverse effects associated with standard antipsychotics, recent surveys indicate that these standard agents continue to be used both in the acute and maintenance treatment of bipolar disorder (Sernyak et al., 1994; Keck et al., 1996; Verdoux et al., 1996). Based on the available studies of standard antipsychotics in patients with bipolar disorder, these agents have traditionally had three primary roles: first, as adjunctive agents in combination with mood stabilizers in the treatment of acute psychotic mania or depression (particularly in the USA); second, an initial treatment for acute mania, followed by initiation of mood-stabilizer treatment when symptoms have begun to abate substantially (particularly in Europe); and, third, as adjunctive maintenance treatment in patients with symptoms refractory to thymoleptics alone (McElroy et al., 1996; Gelenberg and Hopkins, 1996; Keck et al., 1998a).

Acute mania

Only one placebo-controlled, randomized trial of a standard antipsychotic drug in the treatment of acute mania has been reported to our knowledge (Klein and Oaks, 1967). Not surprisingly, chlorpromazine was superior to placebo in reducing manic symptoms in this study. Most other controlled trials of standard antipsychotics were conducted in comparison to lithium (Johnson et al., 1971; Spring et al., 1970; Shopsin et al., 1975). Interpretation of the results of these studies is hampered by the inclusion of patients with schizoaffective disorder in some studies and because of the possibility of failure to find a significant difference between active treatments due to small samples sizes (Keck et al., 1998a). In five controlled studies in which chlorpromazine was compared with lithium, the overall rate of improvement was higher in lithium-treated patients by 3 weeks of treatment (Johnson et al., 1971; Spring et al., 1970; Shopsin et al., 1975). A recent meta-analysis of many of these studies confirmed superior efficacy for lithium (89% responders, 11% non-responders) compared with standard antipsychotics (54% responders, 46% non-responders; $\chi^2 = 13.1$; df $= 1$; $P < 0.001$) (Janicak et al., 1992). The only potential advantage in favour of standard antipsychotics to emerge from these studies was greater efficacy in patients with prominent psychomotor agitation early (first week) in treatment (Prien et al., 1972; Shopsin et al., 1973). This advantage supports the use of antipsychotics as monotherapy during the early phase of treatment of acute mania (Europe).

Two studies comparing chlorpromazine with carbamazepine in the treatment of acute mania found comparable efficacy in the reduction of manic and psychotic symptoms for both agents (Okuma et al., 1979; Grossi et al., 1984). Finally, one study comparing divalproex oral loading with haloperidol in the treatment of patients with acute psychotic mania also found comparable reductions in manic and psychotic symptoms with both agents (McElroy et al., 1996).

Several impressions emerge from these data. First, standard antipsychotics appear to have a more rapid onset of action than lithium in acute mania, but by 3 weeks of treatment lithium exerted greater improvement in core affective symptoms and comparable improvement in psychosis. Second, both valproate and carbamazepine produced reductions in not only manic but also psychotic symptoms similar to comparison standard antipsychotics. This observation suggests that initial monotherapy with either of these agents may produce amelioration of psychosis comparable to standard antipsychotics. However, in neither the USA nor Europe has initial monotherapy of acute psychotic mania with valproate or carbamazepine become commonplace to date. Third, although standard antipsychotics are commonly used adjunctively in the treatment of acute mania, no study has assessed the response of acute mania to antipsychotics, mood stabilizers, or their combination based on the presence or absence of psychotic symptoms.

Acute bipolar depression

To our knowledge, there are no controlled trials of standard antipsychotics in the treatment of acute bipolar depression (with or without psychotic features). One recent case series described three patients with psychotic bipolar depression who experienced depressive relapse when standard antipsychotics were withdrawn or dosage was reduced (Hendrick et al., 1994). Reinstitution of the antipsychotic brought about recovery.

Maintenance treatment

Although standard antipsychotics are commonly used in the maintenance treatment of bipolar disorder, there are several clinical concerns regarding this strategy. First, as described below, there are no definitive data from controlled trials indicating that these agents are effective maintenance treatments. Second, maintenance treatment with standard antipsychotics may exacerbate or precipitate depressive symptoms (Morgan, 1972; Kukopulos et al., 1980; White et al., 1993). Third, standard antipsychotics carry a significant side-effect burden and patients with bipolar disorder may be at higher risk for developing tardive dyskinesia and other neurological side effects than patients with schizophrenia (Mukherjee et al., 1986; Nasrallah et al., 1988; Kane et al., 1992).

Five open-label, mirror-design studies have attempted to assess the efficacy of depot antipsychotics alone or in combination with lithium and/or carbamazepine (Naylor and Scott, 1980; Lowe and Batchelor, 1986, 1990; White et al., 1993; Little John et al., 1994). In all of these studies, significant reductions in the number of manic episodes and overall time affectively ill were found during treatment with depot antipsychotics compared with the preceding treatment interval. These findings appear to underlie the common use of antipsychotics in the maintenance treatment of patients with bipolar disorder in both the USA and Europe. However, these results may have been influenced by improved treatment compliance secondary to the administration of depot agents. In contrast, two open, prospective, comparative maintenance studies of depot flupenthixol found no significant difference in the frequency of affective episodes compared with pretreatment (Ahlfors et al., 1981) and no significant difference compared with placebo when added to lithium (Esparon et al., 1986).

Major depressive disorder with psychotic features

In studies of patients with psychotic unipolar depression, the combination of standard antipsychotics and tricyclic antidepressants has been found to be superior to either class of agents alone (Spiker et al., 1985; Parker et al., 1992). Such combination therapy appears to be common in both the USA and Europe. In general, however, there have been relatively few randomized controlled trials conducted in the treatment of psychotic depression. One study compared amoxapine, an agent with combined antipsychotic and antidepressant activity, with the combination of amitriptyline and perphenazine and found comparable response rates in both treatment groups (Anton and Burch, 1990). In an open trial of fluoxetine in combination with perphenazine, 22 (73%) of 30 patients displayed a $\geq$ 50% reduction of depressive symptoms by the fifth week of treatment (Rothschild et al., 1993). Despite the available evidence indicating the superiority of combined antipsychotic and antidepressant treatment to either class of agents alone, one recent study found that 47% of patients with psychotic depression received either no antipsychotic or treatment for less than 3 weeks (Mulsant et al., 1997).

Remarkably little is known about the optimal duration of antipsychotic treatment in patients with psychotic depression (Rothschild, 1996). The available reports suggest that the risk of depressive or psychotic relapse may be high if antipsychotics are discontinued sooner than 1 year after remission (Avery and Lubrano, 1979; Clower, 1983; Aronson *et al.*, 1988).

New (atypical) antipsychotics in the treatment of mood disorders

Acute mania

There are no published controlled trials of clozapine in the treatment of acute mania. However, data from many open trials in treatment-refractory patients suggest that clozapine may have both acute antimanic effects and efficacy as a mood stabilizer in maintenance treatment (McElroy *et al.*, 1991; Suppes *et al.*, 1992; Zarate *et al.*, 1995; Calabrese *et al.*, 1996). In addition to antimanic activity, clozapine has also been reported to improve mixed affective symptoms and rapid-cycling in bipolar patients without psychosis (Suppes *et al.*, 1996; Frye *et al.*, 1998). Based on these encouraging findings, considerable interest has been generated by the potential thymoleptic as well as antipsychotic effects of other atypical antipsychotics (Keck *et al.*, 1994).

A number of open trials and case reports and one randomized, controlled trial provide preliminary data regarding the use of risperidone in acute mania (Goodnick, 1995; Jacobsen, 1995; Keck *et al.*, 1995; Madhusoodanan *et al.*, 1995; O'Croinin *et al.*, 1995; Diaz, 1996; Kook and Kestrel, 1996; Sajatovic *et al.*, 1996; Schaffer and Schaffer, 1996; Schnierow and Graeher, 1996; Tohen *et al.*, 1996; Tomlinson, 1996; Barkin and Pais, 1997; Bernhard, 1997; Ghaemi *et al.*, 1997; McIntyre *et al.*, 1997; Lane *et al.*, 1998; Segal *et al.*, 1998). Overall, the reports from case series and open trials provide conflicting results regarding risperidone's effects on manic symptoms. Several impressions can be gathered from these reports. First, therapeutic effects in the treatment of manic symptoms have been described with risperidone when administered with mood stabilizers or other antipsychotic agents. Second, possible exacerbation of manic symptoms associated with risperidone treatment has been reported primarily at higher doses and when risperidone was used as monotherapy. The results of a recent double-blind, randomized controlled trial comparing risperidone (6 mg/day), haloperidol (10 mg/day) and lithium (800–1200 mg/day) in the treatmjent of 45 patients with acute mania provide the first controlled data to assess risperidone's effects on manic symptoms (Segal *et al.*, 1998). In this 28-day trial, substantial and comparable reductions in manic symptoms were observed with all three agents. The results of this study must be interpreted with several limitations in mind. First, a larger sample size may have allowed detectable differences in treatment efficacy among the three agents to emerge. Second, adjunctive lorazepam was used throughout the 28-day study period, potentially contributing to some reduction in certain manic symptoms (e.g. sleeplessness, psychomotor agitation). Third, lithium levels were generally at the low end of the therapeutic range. Thus, response rates in the lithium-treated group might have been greater if a higher therapeutic serum concentration had been achieved. The occurrence of extrapyramidal side effects was comparable in the two antipsychotic treatment groups. Nevertheless, these initial controlled data suggest that risperidone may be useful in the treatment of acute mania.

Reports from two open trials (Zarate *et al.*, 1998; McElroy *et al.*, 1998) and one double-blind randomized, placebo-controlled study (Tohen *et al.*, 1997) suggest that olanzapine may be an effective antimanic agent. In the first report, olanzapine produced moderate to marked improvement in 16 (80%) of 20 bipolar manic and 11 (85%) of 13 bipolar mixed patients when administered as monotherapy (15% of cases) or adjunctive treatment to previous regimens (Zarate *et al.*, 1998). In the second case series, olanzapine was added to previous regimens in 14 patients with treatment-resistant bipolar disorder (McElroy *et al.*, 1998). Of these patients, eight (57%) displayed much or very much improvement. In only the second placebo-controlled of an antipsychotic agent in the treatment of acute mania ever conducted, olanzapine (5–20 mg/day) was significantly superior to placebo in reduction of manic symptoms, number of responders, and reduction in measures of psychosis over the 3-week study interval (Tohen *et al.*, 1997). Approximately 50% of patients displayed $\geq$ 50% reduction in manic symptoms, a response rate very similar to those associated with divalproex (Pope *et al.*, 1991; Bowden *et al.*, 1994) and lithium (Bowden *et al.*, 1994) in two other recent placebo-controlled trials. There was no significant difference in response rate according to presence or absence of psychosis, making it unlikely that the olanzapine response was primarily due to the improvement in psychosis. From the results of these studies, olanzapine appears to have promise as a treatment of acute mania.

Presently there are no data available regarding the use of other atypical antipsychotics (e.g. sertindole, quetiapine, ziprasidone) in the treatment of patients with bipolar disorder.

Acute bipolar depression

Although the atypical antipsychotics have substantial pharmacological differences from one another, emerging data suggest that these agents may have thymoleptic properties. There are various pharmacological mechanisms associated with these different agents which may produce antidepressant effects, in particular. These include 5-HT$_{2A}$ receptor antagonism (clozapine, risperidone, olanzapine, quetiapine, ziprasidone), alpha$_2$ antagonism (clozapine, risperidone), significant M$_1$ receptor activity (clozapine, olanzapine), serotonin and norepinephrine reuptake inhibition (ziprasidone), and potent 5-HT$_{1A}$ and 5-HT$_{2D}$ affinity (ziprasidone). However, to date few of these agents have been studied in the treatment of patients with bipolar depression. There are no controlled trials of clozapine in the treatment of the acute or maintenance phase of bipolar depression. Pooled data from three large series revealed that 52% of patients who received clozapine (as adjunctive or monotherapy) for the treatment of syndromal depression (bipolar, unipolar or schizoaffective) responded (Leppig *et al.*, 1989; Banov *et al.*, 1994; Goodnick, 1995).

Several reports suggest that risperidone may exert antidepressant as well as antipsychotic effects (Hillert *et al.*, 1992; Jacobsen, 1995; Keck *et al.*,

1995). However, only one report regarding risperidone's use in bipolar depression has appeared to date (Keck *et al.*, 1995). In this study, both patients with bipolar depression responded to combined treatment with risperidone and a mood stabilizer.

In a retrospective survey of response to olanzapine according to diagnosis, 12 (86%) of 14 patients with bipolar depression were rated as displaying a moderate to marked response (Zarate *et al*, 1998). Two (17%) of the 12 responders received olanzapine as monotherapy, the remainder as adjunctive treatment. There are no data presently available regarding sertindole, quetiapine or ziprasidone in bipolar depression.

Maintenance treatment

There are no controlled trials of any atypical antipsychotic agent as a maintenance treatment for patients with bipolar disorder. A number of open trials suggest that treatment with clozapine as monotherapy may provide effective mood stabilization in patients refractory to standard mood stabilizers (Suppes *et al.*, 1992, 1996; Zarate *et al.*, 1995; Calabrese *et al.*, 1996). In these reports, clozapine was not only effective in providing sustained improvement in affective and psychotic symptoms in most patients, but also in preventing rehospitalization.

Maintenance data regarding other atypical antipsychotics are sparse. One open label study examined the 6-month outcome of 12 patients with bipolar 1 disorder who received adjunctive risperidone (mean 2.75 mg/day) for breakthrough affective episodes (Ghaemi and Sachs, 1997). Of these 12 patients, four discontinued risperidone (two because of lack of efficacy and two because of adverse events), and four of the remaining eight experienced a 10–25 point improvement on Global Assessment of Functioning Scale scores. Of note, none of the 12 patients displayed an exacerbation of manic symptoms. Initial experience with olanzapine as a maintenance treatment for patients with bipolar disorder has been promising. Approximately 80% of patients who displayed a good initial antimanic response to olanzapine remained free of manic or depressive relapses in a 1-year extension study (Tohen, 1998). However, some patients required the addition of lithium or fluoxetine for recurrences of manic or depressive symptoms, respectively. Of note, there were no observed cases of tardive dyskinesia at 1-year follow-up in the 98 patients with bipolar disorder who participated in this open trial.

Major depressive disorder with psychotic features

As described above, there are a number of pharmacological mechanisms by which the different atypical antipsychotics could potentially produce antidepressant effects. A small number of reports have described the use of clozapine in psychotic depression (Wood and Rubinstein, 1990; Naber *et al.*, 1992; Dassa *et al.*, 1993; Banov *et al*, 1994). Two case reports described remission of psychotic and depressive symptoms in patients with treatment-refractory psychotic depression treated with clozapine alone (Wood and Rubinstein, 1990; Dassa *et al.*, 1993). In a survey of 193 treatment-resistant patients who received clozapine at one centre, the response rates were significantly lower in patients who received clozapine for psychotic depression (46%) compared with bipolar mania (73%) (Banov et al., 1994). However, patients with psychotic depression received a lower mean clozapine dose (178 mg/day) than manic patients (325 mg/day). In a second chart review of 644 inpatients who received clozapine at another centre, 55–72% of 54 patients with psychotic depression responded (Naber et al., 1992). Whether patients had unipolar or bipolar psychotic depression was not specified in this report.

Four reports provide preliminary data regarding the efficacy of risperidone in patients with psychotic depression. In the first report, four (57%) of seven patients treated with risperidone (mean 7.4 mg/day) alone displayed marked improvement in psychotic and depressive symptoms (Hillert et al., 1992). In a second case series, four patients with psychotic depression who responded well to risperidone (mean 2.5 mg/day) were described (Jacobsen, 1995). Two received risperidone alone, one in combination with sertraline, and one with imipramine. In a chart review of 144 patients treated with risperidone, all three patients with treatment-refractory psychotic depression responded (Keck et al., 1995). All three were also receiving concomitant antidepressants. The putative antidepressant effects of risperidone have been assessed in one double-blind, randomized controlled trial (Muller-Siecheneder et al., 1998). In this 6-week, multicentre trial, risperidone (mean 6.9 mg/day) was compared with the combination of amitriptyline (mean 180 mg/day) and haloperidol (mean 9 mg/day) in 123 patients with schizophrenia with depressive symptoms, schizoaffective disorder, depressive type, or psychotic depression. Although patients with psychotic depression in both treatment groups ($n = 34$) displayed improvement, combined treatment with amitriptyline and haloperidol was significantly more effective than risperidone on measures of improvement in mood and psychosis. Of note, there were no significant differences in outcome between treatment groups in patients with schizophrenia with depressive symptoms or with schizoaffective disorder, depressive type.

Two preliminary studies suggest that olanzapine may also be useful in the treatment of patients with psychotic depression (Zarate et al., 1998; Rothschild et al., 1998). One retrospective case-control study compared the response of inpatients with psychotic depression to treatment with olanzapine ($n = 15$) or conventional antipsychotics ($n = 15$) (Rothschild et al., 1998). Twelve (80%) of 15 patients in each treatment group also received antidepressants. Ten (67%) of the 15 patients treated with olanzapine were much or very much improved at discharge compared with four (27%) of the 15 patients treated with standard antipsychotics. In their retrospective survey of response to olanzapine by diagnostic group, Zarate et al. found that 39 (68%) of 47 patients with psychotic depression displayed a moderate-to-marked response (Zarate et al., 1998). Four (10%) of the 39 responders received olanzapine as monotherapy.

There are no data currently available regarding the use of sertindole, quetiapine or ziprasidone in the treatment of patients with psychotic depression.

Summary

Antipsychotics represent important therapeutic agents in the treatment of patients with mood disorder complicated by psychotic features. Although conventional antipsychotic medications are effective as acute (and possibly maintenance) antimanic agents, their use in patients with bipolar disorder is associated with several concerns, including lack of antidepressant or mood-stabilizing effects, potential exacerbation of depressive symptoms, and risk of tardive movement disorders. Therefore, conventional antipsychotics have their most clearly delineated role as initial (Europe) or adjunctive (USA) treatment for acute psychotic mania and as maintenance treatment for patients inadequately responsive to, intolerant of, or non-compliant with mood stabilizers. Conventional antipsychotics, in conjunction with antidepressants are an important component of the treatment of patients with psychotic depression across Europe and the USA. The optimal duration of maintenance antipsychotic treatment following remission of psychotic depression has not been carefully studied.

Unlike conventional antipsychotics that appear to have unidirectional antimanic properties and frequent neurological side effects, atypical antipsychotics may have different thymoleptic profiles and are associated with fewer neurological, and with some agents, neuroendocrinological side effects. Thus, the newer antipsychotic agents are potentially useful alternative or adjunctive treatment for patients with psychotic mania and possibly non-psychotic mania, and psychotic depression. The use of these agents in psychotic mood disorders is an important and evolving area of clinical psychopharmacology without clear trends to date in either the USA or Europe. As new antipsychotics become available, each with a distinctive pharmacological profile, careful studies of their potential thymoleptic activity should help to define their roles in the treatment of patients with mood disorders.

References

Ahlfors, U.G., Baastrup, P.C., Denckes, S.J., *et al.* (1981). Flupenthixol decanoate in recurrent manic-depressive illness. *Acta Psychiatr Scand.*, **64**, 226–237.

Andreasen, N.C. (1979a). Thought, language, and communication disorders, I: clinical assessment, definition of terms, and evaluation of their reliability. *Arch. Gen Psychiatry*, **36**, 1315–1321.

Andreasen, N.C. (1979b). Thought, language and communication disorders, II: diagnostic significance. *Arch Gen. Psychiatry*, **36**, 1325–1330.

Anton, R.F. and Burch, E.Z. (1990). Amoxapine versus amitriptyline combined with perphenazine in the treatment of psychotic depression. *Am. J. Psychiatry*, **147**, 1203–1208.

Aronson, T.A., Shukla, S., Gujavarty, K., *et al.* (1988). Relapse in delusional depression: a retrospective study of the course of treatment. *Compr. Psychiatry*, **29**, 12–21.

Avery, D. and Lubrano, A. (1979). Depression treated with imipramine and ECT: The DeCarolis study reconsidered. *Am. J. Psychiatry*, **136**, 559–562.

Banov, M.D., Zarate, C.A., Jr, Tohen, M., *et al.* (1994). Clozapine therapy in refractory affective disorders: polarity predicts response in long-term follow-up. *J. Clin. Psychiatry*, **55**, 295–300.

Barkin, J.S. and Pais, V.M., Jr (1997). Induction of mania by risperidone resistant to mood stabilizers. *J. Clin. Psychopharmacol.*, **17**, 57–58.

Bernhard, R. (1997). Can risperidone be antidepressive and also inhibit aggression? *J. Neuropsychiatr. Clin. Neurosci.*, **9**, 627–628.

Bowden, C. L., Brugger, A.M., Swann, A.C., *et al.* (1994). Efficacy of divalproex vs. lithium and placebo in the treatment of mania. *J. Am. Med. Assoc.*, **271**, 918–924.

Breakey, W.R. and Goodell, H. (1972). Thought disorder in mania and schizophrenia evaluated by Bannister's Grid test for schizophrenic thought disorder. *Br. J. Psychiatry*, **120**, 391–395.

Calabrese, J.R., Kimmel, S.E., Woyshville, M.J., *et al.* (1996). Clozapine for treatment-refractory mania. *Am. J. Psychiatry*, **153**, 759–764.

Carlson, G.A. and Goodwin, F.K. (1973). The stages of mania: a longitudinal analysis of the manic episode. *Arch. Gen. Psychiatry*, **28**, 221–228.

Clower, C.G. (1983). Recurrent psychotic unipolar depression. *J. Clin. Psychiatry*, **44**, 216–218.

Coryell, W., Endicott, J. and Keller, M. (1987). The importance of psychotic features to major depression: course and outcome during a 2-year follow-up. *Acta Psychiatr. Scand.*, **75**, 78–85.

Coryell, W., Leon, A., Winokur, G., *et al.* (1996). The importance of psychotic features to long-term course in major depressive disorders. *Am. J. Psychiatry*, **153**, 483–489.

Coryell, W., Pfohl, B. and Zimmerman, M. (1984). The clinical and neuroedocrine features of psychotic depression. *J. Nerv. Ment. Dis.*, **172**, 521–528.

Coryell, W. and Tsuang, M. (1985). Major depression with mood-congruent or mood-incongruent psychotic features: outcome after 40 years. *Am. J. Psychiatry*, **142**, 479–482.

Dassa, D., Kaladjian, A., Azorin, J.M., *et al.* (1993). Clozapine in the treatment of psychotic refractory depression. *Br. J. Psychiatry*, **163**, 822–824.

Diaz, S. F. (1996). Mania associated with risperidone use (letter). *J. Clin. Psychiatry*, **57**, 41–42.

Esparon, J., Kallaori, J., Naylor, G.J., *et al.* (1986). Comparison of the prophylactic action of flupenthixol with placebo in lithium treated manic-depressive patients. *Br. J. Psychiatry*, **148**, 723–725.

Frances, A., Brown, R., Kocsic, J., *et al.* (1981). Psychotic depression: a separate entity? *Am. J. Psychiatry*, **138**, 831–833.

Frye, M.A., Ketter, T.A., Altshuler, L.L., *et al.* (1998). Clozapine in bipolar disorder: treatment implications for other atypical antipsychotics. *J. Affect. Disord.*, **48**, 91–104.

Gelenberg, A.J. and Hopkins, H.S. (1996). Antipsychotics in bipolar disorder. *J. Clin. Psychiatry*, **57** (Suppl. 9), 49–52.

Ghaemi, S.N. and Sachs, G.S. (1997). Long-term risperidone treatment in bipolar disorder: 6-month follow up. *Int. Clin. Psychopharmacol.*, **12**, 333–338.

Ghaemi, S.N., Sachs, G.S., Baldassano, C., *et al.* (1997). Acute treatment of bipolar disorder with adjunctive risperidone in outpatients. *Can. J. Psychiatry*, **42**, 196–199.

Goodnick, P.J. (1995). Risperidone treatment of refractory acute mania (letter). *J. Clin. Psychiatry*, **56**, 431–432.

Goodwin, F.K. and Jamison, K.R. (1990). *Manic-Depressive Illness*. New York, Oxford University Press.

Grossi, E., Sacchetti, E. and Vita, A. (1984). Carbamazepine vs chlorpromazine in mania: a double-blind trial. In: *Anticonvulsants in Affective Disorders* (H.M. Emrich, T. Okuma and A.A. Muller, eds.), Amsterdam, Excerpta Medica, pp. 177–187.

Harrow, M., Grossman, L.S., Silverstein, M.L., *et al.* (1986). A longitudinal study of thought disorder in manic patients. *Arch. Gen. Psychiatry*, **43**, 781–785.

Harrow, M., Grossman, L.S., Silverstein, M.L., *et al.* (1982) Thought pathology in manic and schizophrenic patients: its occurrence at hospital admission and seven weeks later. *Arch. Gen. Psychiatry*, **39**, 665–671.

Hendrick, V., Altshuler, L.L. and Szuba, M.P. (1994). Is there a role for neuroleptics in bipolar depression? *J. Clin. Psychiatry*, **55**, 533–535.

Hillert, A., Maier, W., Wetzel, H., *et al.* (1992). Risperidone in the treatment of disorders with a combined psychotic and depressive syndrome – a functional approach. *Pharmacopsychiatry*, **25**, 213–217.

Jacobsen, F. M. (1995). Risperidone in the treatment of affective illness and obsessive-compulsive disorder. *J. Clin. Psychiatry*, **56**, 423–429.

Janicak, P.G., Newman, R.H. and Davis, J.M. (1992). Advances in the treatment of manic and related disorders: a reappraisal. *Psychiatr. Ann.*, **22**, 94–98.

Johnson, G., Gerson, S., Burdock, E.I., *et al.* (1971). Comparative effects of lithium and chlorpromazine in the treatment of acute manic states. *Br. J. Psychiatry*, **119**, 267–276.

Kane, J.M., Jeste, D.V., Barnes, T.R.E., *et al.* (1992). *Tardive Dyskinesia: A Task Force Report of the American Psychiatric Association.* Washington, DC, American Psychiatric Association.

Keck, P.E., Jr., McElroy, S.L. and Strakowski, S.M. (1999). Schizoaffective disorder: role of atypical antipsychotics. *Schizophr. Res.* **35** (Suppl.), 5–12.

Keck, P.E., Jr and McElroy, S.L. (1998a). Pharmacological treatment of bipolar disorders. In: *A Guide to Treatments that Work* (P.E. Nathan and J.M. Gorman, eds), New York, Oxford University Press, pp. 249–269.

Keck, P.E., Jr, McElroy, S.L. and Strakowski, S.M. (1998b). Anticonvulsants and antipsychotics in the treatment of bipolar disorder. *J. Clin. Psychiatry*, **59** (Suppl. 6), 74–81.

Keck, P.E., Jr, McElroy, S.L., Strakowski, S.M., *et al.* (1996). Factors associated with maintenance antipsychotic treatment of patients with bipolar disorder. *J. Clin. Psychiatry*, **57**, 147–151.

Keck, P.E., Jr, McElroy, S.L., Strakowski, S.M., *et al.* (1994). Pharmacologic treatment of schizoaffective disorder. *Psychopharmacology*, **114**, 529–538.

Keck, P.E., Jr., Wilson, D.R., Strakowski, S.M., *et al.* (1995). Clinical predictors of acute risperidone response in schizophrenia, schizoaffective disorder, and psychotic mood disorders. *J. Clin. Psychiatry*, **56**, 466–470.

Klein, D.F. and Oaks, G. (1967). Importance of psychiatric diagnosis in prediction of clinical drug effects. *Arch. Gen. Psychiatry*, **16**, 118–126.

Kook, R.J. and Kestrel, C.C. (1996) Probable induction of mania by risperidone (letter). *J. Clin. Psychiatry*, **57**, 174–175.

Kukopulos, A., Reginaldi, D., Laddomana, P., *et al.* (1980). Course of manic-depressive cycle and changes caused by treatments. *Pharmakopsychiatr Neuropsychopharmakol*, **13**, 156–167.

Lane, H.-Y., Lin, Y.-C. and Chang, W.-H. (1998). Mania induced by risperidone: dose related? *J. Clin. Psychiatry*, **59**, 85–86.

Leppig, M., Bosch, B., Naber, D., *et al.* (1989). Clozapine in the treatment of 121 outpatients. *Psychopharmacology*, **99**, 577–579.

Licht, R.W. (1998) Drug treatment of mania: a critical review. *Acta Psychiatr. Scand.*, **97**, 387–397.

Littlejohn, R., Leslie, F. and Cookson, J. (1994). Depot antipsychotics in the prophylaxis of bipolar affective disorder. *Br. J. Psychiatry*, **165**, 827–829.

Lowe, M.R. and Batchelor, D.H. (1986). Depot neuroleptics and manic depressive psychosis. *Int. Clin. Psychopharmacol.*, **1** (Suppl. 1), 53–62.

Lowe, M.R. and Batchelor, D.H. (1990). Lithium and neuroleptics in the management of manic depressive psychosis. *Hum. Psychopharmacol.*, **5**, 267–274.

Lykouras, E., Malliaras, D., Christodoulou, G., *et al.* (1986). Delusional depression: phenomenology in response to treatment. *Acta Psychiatr. Scand.*, **73**, 324–329.

Madhusoodanan, S., Brenner, R., Aranjo, L., *et al.* (1995). Efficacy of risperidone treatment for psychoses associated with schizophrenia, schizoaffective disorder, bipolar disorder, or senile dementia in 11 geriatric patients: a case series. *J. Clin. Psychiatry*, **56**, 514–518.

McElroy, S.L., Dessain, E.C., Pope, H.G., Jr, *et al.* (1991). Clozapine in the treatment of psychotic mood disorders, schizoaffective disorder, and schizophrenia. *J. Clin. Psychiatry*, **52**, 411–414.

McElroy, S.L., Frye, M., Denicoff, K., *et al.* (1998). Olanzapine in treatment-resistant bipolar disorder. *J. Affect. Disord.*, **49**, 119–122.

McElroy, S.L., Keck, P.E., Jr and Strakowski, S.M. (1996). Mania, psychosis and antipsychotics. *J. Clin. Psychiatry*, **57** (Suppl. 3), 14–26.

McElroy, S.L., Keck, P.E., Jr., Stanton, S.P., *et al.* (1996). A randomized comparison of divalproex oral loading versus haloperidol in the initial treatment of acute psychotic mania. *J. Clin. Psychiatry*, **57**, 142–146.

McIntyre, R., Young, L.T., Hasey, G., *et al.* (1997). Risperidone treatment of bipolar disorder. *Can. J. Psychiatry*, **42**, 88–90.

Morgan, H.G. (1972). The incidence of depressive symptoms during recovery from hypomania. *Br. J. Psychiatry*, **120**, 537–539.

Mukherjee, S., Rosen, A.M., Caracci, G., *et al.* (1986). Persistent tardive dyskinesia in bipolar patients. *Arch. Gen. Psychiatry*, **43**, 342–346.

Muller-Siecheneder, F., Muller, M.J., Hillert, A., *et al.* (1998). Risperidone versus haloperidol and amitriptyline in the treatment of patients with a combined psychotic and depressive syndrome. *J. Clin. Psychopharmacol.*, **18**, 111–120.

Mulsant, B.H., Haskett, R.F., Prudic, J., *et al.* (1997). Low use of neuroleptic drugs in the treatment of psychotic major depression. *Am. J. Psychiatry*, **154**, 559–56.

Naber, D., Hogback, R., Perro, C., *et al.* (1992). Clinical management of clozapine patients in relation to efficacy and side effects. *Br. J. Psychiatry*, **160**, 54–59.

Nasrallah, H.A., Churchill, C.M. and Hamdan-Allan, G.A. (1988). Higher frequency of neuroleptic-induced dystonia in mania than schizophrenia. *Am. J. Psychiatry*, **145**, 1455–1456.

Naylor, G.J. and Scott, C.R. (1980). Depot injections for affective disorders (letter). *Br. J. Psychiatry*, **136**, 105.

O'Croinin, F., Zibin, T. and Holt, L. (1995). Hypomania associated with risperidone (letter). *Can. J. Psychiatry*, **56**, 51.

Okuma, T., Inanga, K., Otsuki, S., *et al.* (1979). Comparison of the antimanic efficacy of carbamazepine and chlorpromazine. *Psychopharmacology*, **66**, 211–217.

Parker, G., Roy, K., Hadzi-Pavlovic, D., *et al.* (1992). Psychotic (delusional) depression: a meta-analysis of physical treatment. *J. Affect. Disord.*, **24**, 17–24.

Parker, G., Hadzi-Pavlovic, D., Hickie, I., *et al.* (1991). Distinguishing psychotic and nonpsychotic melancholia. *J. Affect. Disord.*, **22**, 135–148.

Pope, H.G., Jr, McElroy, S.L., Keck, P.E., Jr, *et al.* (1991). Valproate in the treatment of acute mania: a placebo-controlled study. *Arch. Gen. Psychiatry*, **48**, 62–68.

Pope, H.G. and Lipinski, J.F. (1978). Diagnosis in schizophrenia and manic-depressive illness: a reassessment of the specificity of schizophrenic symptoms in the light of current research. *Arch. Gen. Psychiatry*, **35**, 811–828.

Prien, R.F., Caffey, E.M., Jr, Klett, C.J., *et al.* (1972). Comparison of lithium carbonate and chlorpromazine in the treatment of mania: report of the Veterans Administration and National Institute of Mental Health Collaborative Study Group. *Arch. Gen. Psychiatry*, **26**, 146–153.

Rothschild, A.J. (1996). Management of psychotic, treatment-resistant depression. *Psychiatr. Clin. NA*, **19**, 237–252.

Rothschild, A.J., Bates, K.S., Boehringer, K., *et al.* (1998). Olanzapine response in psychotic depression. In: *Abstracts of the 36th Annual meeting of the American College of Neuropsychopharmacology*. Honolulu, HI, December 10, 1997.

Rothschild, A.J., Samson, J.A., Bessette, M.P., *et al.* (1993). Efficacy of the combination of fluoxetine and perphenazine in the treatment of psychotic depression. *J. Clin. Psychiatry*, **54**, 338–342.

Sajatovic, M., DiGiovanni, S.K., Bastain, B., *et al.* (1996), Risperidone therapy in treatment refractory acute bipolar and schizoaffective mania. *Psychopharmacol. Bull.*, **32**, 55–61.

Schaffer, C.B. and Schaffer, L.C. (1996). The use of risperidone in the treatment of bipolar disorder (letter). *J. Clin. Psychiatry*, **57**, 136.

Schatzberg, A.F. and Rothschild, A.J. (1992). Psychotic (delusional) major depression: should it be included as a distinct syndrome in DSM-IV? *Am. J. Psychiatry*, **149**, 733–745.

Schnierow, B. and Graeher, D. (1996). Manic symptoms associated with initiation of risperidone. *Am. J. Psychiatry*, **153**, 1235–1236.

Segal, J., Berk, M. and Brook, S. (1998). Risperidone compared with both lithium and halo-peridol in mania: a double-blind randomized controlled trial. *Clin. Neuropharmacol.*, **21**, 176–180.

Sernyak, M.J., Griffin, R.A., Johnson, R.M., *et al.* (1994). Neuroleptic exposure following inpatient treatment of acute mania with lithium and neuroleptic. *Am. J. Psychiatry*, **151**, 133–135.

Shopsin, B., Gerson, S., Thompson, H., *et al.* (1975). Psychoactive drugs in mania: a controlled comparison of lithium carbonate, chlorpromazine, and haloperidol. *Arch. Gen. Psychiatry*, **32**, 34–42.

Simpson, D.M. and Davis, G.C. (1985). Measuring thought disorder with clinical rating scales in schizophrenic and nonschizophrenic patients. *Psychiatry Res.*, **15**, 313–318.

Spiker, D.G., Weiss, J.C., Dealy, R.S., *et al.* (1985). The pharmacological treatment of delu-sional depression. *Am. J. Psychiatry*, **142**, 430–436.

Spring, G., Schweid, D., Gray, C., *et al.* (1970). A double-blind comparison of lithium and chlorpromazine in the treatment of manic states. *Am. J. Psychiatry*, **126**, 1306–1310.

Suppes, R., McElroy, S.L., Gilbert, J., *et al.* (1992). Clozapine in the treatment of dysphoric mania. *Biol. Psychiatry*, **32**, 270–280.

Suppes, T., Rush, A.J., Webb, A., *et al.* (1996). One year randomized trial of clozapine vs. usual care in bipolar I patients. *Biol. Psychiatry*, **39**, 531.

Tohen, M. (1998). Olanzapine vs. placebo in the treatment of acute mania. In: *Abstracts of the American Psychiatric Association Annual Meeting*. Toronto, Canada, May 31, 1998.

Tohen, M., Sanger, T., Tollefson, G.D., *et al.* (1997). Olanzapine vs. placebo in the treatment of acute mania. In: *Abstracts of the 36th Annual Meeting of the American College of Neuropsychopharmacology*. Honolulu, HI, December 10, 1997.

Tohen, M., Tsuang, M.T. and Goodwin, D.C. Prediction of outcome in mania by mood-congruent or mood-incongruent psychotic features. *Am. J. Psychiatry*, **149**, 1580–1584.

Tohen, M. and Zarate, C.A., Jr. (1998). Antipsychotic agents and bipolar disorder. *J. Clin. Psychiatry*, **59** (Suppl. 1), 38–48.

Tohen, M., Zarate, C.A., Jr, Centorrino, F., *et al.* (1996). Risperidone in the treatment of mania. *J. Clin. Psychiatry*, **57**, 249–253.

Tomlinson, W.G. (1996). Risperidone and mania. *Am. J. Psychiatry*, **153**, 132–133.

Verdoux, H., Gonzales, B., Takei, N., *et al.* (1996). A survey of prescribing practice of anti-psychotic maintenance treatment for manic-depressive outpatients. *J. Affect. Disord.*, **57**, 147–151.

White, E., Cheung, T. and Silverstone, T. (1993). Depot antipsychotics in bipolar affective disorder. *Int. Clin. Psychopharmacol.*, **8**, 119–122.

Wood, M.J. and Rubinstein, M. (1990). An atypical responder to clozapine. *Am. J. Psychiatry*, **147**, 369.

Zarate, C.A., Jr, Narendran, R., Tohen, M., *et al.* (1998). Clinical predictors of acute response with olanzapine in psychotic mood disorders. *J. Clin. Psychiatry*, **59**, 24–28.

Zarate, C.A., Jr, Tohen, M. and Baldessarini, R.J. (1995). Clozapine in severe mood disorders. *J. Clin. Psychiatry*, **56**, 411–417.

17

Future directions in novel antidepressants and mood stabilizing agents

Siegfried Kasper and Alan Schatzberg

Key points

- Newer antidepressants are as effective as first generation antidepressants, but exhibit fewer side effects.
- Newer antidepressants have a more favourable risk/benefit profile, e.g. intoxication in overdose.
- Newer antidepressants effectively open the possibility for the necessary long-term treatment perspective in depression.
- In addition to lithium, anticonvulsants are effective mood stabilizers for long-term treatment of bipolar disorder.
- Antidepressants with novel mechanisms of actions (e.g. peptide antagonism) are actively being developed.
- Mood stabilizers should preferably be used for bipolar depression as well as mania. Antidepressants and typical antipsychotics may worsen the outcome of bipolar disorder.

Introduction

Whereas antidepressants (AD) of the first generation were developed primarily on the basis of their chemical structure (e.g. tricyclic antidepressants, TCA), the newer generation of antidepressants have been developed strictly on the basis of their mechanism of action (e.g. selective serotonin or noradrenaline reuptake inhibitors). Although there was no evidence that the elderly antidepressants like imipramine are psychostimulants or a 'happy pill', this notion is still often discussed in the media, over 40 years after the introduction of antidepressants for treatment of depression.

When Kuhn (1957, 1958) first described the antidepressant effect of imipramine, he based his assumption only on clinical observation. There were no standardized diagnostic criteria, no psychometric instruments, like the Hamilton Depression Rating Scale (HAM-D) and no computer to establish statistical significance levels and confidence intervals. Subsequent development resulted in a refined methodology, which is now the basis for internationally accepted drug development programmes with the possibility of having the medications available in Europe and world-wide (European Community, 1994). Whereas the methodology and the quality of the studies are nowadays acceptable throughout different health authorities world-wide, pricing of the product is the limiting factor for the availability of medication in the individual countries.

One of the aims for developing new antidepressants was to have a better tolerability profile compared to the older AD, specifically also toxicity in overdose (Cassidy and Henry, 1987). To achieve this goal a more circumscribed mechanism of action was studied. Specifically, it was targeted to eliminate anticholinergic (dry mouth, constipation, cognitive dysfunction), antihistaminergic (sedation, weight gain), as well as alpha1-adrenolytic (orthostatic hypotension) mediated side effects (Montgomery and Kasper, 1995). A beneficial side-effect profile is of specific importance in treatment of depression in the elderly (Salzman, 1993).

Antidepressants of the first generation

Soon after antidepressants had been shown to be effective in open trials, randomized controlled trials (RCT) with the use of placebo were introduced in depression research. Morris and Bech (1974) published the first comprehensive review of RCT. The authors noticed that there were many differences, e.g. diagnostic assessment of depression, the control treatment, the definition of response and the statistical analysis, which makes it difficult to compare the individual studies. Interestingly, the first trial conducted in a setting of general practice (GP) was published in 1970 (Porter, 1970). This is of importance since more than 80% of the prescriptions come from these doctors.

Overall, the RCT indicated that TCAs as well as monoamine oxidase inhibitors (MAOI) are significantly superior to placebo, but with a burdensome side-effect profile. The largest long-term study with antidepressants has been performed with imipramine (Frank et al., 1990), which indicated that the dose which had proven to be effective in the short-term treatment should also be used for continuation and prophylactic treatment (Frank et al., 1993). Furthermore, this study elegantly demonstrated the superiority of antidepressive medication over placebo and interpersonal psychotherapy.

The necessity of long-term treatment of depression soon underlined the importance for a low side-effect profile of antidepressants which was the lead for the development of newer antidepressants.

Newer antidepressants

Compared to the RCTs carried out with TCAs, newer antidepressants have been studied with a more refined methodology, since DSM-III to DSM-IV diagnoses of major depression as well as standardized research instruments were more accepted (Bech, 1981). These methodological standardizations facilitated the use of meta-analysis like the ones of Loonen and Zwanikken (1990), Bech and Cialdella (1992) or Anderson and Tomenson (1994).

Selective Serotonin Reuptake Inhibitors (SSRIs)

To date there are five SSRIs available world-wide: citalopram, fluoxetine, fluvoxamine, paroxetine and sertraline (Kasper and Heiden, 1995). While they all have the serotonin-reuptake inhibition as the common mechanism of action, they differ in pharmacokinetic properties (Brøsen and Rasmussen, 1996, see also Leonard and Richelson, Chapter 8). RCT indicated that the SSRIs are superior to placebo in their antidepressant efficacy and not different from TCA, with the possible exception in severe depression, if clomipramine is used as a comparator (DUAG, 1986, 1990). The long-term studies with SSRIs support the notion that SSRIs are effective in preventing relapse (e.g. in the first 4–6 months after acute episode) and recurrence (6 months after remission has been achieved) (Kasper, 1993).

With regard to side effects, SSRIs have a more favourable side-effect profile compared to TCAs and their side effects mitigate after 2–3 weeks, whereas those of amitriptyline persist (Rheimherr *et al.*, 1990).

Selective Noradrenaline Reuptake Inhibitor (SNRI)

Recently reboxetine has been introduced in Europe and will soon be available in the USA, which has a specific noradrenaline reuptake mechanism (Dubini *et al.*, 1997). Besides antidepressant efficacy this compound promises specifically to improve social functioning compared with SSRIs (Kasper, 1999).

Dual and receptor-specific acting antidepressants

After the success of the SSRIs researchers set out to develop compounds which exert additionally to serotonin, a norepinephrine reuptake blocking property (= SNRIs). Antidepressants with this mechanism of action have been termed dual acting antidepressants. Venlafaxine (Lecrubier *et al.*, 1997; Burnett and Dinan, 1998) and milnacipran (Briley *et al.*, 1996) fall into this class and based on data available from basic science it seems that venlafaxine is more a 5-HT than a NA-reuptake inhibitor and milnacipran the opposite. Both compounds have been shown to be significantly superior to placebo and equally effective as TCAs (Benkert *et al.*, 1996; Kasper, 1997). However, compared with SSRIs a significantly superior efficacy has been demonstrated in severely depressed patients. The side-effect profile of the SNRIs is linked to their pharmacodynamic properties with nausea and agitation found to be the most frequent.

Mirtazapine is a specific acting antidepressant, which enhances noradrenaline as well as serotonin neurotransmission via blockade of the presynaptic autoreceptor sites (Kasper *et al.*, 1997). Additionally it exerts its antidepressant properties via blockade of post-synaptic 5-HT$_2$ and 5-HT$_3$ receptors. RCTs demonstrated superior efficacy to placebo and comparable efficacy to TCAs, including clomipramine. Superior antidepressant properties have been demonstrated to fluoxetine. Nefazodone is another newly introduced compound with a combined serotonergic mechanism of action (5-HT reuptake inhibition, 5-HT$_2$ blockade) which offers the benefit of not having sexual side effects (Baldwin and Birtwhistle, 1998). However, the necessity for a dosing-in regimen as well as other side effects (like light-headedness), suggests that this compound does not have an overall advantage over SSRIs (Feighner et al., 1998).

Moclobemide, a reversible inhibitor of MAO-A is marketed in Europe but not the USA (Lecrubier and Guelfi, 1990; Angst and Stabl, 1992). This compound can be viewed as efficacious in mild to moderate, but not severe depression. However, specific studies in this indication have not been carried out.

St John's wort as an antidepressant

Since ancient times preparations of St John's wort ('Johanniskraut') have been used for their antidepressant treatment properties (Müller and Kasper, 1997). In Germany this treatment modality comprises as much as 40% of the antidepressant market. Recently it has been demonstrated for one standardized formulation (LI-160, Lichtwer), that the pharmacodynamic properties include serotonin, noradrenaline and dopamine reuptake inhibition together with GABA-ergic effects (Müller et al., 1997). There are a number of RCTs with LI-300 and quite a few ones to come, which indicate the superiority over placebo and no difference to TCAs. However, the quality of these trials by and large is not comparable to synthetic antidepressants with regard to sample size, dosage of reference compound etc. The trials currently being performed will answer these questions in the near future. For example in the USA, the National Institutes of the Health are sponsoring a 300 patient double-blind, multicentre trial comparing St John's wort, sertraline, and placebo in depressed outpatients. Compared to synthetic antidepressants LI-160 has significantly less side effects and this is most probably one of the reasons for the high prescription rates.

Novel antidepressants

Currently, efforts at developing new antidepressants are pursuing drugs with novel mechanisms of actions. In particular, a number of strategies have focused on agents that block receptors for brain peptides. These approaches have been built upon theories that alterations in the activity of specific brain peptides could play a major role in stress responses or in the development of symptoms of anxiety or depression.

The most advanced of these pharmacological approaches is the use of substance P antagonists. Substance P is a neurokinin peptide with wide distribution in brain (Pernow, 1983). It was identified in the early 1930's by von Euler and its amino acid sequence was identified some 40 years later (Wahlestedt 1998). Its potential role as a neurostransmitter in the brain was demonstrated in 1975. In the late 1980s, a neurokinin receptor (NK_1) which preferred substance P was cloned and early antagonists, that were large molecules and had less availability than was optimal, were developed. Recently a number of companies have developed relatively small molecules with better availability and these are under active clinical investigation for their potential efficacy in depression. One compound – MK-869 – has been tested in major depression and has been reported to be effective (Kramer *et al.*, 1998).

Initially, substance P antagonists were tested as pain modulators but studies were remarkable in their consistent lack of efficacy for this indication. The mapping of substance P in mammalian brain pointed to high concentrations in areas (e.g. the amygdala) thought to be involved in stress modulation, anxiety, or depression and this led investigators to explore the possible use of NK_1 antagonists in animal models of stress. Kramer and colleagues have described elegantly that MK-869 – an NK_1 antagonist – can exert significant suppression effects on separation-induced vocalizations in a gerbal model of stress. In addition, NK_1 antagonists have been reported to have potent antiemetic effects.

MK-869 has been tested in a multicentre trial in which 300 mg/day of the agent was compared with paroxetine (20 mg/day) and placebo in 213 patients (Kramer *et al.*, 1998). Both drugs separated from placebo in reducing total scores on the Hamilton Depression Rating Scale (HDRS) and the Hamilton Anxiety Rating Scale (HARS) and there was a suggestion – though not statistically significant – of possible superiority of MK-869 over paroxetine on anxiety measures at the conclusion of study. MK-869 did not appear to produce more rapid effects.

The drug's side-effect profile appeared relatively benign. Principal side effects appeared to be irritability, nausea, and fatigue. The drug appeared to produce significantly less sexual dysfunction than did the SSRIs.

Subsequent to this report, the manufacturer of MK-869 has decided to suspend development of this particular compound in favour of much more potent second-generation antagonists that can be prescribed at lower doses. In addition, a number of pharmaceutical companies with small molecule antagonists in their portfolios have also started investigation of their compounds in major depression. This approach is innovative and opens new avenues for treatment.

Another recent approach has been to develop antagonists for corticotrophin releasing hormone (CRH). This peptide, found in the hypothalamus and hippocampus, has been reported to play an initiating role in the hypothalamic–pituitary–adrenal (HPA) axis response to stress. The peptide stimulates the pituitary to release adrenocorticotrophin hormone (ACTH) which in turn stimulates the adrenal gland to secrete cortisol. Cortisol feeds back at the levels of the brain and pituitary to inhibit further stimulation of CRH and ACTH and ultimately to decrease its own release. Potential antagonism of the stress-induced increases in HPA axis activity underlie early attempts to develop CRH antagonists as antidepressants. However, more recent studies have concentrated on CRH outside of the HPA axis (e.g. in the amygdala) which is not responsive to negative feedback by cortisol. CRH outside the HPA axis may play an important role in general stress responsivity and the pathogenesis of anxiety and depressive disorders.

Early prototypes, e.g. a helical CRH, were potent antagonists but, again, their large structures led to poor bioavailability or permeability of the blood–brain barrier. Studies in rats required intracerebral administration. More recently a number of antagonists have been developed and these are generally smaller and enjoy greater permeability into brain. Several prototypes have passed phase I screening for safety and are now headed for early dose finding phase II efficacy studies.

A third approach has been to develop drugs that act as antagonists of the sigma receptor. The sigma receptor was thought for many years to be linked to opioid systems but over time data emerged to indicate that this receptor has less to do with opioids than was originally thought. More recently a number of studies have pointed to some sigma antagonists as exerting effects on other systems such as glutamate, GABA-B acetylcholine and neuropeptides. Sigma antagonists may increase release of norepinephrine from pre-synaptic terminals and are effective in several animal models used to determine possible antidepressant properties. Still, the exact mechanisms of action *vis-à-vis* relief of depression is unclear.

Sigma antagonists were originally studied in schizophrenia with relatively limited efficacy in positive symptoms. Recently, one such compound, igmesine, has begun to be studied in major depression. Results are not yet available. Still, sigma antagonists represent a novel approach to antidepressant therapy.

Emerging opportunities with mood stabilizers

Whereas for a long time only lithium was available for long-term treatment of bipolar disorder (BP), valproic acid, carbamazepine and as an add-on therapy clonazepam are now available. The side-effect profile and toxicity of lithium are not the only reason why further developments were necessary. Based on the kindling hypothesis of Post *et al.* (1992) it is likely that in BP-patients who respond in a later stage of their illness this response is more likely to be due to anticonvulsants than to lithium. Within the group of mood stabilizers in the USA, valproic acid and, in Europe, carbamazepine are predominantly used as monotherapy or combination therapy together with lithium. There is some indication that carbamazepine has a favourable profile in schizoaffective disorders (Stuppäck *et al.*, 1994) whereas valproic acid is specifically beneficial in rapid-cycling (Calabrese *et al.*, 1993). Both compounds have limiting side effects, such as weight gain or changes in plasma levels of concomitant medication (carbamazepine lowers and valproic acid increases levels of concomitant medication).

Further candidates for treatment of bipolar disorder under current investigation are lamotrigine, topiramate and gabapentin which do not, for instance, have the side effect of weight gain and one of them, lamotrigine, appears to be effective for treatment of acute depression in bipolar patients (Calabrese *et al.*, 1999). These agents are likely to have a substantial role in the management of affective disorders over the coming years.

Conclusion

The introduction of TCAs in the 1950s was the first revolution of antidepressant therapy followed by the SSRIs in the late 1980s. The relative lack of side effects of the SSRIs and their efficacy in disorders other than major depression (including anxiety disorders and eating disorders) made them widely prescribed and accepted medications. The SSRIs fostered a mechanism-based approach to antidepressant research which will hopefully lead to antidepressants with more distinct mechanisms of action, e.g. substance P antagonists (Kramer *et al.*, 1998). More effective and better tolerated antidepressant medications improve patients' quality of life, foster greater acceptance of the disease in our society, and ultimately provide wider benefit for patients (Currie *et al.*, 1993).

References

Anderson, I.M. and Tomenson, B.M. (1994). The efficacy of selective serotonin re-uptake inhibitors in depression: a meta-analysis of studies against tricyclic antidepressants. *J. Psychopharmacol.*, **8**, 238–249.

Angst, J. and Stabl, M. (1992). Efficacy of moclobemide in different patient groups: a meta-analysis of studies. *Psychopharmacology*, **106**, 109–113.

Baldwin, D.S. and Birtwhistle, J. (1998). Antidepressant drugs and sexual function: improving the recognition and management of sexual dysfunction in depressed patients. In: *Antidepressant therapy at the dawn of the Third Millennium* (M. Briley and S.A. Montgomery, eds), London, Martin Dunitz, pp. 231–253.

Bech, P. (1981). Rating scales for affective disorders: their validity and consistency. *Acta Psychiatr Scanad.*, **64** (Suppl. 295), 1–101.

Bech, P. and Cialdella, P. (1992), Citalopram in depression: meta-analysis of intended and unintended effects. *Int. Clin. Psychopharmacol.*, **6** (Suppl. 5), 45–54.

Benkert, O., Gründer, G., Wetzel, H., *et al.* (1996). A randomized double-blind comparison of a rapidly escalating dose of venlafaxine and imipramine in inpatients with major depression and melancholia. *J. Psychiatr. Res.*, **30**, 441–451.

Brøsen, K. and Rasmussen, B.B. (1996). Selective serotonin reuptake inhibitors: In: *Pharmacokinetics and Drug Interactions*, 2nd edn. Chichester, John Wiley, pp. 87–108.

Briley, M., Prost, J. and Moret, C. (1996). Preclinical pharmacology of milnacipran. *Int. Clin. Psychopharmacol.*, **11**, 9–14.

Burnett, F.E. and Dinan, T.G. (1998). The clinical efficacy of venlafaxine in the treatment of depression. *Rev. Contemp. Pharmacother.*, **9**, 303–320.

Calabrese, J.R., Woyshville, M.J., Kimmel, S.E., *et al.* (1993). Mixed states and bipolar rapid cycling and their treatment with VPA. *Psychiatr. Ann.*, **23**, 70–78.

Calabrese, J.R., Bowden, C.L., Sachs, G.S., *et al.* (1999). A double-blind placebo controlled study of lamotrigine monotherapy in outpatients with Bipolar I depression. *J. Clin. Psychiatry*, **60**, 79–88.

Cassidy, S. and Henry, J. (1987). Fatal toxicity of antidepressant drugs in overdose. *Br. Med. J.*, **295**, 1021–1024.

Currie, D.J., Fairweather, D.B. and Hindmarch, I. (1993) Social aspects of treating depression. In: *Health Economics of Depression* (B. Jönsson and J. Rosenbaum, eds), Chichester, Wiley, pp. 129–139.

Danish University Antidepressant Group (DUAG) (1986). Citalopram: clinical effect profile in comparison with clomipramine: a controlled multicenter study. *Psychopharmacology*, **90**, 131–138.

Danish University Antidepressant Group (DUAG) (1990). Paroxetine: a selective serotonin reuptake inhibitor showing better tolerance but weaker antidepressant effect than clomipramine in a controlled multicenter trial. *J. Affect. Dis.*, **18**, 289–299.

Dubini, A., Bosc, M. and Polin, V. (1997). Noradrenaline-selective versus serotonin-selective antidepressant therapy: differential effects on social functioning. *J. Psychopharmacol.*, **11** (Suppl. 4), 17–23.

European Community (1994). Guidelines on psychotropic drugs: antidepressant medical products. *Eur. Neuropsychopharmacol*, **4**, 62–65.

Feighner, J.P., Bennett, M.E. and Roberts, D.L. (1998). A double-blind trial of nefazodone versus placebo in depressed patients. *Int. J. Clin. Psychopharmacol.* (in press).

Frank, E., Kupfer, D.J. and Perel J.M. (1990). Three-year outcomes for maintenance therapies in recurrent depression. *Arch. Gen. Psychiatry*, **47**, 1093–1099.

Frank, E., Kupfer, D.J., Perel, J.M. *et al.* (1983). Comparison of full-dose versus half-dose pharmacotherapy in the maintenance treatment of recurrent depression. *J. Affect. Dis.*, **27**, 139–149.

Kasper, S. (1993). The rationale for long-term antidepressant therapy. *Int. Clin. Psychopharmacol.*, **8**, 225–235.

Kasper, S. (1997). The place of milnacipran in the treatment of depression. *Hum. Psychopharmacol.*, **12**, S135–S141.

Kasper, S. (1999). From symptoms to social functioning: differential effects of antidepressant therapy. *Int. Clin. Psychopharmacol.* **14** (Suppl. 1), S27–S31.

Kasper, S. and Heiden, A. (1995) Do SSRIs differ in their antidepressant efficacy? *Hum. Psychopharmacol.*, **10**, 163–171.

Kasper, S., Praschak-Rieder, N., Tauscher, J., *et al.* (1997). A risk-benefit assessment of mirtazapine in the treatment of depression. *CNS Drug Safety*, **17**, 251–264.

Kramer, M.S., Cutler, N., Feighner, J. *et al.* (1998). Distinct mechanism for antidepressant activity by blockade of central substance P receptors. *Science*, **281**, 1640–1645.

Kuhn, R. (1957). Über die Behandlung depressiver Zustände mit einem Iminodibenzylderivat (G 22355). *Schweiz Med. Wochenschr.*, **87**, 1135–1140.

Kuhn, R. (1958). The treatment of depressive states with G 22355 (imipramine hydrochloride) *Am. J. Psychiatr.*, **115**, 459–464.

Lecrubier, Y. and Guelfi, J.D. (1990). Efficacy of reversible inhibitors of monoamine oxidase A in various forms of depression. *Acta Psychiatr. Scand.*, **82** (Suppl. 1), 74–87.

Lecrubier, Y., Moon, C.A.L. and Schifano, F. (1997). Efficacy of venlafaxine in depressive illness in general practice. *Acta Psychiatr. Scand.*, **95**, 485–493.

Loonen, A.J.M. and Zwanikken, G.J. (1990). Continuation and maintenance therapy with antidepressive agents. An overview of research. *Pharm. Weekbl. (Scientific Edition)*, **12**, 128–141.

Montgomery, S.A. and Kasper, S. (1995). Comparison of compliance between serotonin reuptake inhibitors and tricyclic antidepressants: a meta-analysis. *Int. Clin. Psychopharmacol.*, **9** (Suppl. 4), 33–40.

Morris, J.B. and Bech, A.T. (1974). The efficacy of antidepressant drugs. *Arch. Gen. Psychiatry*, **30**, 667–674.

Müller, W.E. and Kasper, S. (eds) (1997). Hypericum extract (LI 160) as a herbal antidepressant. *Pharmacopsychiatry*, **30** (Suppl.), 71–134.

Müller, W.E., Rolli, M., Schäfer, C., *et al.* (1997). Effects of hypericum extract (LI 160) in biochemical models of antidepressant activity. *Pharmacopsychiatry*, **30** (Suppl.), 102–107.

Pernow, B. (1983). Substance P. *Pharmacol. Rev.*, **35**, 85–141.

Porter, A.M.W. (1970). Depressive illness in a general practice. A demographic study and a controlled trial of imipramine. *Br. Med. J*, **1**, 773–778.

Post, R.M., Leverich, G.S., Altshuler, L.L., *et al.* (1992). Lithium-discontinuation-induced refractoriness: preliminary observations. *Am. J. Psychiatry*, **149**, 1727–1729.

Reimherr, F.W., Chouinard, G., Cohn, C.K., *et al.* (1990). Antidepressant efficacy of sertraline: a double-blind placebo- and amitriptyline-controlled multicenter comparison study in outpatients with major depression. *J. Clin. Psychiatry*, **12** (Suppl. 1), 18–27.

Salzman, C. (1993). Pharmacological treatment of depression in the elderly. *J. Clin. Psychiatry*, **54** (Suppl. 2), 23–28.

Stuppäck, C.H., Barnas, C., Schwitzer, J., *et al.* (1994). Carbamazepine in the prophylaxis of major depression. A 5-year follow up. *J. Clin. Psychiatry*, **55**, 146–150.

Wahlestedt, C. (1998). Reward for persistence in substance P research. *Science*, **281**, 1624–1625.

Key Issues in Clinical Psychopharmacology

18

Drug interactions

David King

Key points

- Clinically important drug–drug interactions are those which involve drugs with a narrow therapeutic index (e.g. lithium, tricyclic antidepressants, antipsychotics, phenytoin, warfarin, and digoxin).
- Such interactions are more frequent in patients with comorbidity and/or those requiring polypharmacy, e.g. the elderly.
- Inhibition of cytochrome P450 isoenzymes by the selective serotonin reuptake inhibitors can lead to pharmacokinetic interactions with serious clinical consequences.
- Tricyclic antidepressants and selective serotonin reuptake inhibitors should not be combined unless facilities for drug plasma level and ECG monitoring are available.
- The cardiotoxicity of antipsychotics (particularly pimozide, sertindole and thioridazine) is increased by combinations with quinidine-like antiarrhythmics or the antihistamines, astemizole and terfenadine.
- A desk reference source or a physician's manual should always be consulted before an unfamiliar drug combination is prescribed.

Introduction

Potential psychotropic drug–drug interactions are a minefield which can either cause practising clinicians to be unnecessarily fearful and overcautious on the one hand, or cynical on the other. The latter reaction is understandable since the majority of these interactions are in fact theoretical and it has even been suggested that in the future they will be predicted by computer modelling techniques. Furthermore, not all drug interactions are hazardous and some may even be beneficial and are exploited to enhance drug effects (e.g. penicillin and probenecid; L-dopa and carbidopa). Others, if recognized and understood, can be allowed for by dose adjustment if the combination is essential in certain clinical situations (e.g. lithium and diuretics). It must also be remembered that drug interactions represent only one of a variety of factors which modify a patient's response to medication. Other factors such as dose, diet, age, concurrent disease and individual idiosyncracy are often at least, if not more, important. Recently, for example, there has been a great deal of concern about the significance of the inhibition of hepatic cytochrome P450 enzymes by the selective serotonin reuptake inhibitors (SSRIs) and their potential for drug interactions (see below). Nevertheless, even if such a drug were to inhibit such a drug metabolizing enzyme completely, the result would be no different from that of a patient with a poor metabolizing genotype with a genetic deficiency of that enzyme system (55–60% of Europeans are slow acetylators of isoniazid, about 10% are poor metabolizers of debrisoquine, and 5–10% have deficient CYP 2D6 oxidation, see Table 18.1). Thus, this interaction produces a greater sensitivity to adverse effects, similar to those with the poor metabolizing genotype, rather than a qualitatively different toxic reaction.

Nevertheless, a working knowledge of drug–drug interactions is important in clinical psychiatry because of the high potential for polypharmacy (sometimes justified by the high incidence of comorbidity, sometimes because of the frequency of covert drug abuse), and the tendency to use higher than recommended doses in treatment-refractory patients. This chapter will, therefore, focus on clinically important interactions – 'interactions that matter'. These are interactions that are potentially hazardous, where a dosage adjustment should be made, are well established and of clinical significance. Essentially these are interactions that involve a drug(s) with important toxic effects such as lithium, monoamine oxidase inhibitors (MAOIs), clozapine, warfarin, or digoxin, and which have a low therapeutic ratio.

For a more comprehensive treatment of the subject UK readers should have access to *Drug Interactions* (Stockley, 1995) and for those in the USA to *Drug Interactions in Psychiatry* (Ciraulo *et al.*, 1995). In addition, before prescribing a drug combination with which one is not familiar it is prudent to consult an up-to-date handbook such as the *British National Formulary* or the *Psychotropic Drug Directory* (Bazire, 1997) in the UK, or *the Clinical Handbook of Psychotropic Drugs* (Bezchlibnyk-Butler and Jeffries, 1995) in the USA. This chapter will take the form of a description of the mechanisms underlying drug–drug interactions with a few well known examples, followed by some Tables classifying these according to the principal drug groups involved.

Mechanisms of drug interaction

Drug–drug interactions can be either pharmacodynamic or pharmacokinetic in nature. In the latter the altered response can be related to altered circulating blood levels of the drug(s) involved, while with the former an interaction at the receptor level is inferred.

Table 18.1 CYP450 enzyme inhibition

Enzyme	Genetic polymorphisms Frequency of poor metabolizers	Substrates
CYP2D6	5–10% Caucasians	Desipramine
	3% Blacks	
	1% Asians	Nortriptyline
	1% Arabs	
CYP2C19	3–5% Caucasians	Diazepam
	15–20% Asians	

Adapted from DeVane (1998b)

1. Pharmacokinetic interactions

Most CNS drugs are lipid soluble, readily absorbed from the gut and have a high apparent volume of distribution. They are also highly bound to plasma proteins, extensively metabolized, some but not all metabolites being active, with high 'first-pass' metabolism. The serum levels are thus subject to wide, genetically determined, individual variation and readily affected by enzyme induction or inhibition. This seems to have little consequence for therapeutic effects (for which brain receptor occupancy levels are more relevant), but may have important consequences for adverse effects.

1.1 Drug absorption

Absorption can be impaired by analgesics, chelating agents and anticholinergics (which delay gastric emptying and reduce peristalsis, preventing efficient mixing in the gut). Thus antacids reduce the absorption of phenothiazines (probably by a chelating effect) but this effect can be minimized by separating the doses by a couple of hours.

The interaction with anticholinergics is more complex and controversial. Theoretically both pharmacokinetic and pharmacodynamic effects may be involved. Johnstone *et al.* (1983) reported a reduced antipsychotic effect of oral flupenthixol in 16 acute schizophrenic patients given procyclidine (5 mg daily) in comparison with 18 given placebo, without any associated change in flupenthixol blood levels. In contrast, Bamrah *et al.* (1986) found no change in symptom severity in 25 chronic schizophrenic patients when they were given procyclidine (5–15 mg/day), but reductions occurred in the blood levels of both oral and depot antipsychotic drugs. They therefore concluded that liver enzyme induction was the most important mechanism underlying the interaction. The difference between these two studies may be due to differences between acute and chronic patients, but the effect on symptomatology is small and clinically insignificant. A more important interaction is the pharmacodynamic additive effect in combination with either tricyclic antidepressants or phenothiazine antipsychotics, leading to increased anticholinergic adverse effects.

1.2 Displacement from protein binding sites

In spite of being highly protein bound, few important interactions between antidepressant or antipsychotics and other highly protein bound drugs have been documented. Normally there is no problem with tricyclic antidepressants and warfarin, although occasional control problems have been reported (SSRIs possibly enhance the anticoagulant effect of warfarin by enzyme inhibition and fluoxetine (Hanger and Thomas, 1995), fluvoxamine (Benfield and Ward, 1986) and paroxetine (Askinazi, 1996) have been associated with increased bleeding time when given with warfarin.) There has been one report of increased drowsiness and confusion with the combination of indomethacin and haloperidol.

1.3 Altered hepatic metabolism

The activity of the hepatic enzymes involved in biotransformation may be increased by chronic exposure to some drugs (enzyme induction) and reduced by others (enzyme inhibition). A few drugs show biphasic activity in that initially they inhibit enzyme activity, but with continued dosage they act as enzyme inducers. Such an effect has been seen with glutethimide and phenylbutazone which act in this way on the metabolism of hexobarbitone.

Well known *enzyme inducers* are :

1 Barbiturates
2 Alcohol
3 Phenylbutazone
4 Phenytoin
5 Carbamazepine.

The antipsychotics as a group cannot be regarded as either inducers or non-inducers of hepatic enzymes since, while chlorpromazine and flupenthixol are enzyme inducers, fluphenazine is not (Salem *et al.*, 1982). Tricyclic anti-depressant blood levels are reduced by enzyme inducers such as barbiturates and carbamazepine.

Well known *enzyme inhibitors* are:

1 Disulfiram
2 MAOIs
3 Cimetidine
4 SSRIs.

The effect of an interaction with these drugs is effectively to increase the dose of the other drug. The SSRIs may inhibit different enzyme systems from those by which they are metabolized.

1.3.1 Cytochrome P450 enzyme inhibition

The cytochrome P450 system is a 'super-family' of microsomal hepatic enzymes which are responsible for the oxidation of xenobiotics, including many drugs. Molecular biology has revealed that there are 14 P450 gene families in humans which can be further classified according to the homology of their protein sequences. The four isoenzymes of greatest interest for psychotropic drug interactions are CYP 450 1A2, CYP 450 2D6, CYP 450 2C, and CYP 450 3A4. Indeed, in a Medline Search for 1995–98, using the key words 'interaction', 'humans' and each of 17 new antidepressants and antipsychotics (risperidone, olanzapine, sertindole, zotepine, quetiapine, ziprasidone, sertraline, fluvoxamine, fluoxetine, paroxetine, citalopram, venlafaxine, nefazodone, mirtazepine, tianeptine, reboxetine and moclobemide), 29 articles were found, all of which concerned possible interactions due to the inhibition of one or more of these isoenzymes by SSRIs.

Table 18.2 lists the four principal isoenzymes and some of their clinically relevant substrates and inhibitors. A given drug may be metabolized by more than one isoenzyme and an SSRI may or may not inhibit its own metabolism, e.g. paroxetine is metabolized by at least two pathways and inhibits one of these (CYP 450 2D6). Most SSRIs are metabolized by CYP 450 2D6. Both fluoxetine and paroxetine inhibit their own metabolism at

Table 18.2 Newer antidepressants and the cytochrome P450 system

Substrates	Inhibitors
CYP450 1A2	
Caffeine	Fluvoxamine
Theophylline	
Clozapine	
Haloperidol	
CYP450 2D6	Fluoxetine
Amitriptyline	Norfluoxetine
Desipramine	Sertraline
Nortriptyline	Paroxetine
Thioridazine	
Haloperidol	
Risperidone	
CYP450 2C	
Warfarin	Fluvoxamine
Phenytoin	Fluoxetine
Diazepam	Sertraline
CYP450 3A4	
Terfenadine	Fluvoxamine
Astemizole	Fluoxetine
Carbamazepine	Sertraline
Aprazolam	Nefazodone
Triazolam	
Reboxetine	

Adapted from Nemeroff *et al.* (1996).

high doses and therefore show non-linear pharmacokinetics with regard to dose increases (Preskorn, 1993).

Two questions arise concerning the inhibition of CYP 450 enzymes by SSRIs: what is its clinical importance? and are there differences between individual SSRIs?

The clinical importance arises as a result of increases in blood levels of tricyclic antidepressants or antipsychotics when combined with SSRIs. Most studies, however, have been carried out on *in vitro* hepatic microsomal enzyme preparations or demonstrate increases in a 'marker' drug such as desipramine in healthy volunteers. Some of these are to the extent of converting extensive metabolizer phenotypes to poor metabolizers. Few systematic studies have reported important *pharmacodynamic* effects. Nevertheless, some serious consequences have been documented in case reports such as *torsades de pointes* with terfenadine (metabolized by CYP 450 3A4) and ketoconazole (Monahan *et al.*, 1990), which has led to terfenadine being made a prescription-only medicine in the UK and its removal from the USA market being considered by the FDA. Other serious adverse effects such as seizures and cardiac arrhythmias (QTc abnormalities) have also been reported with the SSRIs, particularly fluoxetine, and tricyclic antidepressants (Preskorn *et al.*, 1990; Taylor and Lader, 1996). Furthermore, it is possible that some of these interactions are being missed by clinicians who have not been aware of their possibility. There would now seem to be sufficient evidence to recommend that SSRIs and tricyclics should not be combined unless facilities for the monitoring of tricyclic plasma levels and ECGs are available (Taylor and Lader, 1996). Important interactions between fluvoxamine and clozapine (DeVane, 1998a) or caffeine (see Table 18.2) should also be anticipated. Thus the laboratory-based studies in this area have led to predictions of important clinical consequence.

In spite of the title of Preskorn's (1998) paper: 'Debate resolved', the issue of the significance of the difference in potency of CYP 450 2D6 inhibition between SSRIs remains somewhat controversial. It would appear that *all* the SSRIs inhibit CYP 450 2D6 isoenzymes to some extent and that the differences between them are, therefore, of degree rather than absolute; quantitative rather than qualitative (Table 18.3). Furthermore, the effect is dose-dependent and steady state levels of sertraline were reported to have a six-fold variation in one small series of 13 subjects (DeVane, 1998a). Only fluoxetine and paroxetine, however, at therapeutic doses convert approximately two-thirds of extensive metabolizers to poor metabolizers (Preskorn, 1998). Thus fluoxetine and paroxetine appear to be the most important inhibitors of CYP 450 2D6, with sertraline having an intermediate dose-dependent effect, and fluvoxamine, citalopram and the newer drugs nefazodone, venlafaxine and reboxetine having little or no effect (see Tables 18.2 and 18.3). Fluvoxamine and nefazodone, however, are important inhibitors of CYP 450 3A4 with corresponding implications for combinations with terfenadine, astemizole, carbamazepine and the benzodiazepines (Nemeroff *et al.*, 1996). Interestingly, the new noradrenaline reuptake inhibitor, reboxetine, although apparently metabolized by CYP 450 3A4, neither inhibits nor induces this isoenzyme nor any of the others tested so far (Dostert *et al.*, 1997).

Finally, apart from potential interactions due to enzyme inhibition, it must be remembered that combining any two drugs that are substrates for the same enzyme (see Table 18.2) increases the likelihood of competitive enzyme inhibition (DeVane, 1998b).

Drug plasma level monitoring can be of value in the investigation of some pharmacokinetic interactions such as those between tricyclics and the

Table 18.3 Newer antidepressants and P450 enzyme inhibitory potential

Drug	CYP1A2	CYP2C	CYP2D6	CYP3A4
Fluvoxamine	+ + + +	+ +	0	+ + +
Fluoxetine	0	+ +	+ + + +	+ +
(metabolite)			(+ + + +)	(+ + +)
Sertraline	0	+ +	+	+ +
(metabolite)		(+ +)	(+ +)	(+ +)
Paroxetine	0	0	+ + + +	0
Citalopram	0	0	0	0
Nefazodone	0	0	0	+ + + +
Venlafaxine	0	0	0	0
(metabolite)			(+)	
Bupropion	0	0	0	0
Mirtazapine	0	0	0	0

Note: 0 = unknown or insignificant; + = mild and usually insignificant; + + = moderate and possibly significant; + + + = moderate and usually significant; + + + + = potent.
From: DeVane (1998b)

SSRIs, but should not be used indiscriminately. The clinical and pharmacological considerations that help to increase the value of such monitoring are listed in Table 18.4.

1.4 Interactions during excretion

Drug–drug interactions can occur during the renal elimination of drugs either due to effects on urinary pH or due to competition for active transport systems in the kidney tubule. Most antidepressants and antipsychotics are weak bases, like amphetamine, and their clearance is increased in acid urine (which increases the proportion of the ionized form of the drug) and, conversely, decreased in alkaline urine. This is the converse of the situation with the barbiturates (weak acids) with the clinical consequence that alkalizing the urine following a suspected barbiturate overdose will *decrease* the excretion of tricyclics and phenothiazines.

More important are the potential interactions with lithium which is not metabolized and depends entirely on intact renal function for its elimination. The well known interactions with thiazide diuretics and non-steroidal anti-inflammatory drugs (NSAIDs) are due to decreased lithium clearance. This is because the kidney does not distinguish between sodium and lithium at the proximal renal tubule where both are reabsorbed. Thiazide and loop diuretics, however, reduce sodium reabsorption in the proximal part of the distal tubule and, as a consequence, increase reabsorption of *both* sodium and lithium in the proximal tubule. Lithium excretion is also reduced by ACE inhibitors.

2. Pharmacodynamic interactions

Pharmacodynamic interactions which result in direct clinical effects can generally be predicted from the known pharmacological properties of the drugs being combined and some of the most common have been listed in Table 18.5. Alcohol and most antihistamines potentiate the sedative effects of all other centrally acting drugs.

Most interactions with the MAOIs, including the 'cheese reactions' can be regarded as pharmacodynamic. The inhibition of monoamine oxidase

Table 18.4 Value of drug plasma level monitoring

Clinical considerations
- Drug overdose
- Investigation of severe ADR (death, toxicity)
- Complex drug–drug interactions
- Investigation of non-response
- Compliance problems

Pharmacological considerations
- Narrow therapeutic index
- Good dose/response relationship
- Linear plasma/tissue level relationship

Table 18.5 Important pharmacodynamic drug–drug interactions with psychotropic drugs

Drug (1)	Drug (2)	Mechanism	Effect
MAOIs	MARIs	Potentiation of NA	Hypertension
	SSRIs	Potentiation of 5-HT	Serotonin syndrome
	Ephedrine etc	Potentiation of NA	Hypertension
	Tyramine foods etc	Potentiation of NA	Hypertension
	General aesthetics, analgestics etc	Reduced hepatic metabolism	Prolongation of effects
	Pethidine	Reduced hepatic metabolism	Coma, hypotension pyrexia
MARIs ('Tricyclics')	Anticholinergics	Potentiation	Delirium; cardiotoxicity
	MAOIs	Potentiation of NA	Hypertension
	Adrenaline (in local anesthetics)	Potentiation	Hypertension; seizures
	Isoprenaline	Potentiation	Seizures
	Anticonvulsants	Decreased convulsive threshold	Seizures
	Adrenergic neuron antagonists	Neutralization	Uncontrolled hypertension
Antipsychotics	Alcohol, benzodiazines antihistamines, opiates	CNS depression	Increased sedation
	Anticholinergics	Potentiation	Delirium, cardiotoxicity
	Lithium	(?) Increased intracellular Li	Increased possibility of neurotoxic reactions
	L-dopa, dopaminergics	Dopamine receptor antagonism	Reduced efficacy of drug (2)
	Anticonvulsants	Reduced convulsive threshold	Reduced efficacy of drug (2)
	ACE inhibitors	Potentiation	Hypotension
	Adrenergic neuron blockers	Neutralization	Uncontrolled hypertension
Pimozide, Sertindole, Thioridazine	Quindine, procainamide disopyramide, astemizole terfenadrine	QTc prolongation	Cardiac arrhythmias, inc. torsades de pointes
Clozapine	Carbamazepine, co-trimoxazole, sulphonamides, azapropazone	Myelosuppression	Increased risk of agranulocytosis

(MAO) in the gut wall and the mixed hepatic oxidases gives rise to higher levels of circulating pressor amines, on the one hand, and a variety of drugs normally oxidized in the liver, on the other. Inhibition of presynaptic mitochondrial MAO increases the available noradrenaline in synaptic vesicles. A serotonin syndrome (pyrexia, tremor and convulsions) is potentially hazardous when MAOIs and SSRIs are combined (Committee on Safety of Medicines, 1989) but the MAOI and lithium combination, initially suspected of causing similar problems on theoretical grounds, has not been found to be a problem in clinical practice. MAOI and tricyclic antidepressant combinations, once advocated in treatment-refractory cases, were potentially hazardous especially with either tranylcypromine or clomipramine, and have now been largely superseded by other adjunctive agents such as lithium.

Combinations of tricyclic antidepressants with anticholinergic drugs are ill advised, leading to delirium especially in the elderly, but are still occasionally found in clinical practice. Tricyclic combinations with the adrenergic neuron blocking agents (guanethidine, bethanidine and debrisoquine), which neutralize the hypotensive effect of these drugs, are now rarely encountered since the latter have become obsolete. The precipitation of seizures by tricyclics in epileptic patients due to a reduction of the convulsive threshold is more of a type A (dose-dependent) adverse drug reaction than an interaction.

Antagonism of the actions of anticonvulsants and antiparkinson drugs can be anticipated with antipsychotic drugs. Clozapine, while having less effect on parkinsonism, has, however, a greater effect on the precipation of seizures. The new 'atypicals' likewise have less effect on parkinsonism but their effects on seizures do not, as yet, appear to have been reported to the same extent as clozapine. The antipsychotic and lithium combination was associated with some alarm following four widely quoted case reports (Cohen and Cohen, 1974). Subsequent systematic reviews, however, suggested that these could have been explained either by toxic lithium levels alone or the occurrence of the neuroleptic malignant syndrome (Baastrup et al., 1976; Juhl et al., 1977; Spring and Frankel, 1981). Nevertheless, since antipsychotics, especially thioridazine, are known to increase intracellular lithium levels (Pandey et al., 1979; Ostrow et al., 1980) caution, especially with high doses, is advisable when using this combination. An interesting possible beneficial interaction between chlorpromazine and propranolol was eventually explained by a pharmacokinetic mechanism. Addition of the β-adrenoceptor antagonist was apparently associated with an increase in circulating antipsychotic blood levels, presumably as a result of competitive enzyme inhibition (Peet et al., 1981). Other pharmacokinetic interactions involving antipsychotic drugs have been mentioned in an earlier section. Table 18.2 shows that several of these antipsychotic drugs will have increased blood levels in combination with CYP 450 2D6 inhibitors but that clozapine (as well as haloperidol) blood levels are increased by CYP 450 1A2 inhibition.

Perhaps the most important pharmacodynamic interaction with antipsychotics is the potential additive cardiotoxicity with other drugs that prolong the QTc interval such as quinidine, procainamide, amiodarone, disopyramide and the antihistamines, astemizole and terfenadine. There is some controversy as to whether this risk applies only to some or all antipsychotics but, at the present time, the particular antipsychotics identified by most authorities are pimozide (which is also a calcium antagonist), sertindole and thioridazine. Haloperidol and amiodarone combinations should also be avoided.

While the UK CSM yellow card reporting system can be useful in identifying the profile of adverse drug reactions associated with psychotropic drugs, it cannot indicate how many of these are associated with comorbid conditions or drug combinations. There is, however, some indication that sudden deaths (Royal College of Psychiatrists, 1997) or increased mortality (Waddington et al., 1998) in patients on antipsychotic medication may be more likely in association with polypharmacy.

Finally, clozapine should not be used with potentially myelosuppressive drugs, such as carbamazepine, co-trimoxazole, sulphonamides, chloramphenicol and the analgesic azapropazone, because of the increased risk of agranulocytosis. This is also a further reason for avoiding the combination of clozapine with depot antipsychotics (which also have myelosuppressive potential).

References

Askinazi, C. (1996). SSRI treatment of depression with comorbid cardiac disease. *Am. J. Psychiatry*, **153**, 135–136.

Baastrup, P.C., Hollnagel, P., Sørensen, R., *et al.* (1976). Adverse reactions in treatment with lithium carbonate and haloperidol. *J. Am. Med. Assoc.*, **236**, 2645–2646.

Bamrah, J.S., Kumar, V., Krska, J., *et al.* (1986). Interactions between procyclidine and neuroleptic drugs. *Br. J. Psychiatry*, **149**, 726–733.

Bazire, S. (1977). *Psychotropic Drug Directory*, Salisbury, Wiltshire, Quay Books Division: Mark Allen Publishing Ltd.

Benfield, P. and Ward, A. (1986). Fluvoxamine - a review of its pharmacodynamic and pharmacokinetic properties, and therapeutic efficacy in depressive illness. *Drugs*, **32**, 313–334.

Bezchlibnyk-Butler, K.Z. and Jeffries, J.J. (eds) (1995). *Clinical Handbook of Psychotropic Drugs*, 5th revised edn. Seattle, Toronto, Hogrefe & Huber Publishers.

British National Formulary (1998). London, British Medical Association and the Royal Pharmaceutical Society of Great Britain.

Ciraulo, D.A., Shader, R.I., Greenblatt, D.J., *et al.* (eds) (1995). *Drug Interactions in Psychiatry*, Baltimore, Williams & Wilkins.

Cohen, W.J. and Cohen, N.H. (1974). Lithium carbonate, haloperidol, and irreversible brain damage. *J. Am. Med. Assoc.*, **230**, 1283–1287.

Committee on Safety of Medicines (1989). *Current Problems*. No 26.

DeVane, C.L. (1998a). Clinical implications of dose-dependent cytochrome P-450 drug-drug interactions with antidepressants. *Hum. Psychopharmacol.*, **13**, 329–336.

DeVane, C.L. (1998b). Principles of pharmacokinetics and pharmacodynamics. In *Textbook of Psychopharmacology*, 2nd edn (A.F. Schatzberg and C.B. Nermeroff, eds), Washington, DC, American Psychiatric Press Inc., pp. 155–169.

Dostert, P., Benedetti, M.S. and Poggesi, I. (1997). Review of the pharmacokinetics and metabolism of reboxetine, a selective noradrenaline reuptake inhibitor. *Eur. Neuropsychopharmacol.*, **7** (Suppl. 1), S23–S35.

Hanger, H.C., and Thomas, F. (1995). Fluoxetine and warfarin interactions. *NZ Med. Journal*, **108**, 157.

Johnstone, E.C., Crow, T.J., Ferrier, I.N., *et al.* (1983). Adverse effects of anticholinergic medication on positive schizophrenic symptoms. *Psychol. Med.*, **13**, 513–527.

Juhl, R.P., Tsuang, M.T. and Perry, P.J. (1977). Concomitant administration of haloperidol and lithium carbonate in acute mania. *Dis. Nervous System, Sept.*, 675–676.

Monahan, B.P., Ferguson, C.L., Killeavy, E.S., *et al.* (1990). Torsades de pointes occurring in association with terfenadine use. *J. Am. Med. Assoc.*, **264**, 2788–2790.

Nemeroff, C.B., DeVane, C.L. and Pollock, B.G. (1996). Newer antidepressants and the cytochrome P450 system. *Am. J. Psychiatry*, **153**, 311–320.

Ostrow, D.G., Southam, A.S. and Davis, J.M. (1980). Lithium-drug interactions altering the intracellular lithium level: an *in vitro* study. *Biol. Psychiatry*, **15**, 723–739.

Pandey, G.N., Goel, I. and Davis, J.M. (1979). Effect of neuroleptic drugs on lithium uptake by the human erthyrocyte. *Clin. Pharmacol. Ther.*, **26**, 96–102.

Peet, M., Middlemiss, D.N. and Yates, R.A. (1981). Propranolol in schizophrenia II. Clinical and biochemical aspects of combining propranol with chlorpromazine. *Br. J. Psychiatry*, **139**, 112–117.

Preskorn, S., Beber, J.H., Faul, J.C., *et al.* (1990). Serious adverse effects of combining fluoxetine and tricyclic antidepressants. *Am. J. Psychiatry*, **147**, 532.

Preskorn, S.H. (1993). Pharmacokinetics of antidepressants: why and how they are relevant to treatment. *J. Clin. Psychiatry*, **54** (9, Suppl.), 14–34.

Preskorn, S.H. (1998). Debate resolved: there are differential effects of serotonin selective reuptake inhibitors on cytochrome P450 enzymes. *J. Psychopharmacol.*, **12**, S89–S97.

Royal College of Psychiatrists (1997). Working Party Report on the Association between antipsychotic drugs and sudden death, *College Report* no. *CR 57*.

Salem, S.A.M., King, D.J. and McDevitt, D.G. (1982). Induction of microsomal enzyme activity by flupenthixol in chronic schizophrenics. *Psychopharmacology*, **78**, 147–149.

Spring, G. and Frankel, M. (1981). New data on lithium and haloperidol incompatibility. *Am. J. Psychiatry*, **138**, 818–821.

Stockley, I. (1995). *Drug Interactions*, Oxford, Blackwell Scientific.

Taylor, D. and Lader, M. (1996). Cytochromes and psychotropic drug interactions. *Br. J. Psychiatry*, **168**, 529–532.

Waddington, J.L., Youssef, H.A. and Kinsella, A. (1998). Mortality in schizophrenia: antipsychotic polypharmacy and absense of adjunctive anticholinergics over the course of a 10-year prospective study. *Br. J. Psychiatry*, **173**, 325–329.

19

Psychotropic drugs during pregnancy

Sheila Marcus and Rajiv Tandon

Key points

- Pregnancy does not have a protective effect against major psychiatric illness.
- Untreated major mental illness in the pregnant mother may have adverse effects on obstetrical outcome and fetal development.
- All psychotropic medications diffuse readily across the placenta.
- Psychotropic medication use during pregnancy can adversely affect the fetus in one of three ways: (1) have a teratogenic effect, related to first-trimester exposure; (2) neonatal behavioural and physical syndromes, usually related to late third-trimester exposure; and (3) long-term behavioural effects, often but not invariably related to third-trimester exposure.
- Mood stabilizers (lithium, carbamazepine, valproic acid) and benzodiazepines appear to be associated with some increase in teratogenic risk. SSRIs, tricyclic antidepressants, and most antipsychotics appear not to be associated with increased teratogenic risk, although available data are limited. Information about long-term behavioural effects, if any, of prenatal exposure to psychotropic agents is sparse.
- No psychotropic medications are approved for use during pregnancy by the US Food and Drug Administration or any drug regulatory body in Europe.
- Use of psychotropic medications during pregnancy is often appropriate and requires careful balancing of the risks of prenatal exposure against the risks to the mother and the fetus of not adequately treating the major mental illness.
- Care should be carefully coordinated between patient, family, psychiatrist and obstetrician.

Introduction

Psychiatric illnesses occur frequently in women of child-bearing age. Pregnancy, once thought to be a 'honeymoon' from psychiatric illness is a time when up to 10% of women may experience depression (Gotlib *et al.*, 1989). Psychotic illnesses may be exacerbated in pregnancy and significantly reduce a woman's capacity to maintain a healthy pregnancy (McNeil *et al.*, 1984). Many women are using psychotropics at the time of conception. At no time is a decision to use or discontinue medications more challenging than during early pregnancy; nor is there a time when the stakes are so high. As all psychotropics cross the placental barrier, the woman's health and management of her illness must be balanced against the risk of the infant's *in utero* exposure to medication. Untreated psychiatric illness has adverse consequences of its own; resulting in poor nutrition, inability to obtain medical care, substance abuse, and dangerous or risk-taking behaviour. Maternal suicide, fetal abuse, and infanticide may be the most disastrous consequences of untreated illness. Thus, the specific risks to the fetus of *in utero* medication exposure must be balanced against the substantial risks of untreated illness. At such times the clinician is called upon to assist a woman and her family with making thoughtful treatment decisions both to optimize her health and that of her baby.

This chapter will discuss the course and treatment of psychotic and major mood disorders through pregnancy. After a discussion of some general principles pertaining to psychotropic medication use during pregnancy, treatment strategies for these illnesses with guidelines for use of psychotropic medications will be highlighted. Pharmacological strategies should be combined with psychosocial and behavioural interventions to maximize care and these adjuvant strategies will be outlined. Available data on the risks and potential sequelae of using various psychotropic medications during pregnancy will be summarized.

General principles

The benefits of continuing psychotropic medication during pregnancy

Psychotic and major mood disorders can begin in pregnancy and pre-existing major mental disorders continue through pregnancy. Historically, clinicians have had great reservations about using psychotropic medications during pregnancy. However, discontinuing maintenance psychotropic medications at any time, including pregnancy, results in high rates of relapse in patients suffering from schizophrenia (Gilbert *et al.*, 1995) and major mood disorders (DeQuardo and Tandon, 1981; Suppes *et al.*, 1991; Kupfer *et al.*, 1992). Unfortunately, few studies have been conducted on the specific risk of recurrence of these disorders when medications are withdrawn during pregnancy.

Untreated psychiatric illness can have adverse effects on both the mother and the fetus. Relapses increase the risk of chronicity and treatment resistance in both schizophrenia (Wyatt, 1991; DeQuardo, 1998) and major mood disorders (Greden and Tandon, 1995). Suicidality associated with psychotic exacerbations in schizophrenia and depression represents another significant risk of not effectively treating these illnesses.

The specific risks to the fetus of untreated psychiatric illness in the mother are ill-defined. Untreated schizophrenia has been found to be associated with an increased occurrence of perinatal death (Rieder *et al.*, 1975) and significant depressive symptomatology has been found to be associated with low-birthweight and an increased risk of preterm delivery (Steer *et al.*, 1992). Hypercortisolaemia is observed in about 50% of patients with major depression and exacerbations of schizophrenic illness (Carroll *et al.*, 1980; Tandon *et al.*, 1991); elevated maternal glucocorticoids and concurrent symptoms of stress pose a risk to the developing fetus. In animal models there is evidence that maternal stress is associated with fetal death and low birthweight

(Istvan, 1986). The potential risks of withholding pharmacology during gestation are summarized by Miller (1991) and include: (1) malnutrition, secondary to loss of appetite or impaired judgment; (2) attempts at premature self-delivery; (3) fetal abuse or neonaticide; (4) inability to participate in obstetric care; and (5) precipitous delivery when patient is unable to identify labour.

The costs of continuing psychotropic medication during pregnancy

In the early 1960s, thalidomide consumption by the pregnant mother during the first half of the first trimester of pregnancy was linked to the development of congenital limb defects in the fetus. The thalidomide tragedy dramatically altered the way in which medication use during pregnancy was viewed. Until that time, the placenta had been viewed as a barrier that protected the fetus from exposure to potential toxins. Since that time, it has become clear that the placenta functions more like a diffusion medium across which most agents can travel from mother to fetus; in fact, all currently-used psychotropic medications do cross the placenta and are therefore, potential teratogens.

The US Food and Drug Administration (FDA) uses a specific system to classify the degree of known risk to the fetus of intrauterine exposure to different medications (Table 19.1); other regulatory authorities utilize a similar though often less formal system.

Psychotropic medications potentially can have three kinds of adverse effects on the fetus:

1   they can be teratogenic, i.e., they can increase the risk of specific organ malformations. Teratogenic effects are associated with exposure to the drug in the first 12 weeks of pregnancy, when organogenesis occurs. A medication is considered teratogenic when prenatal exposure is asso-

Table 19.1 US Food and Drug Administration (FDA) categorization of risk of medication-use during pregnancy

Category	Definition of Risk
A	Controlled studies show no risk to humans. *Well-controlled studies in pregnant women demonstrate no risk to the fetus*
B	No evidence of risk in humans, but data inadequate. *Either animal studies show risk but human studies do not show risk, or animal studies show no risk and no well-controlled human studies conducted*
C	Risk cannot be ruled out. *Well-controlled human studies lacking and animal studies either lacking or show risk*
D	Positive evidence of risk, but risk may be outweighed by potential benefit. *Some evidence of risk in human studies (investigational or post-marketing data)*
X	Contraindicated in pregnancy. *Studies in humans and/or animals show clear evidence of significant fetal risk*

ciated with a significant increase in the risk of congenital deformities above a baseline risk of 2.0–2.5% (Nelson and Holmes, 1989).

2   they can contribute to neonatal toxicity, i.e., they can increase the risk of various physical and behavioural syndromes in the first few weeks of life. Such effects can be related to continuing effects or withdrawal effects in the neonate, who is born with the implicated drug in his/her system. Obviously, this kind of toxicity is related to late third-trimester exposure to the putative drug and is generally manifest for a brief period of time.

3   they can contribute to long-term behavioural or neurological effects in children. These effects are the least clearly defined.

Although estimates of the teratogenic effects of various psychotropic medications are imprecise, the FDA has assigned risk categories B, C, D, and X to different psychotropic medications (Table 19.2). Certain benzodiazepines have received the X (completely contraindicated) designation. Lithium, carbamazepine, sodium valproate, most tricyclic antidepressants, and other benzodiazepines (other than clonazepam) have received the D designation, which indicates evidence of fetal risk, but not blanket contraindication of the agent during pregnancy. Selective serotonin reuptake inhibitors (SSRIs), desipramine, venlafaxine, mirtazapine, nefazodone, clonazepam, most conventional and atypical antipsychotics have received the C designation, which denotes that while there is no clear evidence of fetal risk from the agent, it cannot be clearly ruled out. Bupropion, clozapine, and buspirone have received the B designation, which denotes the absence of risk with the caveat of limited data.

Clinical features and course of major psychiatric disorders through pregnancy

Major depression

Major mood disorders are so ubiquitous as to have earned the reputation as the common cold of psychiatry. The illness is particularly prevalent among

Table 19.2 US Food and Drug Administration (FDA) categorization of risk of various psychotropic medications during pregnancy

Category	Psychotropic Medications
A	None
B	Bupropion, clozapine, buspirone
C	All other antipsychotics (conventional and atypical), various antiparkinsonian agents, SSRIs, desipramine, clomipramine, MAOIs, venlafaxine, trazodone, nefazodone, mirtazapine, clonazepam, chloral hydrate, zolpidem, carbamazepine
D	Other tricyclic antidepressants, lithium, sodium valproate, diazepam, alprazolam
X	Triazolam, temazepam, flurazepam, quazepam

women, and it is estimated that up to 21% of women will suffer an episode of depression within their lifetime (Kessler *et al.*, 1993). Most women will have an onset during child-bearing years and the prevalence of depression in pregnancy is roughly 10% (Cohen *et al.*, 1989). The DSM-IV criteria for major depression have considerable overlap with symptoms of pregnancy itself. Appetite and sleep change, fatigue and diminished energy are the rule. These overlaps lead to difficulties in diagnosing depression during pregnancy and contribute to lack of consensus about the prevalence and course of depression in pregnancy (Altshuler *et al.*, 1998).

Much has been written about recurrence of depressive illness following discontinuation of medication and relapse rates have been estimated as high as 50% within 6 months of medication withdrawal (Frank *et al.*, 1990). There are no studies specific to pregnancy, however. Prenatal depressive symptoms are thought to be strong predictors of postpartum depression (O'Hara and Swain, 1996) affecting 12–16% of pregnancies during the 6–12 weeks after delivery. A number of studies have examined risk factors for the occurrence of depression in pregnant and lactating women. Social support and contented marital relationships appear to be protective from depression. Factors which appear to confer heightened risk for depression in pregnancy include: (1) prior history of mood disorder; (2) family history of mood disorder; (3) marital conflict; (4) younger age; and (5) limited social support with greater number of children (O'Hara, 1986; Altshuler *et al.*, 1998).

Bipolar disorder

Bipolar disorder has a lifetime prevalence of about 1.7% in women (Kessler *et al.*, 1993). The course of bipolar disorder in women differs from that in men in that women are more prone to rapid-cycling, and experience more depressions and dysphoric mania (Faedda *et al.*, 1993; Burt and Hendrick, 1997). There is ample evidence to suggest that there is a high rate of relapse when medications for treatment of bipolar illness are discontinued (Frank *et al.*, 1990). There is little information about the natural course of bipolar disorder during pregnancy. While admissions for bipolar illness may drop somewhat during pregnancy (Altshuler *et al.*, 1998), there is substantial evidence to suggest that the postpartum period is a time of extreme vulnerability to relapse (Kendell *et al.*, 1987).

Schizophrenia

Schizophrenia is the prototypic psychotic disorder, which is distinguished by the presence of psychotic symptoms or impaired reality testing in one of several domains (perception, thought content, etc.). The onset of this disorder is generally in adolescence or early adulthood, although a significant number of patients exhibit significant 'premorbid' dysfunction prior to manifesting frank psychotic symptoms. Although delusions and hallucinations appear as its most prominent features, neurocognitive impairment and negative symptoms such as apathy, asociality, anhedonia, and alogia contribute to much of the debilitation associated with the illness. There is marked variability in the course of the illness, with some patients returning to virtually normal function and others exhibiting unrelenting deterioration, with a majority showing an intermediate trajectory. The illness is chronic, generally life-long, and is characterized by periodic psychotic exacerbations and frequently incomplete remissions. Negative symptoms and cognitive impairment are particularly prominent during these remissions (Tandon, 1995).

The effect of pregnancy on the course of schizophrenic illness is not clearly delineated. Although it was earlier believed that pregnancy reduced the severity of psychotic symptomatology and the risk of a psychotic relapse in women suffering from a schizophrenic illness, many reports continue to document psychotic exacerbations during pregnancy (McNeil et al., 1984). While higher levels of oestrogen present during pregnancy can have a beneficial effect, the physiological and psychological stresses during pregnancy can have an adverse effect. Delusions can become bizarre and may be related to body changes and fetal movements. Auditory hallucinations may be related to the pregnancy as well; for example, the patient can 'hear' second person auditory hallucinations directing the patient to get rid of the fetus. Agitation and disorganization can increase. Psychotic denial of pregnancy can represent a major problem.

Review of psychotropic agents

There are significant methodological difficulties in examining risks of psychotropic agents in pregnancy. Confounding factors include use of other medications, impact of other illnesses for which the medications were prescribed, use of alcohol and nicotine, genetic factors, maternal age, time of gestation and other environmental and psychosocial factors (Altshuler et al., 1996). Current views are summarized.

Selective serotonin reuptake inhibitors

Teratogenicity

Data on the use of SSRIs during pregnancy suggests that they are relatively safe. One prospective, controlled, multicentre study (Kulin et al., 1996) studied 267 women using sertraline, paroxetine, and fluvoxamine throughout pregnancy. Exposure to the SSRIs did not appear to increase the risk for major malformations. Moreover, there was no evidence of prematurity or low birthweight in infants exposed. Another study noted no increase in the risk of congenital malformations or perinatal toxicity in patients receiving tricyclic antidepressants or fluoxetine (Patuszak et al., 1993). In both Eli Lilly's patient register for fluoxetine and that of Smith Kline Beecham for paroxetine there do not appear to be any increases in the pattern and type of congenital anomalies compared to the general population. Animal studies with fluvoxamine, paroxetine and sertraline have similarly failed to show an increased risk of fetal anomalies (Solvay, Smith Kline Beecham and Pfizer pharmaceuticals).

Behavioural toxicity

There has only been one study to date exploring behavioural toxicities. This preliminary study involving prenatal exposure to fluoxetine and tricyclic agents failed to show any adverse neurobehavioural effects on language, IQ, or behaviour in children up to the age of 5 years (Nulman et al., 1997).

Neonatal effects

There are anecdotal reports of possible cases of irritability and colic in infants exposed to fluoxetine prenatally and through lactation (Altshuler et al., 1996). Similarly there has been a case report of jitteriness and increased respiratory rate in one infant exposed to paroxetine in the third trimester (Smith Kline Beecham product information).

Tricyclic antidepressants

Metabolism

Increases in tricyclic antidepressant dosages are necessitated in the second and third trimesters of pregnancy to maintain antidepressant effect and achieve therapeutic serum levels (Wisner and Perel, 1996). Effects are thought to be due to decreased serum albumin with diminished protein binding of the medication leading to increased renal clearance (Mortola, 1989).

Teratogenicity

There are multiple studies assessing the effect of in utero exposure to tricyclic antidepressants. The bulk of the evidence seems to suggest that the tricyclic agents do not contribute to teratogenicity when used in pregnancy. A comprehensive review and analysis of the literature from 1966 to 1995 did not reveal an association between fetal exposure to tricyclic antidepressants and rates or clustering of congenital malformation in the 414 cases of first trimester exposure described (Altshuler et al., 1996).

Behavioural toxicity

Animal studies have suggested the possibility of behavioural toxicity, but a more recent human study (Nulman et al., 1997) revealed that in utero exposure to the tricyclic agents did not affect global IQ (mean IQ = 118 + 17), language development or behavioural development in children followed through their preschool years.

Neonatal effects

There are documented perinatal syndromes associated with the use of tricyclic agents used in late third trimester and in labour and delivery. These withdrawal syndromes include: jitteriness, cyanosis, tachypnoea, tachycardia, irritability and convulsions (Wisner and Perel, 1996). Rare anticholinergic symptoms including urinary retention and bowel obstruction have also been reported (Schearer *et al.*, 1972; Falterman and Richardson, 1980). One study described neonatal withdrawal seizures in two infants (Cowe *et al.*, 1982).

Other antidepressant agents

Monoamine oxidase inhibitors have been associated with growth retardation and fetal death in animal studies (Compendium of Drug Therapy, 1984). In one small human study of 21 mother–infant pairs there was a higher rate of congenital anomalies in infants (Wisner and Perel, 1996). Because of the risk of hypertensive crisis in the event that tocolytic agents are necessary to forestall labour, MAOIs are contraindicated in pregnancy.

To our knowledge, there are no clinical trials involving bupropion, venlafaxine, trazodone, or mirtazapine during pregnancy that are currently available for review. Animal studies with bupropion have revealed no evidence of impaired fertility or fetal harm (Glaxo Wellcome Pharmaceuticals product information).

Alternative therapies

Though there have been double-blind placebo-controlled studies involving St John's wort (*Hypericum perforatum*) that suggest efficacy in mild–moderate depression (Wheatley, 1997), they have not been studied in pregnancy. Variability in percentage of psychoactive substance in the various preparations, as well as contaminants, confound studies exploring efficacy. Additional research in this area is necessary as many women willingly medicate themselves with herbal remedies considering them more natural and not considering potential toxicity in pregnancy.

Mood stabilizers

Lithium

Metabolism

Physiological changes in pregnancy increase the metabolism of lithium. A higher glomerular filtration rate coupled with an increase in plasma volume often leads to significant increases in lithium requirements (30–50%) in the third trimester. Rapid fluid losses at the time of delivery may precipitate toxicity in the immediate postpartum period, therefore close monitoring of lithium levels are essential in third trimester and postpartum (Schou *et al.*, 1973; Wisner and Perel, 1996).

Teratogenicity

Lithium is known to cross the placenta freely and maternal and fetal plasma concentrations are similar (Mortola, 1989). Lithium has been well studied in pregnancy and the Register of Lithium Babies was established in 1968 to collect information on first trimester exposures. Early analysis of the Register had suggested a 400-fold increase in the expected frequency of Ebstein's anomaly. However, the anomalies were markedly over-represented in the register due to increased reporting of the abnormal babies. Two more recent studies (Elia *et al.*, 1987; Cohen *et al.*, 1994) more conservatively estimate the incidence at 0.1%; or 10–20 times the rate in the general population. Other studies (Kallen and Tandberg, 1983; Kerns, 1986) found a relationship between first trimester lithium exposure and general cardiovascular anomalies in about 7% of bipolar women exposed to lithium. Women with bipolar illness who did not receive lithium were at no increased risk. Overall the risk of major congenital anomalies in women with first trimester exposure to lithium appears to be between 4 and 12%, relative to the general population rate of 2–4% (Cohen *et al.*, 1994).

Behavioural toxicity

Behavioural toxicity of lithium has been suggested in animal studies (Kerns, 1986), however a follow-up study of cases reported to the Register of Lithium Babies did not find any evidence of behavioural toxicity (as assessed by maternal report and formal clinical and neuropsychological evaluation) in lithium exposed children (Schou, 1976). Major developmental milestones were also achieved in a timely fashion in a small group of lithium exposed children as reported in another study (Jacobson *et al.*, 1992).

Neonatal effects

Lithium is associated with several perinatal syndromes, and toxicity in the neonate may result from levels that are not toxic to the mother. Clinical manifestations include flaccidity, cyanosis, lethargy, poor sucking and abnormal reflexes. Lithium may also cause reversible inhibition of thyroid function, cardiac arrhythmias and reversible diabetes insipidus. Increases in prematurity and perinatal mortality have also been reported (Woody *et al.*, 1971; Karlsson *et al.*, 1975; Wilson *et al.*, 1983; Yoder *et al.*, 1984).

Carbamazepine and valproic acid

Metabolism

Carbamazepine crosses the placenta freely and cord serum concentrations approximate those in maternal serum (Wiebyl *et al.*, 1979). Neonatal metabolism of carbamazephine is also equal to adult metabolism (Rane *et al.*, 1975).

Teratogenicity

Most studies in children exposed to anticonvulsants during pregnancy involved patients being treated for epilepsy rather than for psychiatric disorders. Women with seizure disorders have higher rates of congenital malformations, independent of their medication status. Nonetheless, the incidence of malformations in neonates with anticonvulsant exposure during pregnancy remains higher than rates for comparison groups, after control for effect of maternal epilepsy (Altshuler *et al.*, 1996). Prenatal exposure to valproic acid has been associated with a 1–5% risk of spina bifida (Lammer *et al.*, 1987; Lindhout *et al.*, 1992; Omtzigt *et al.*, 1992). One study found that the risk of spina bifida was positively correlated to higher maternal serum levels of valproate. Additionally, the study demonstrated evidence that clearance of valproate from the fetal compartment was diminished allowing valproate to accumulate in the fetus (Omtzigt *et al.*, 1992).

The incidence of spina bifida in carbamazepine exposed children is 0.5–1% (Altshuler *et al.*, 1996). Many minor malformations including fingernail hypoplasia, developmental delays and craniofacial anomalies, have also been reported (Jones *et al.*, 1989).

Behavioural teratogenicity

The data on behavioural teratogenicity related to anticonvulsant exposure are difficult to interpret due to the influence of factors such as parental IQ, impact of seizure disorders in pregnancy, maternal blood levels of anticonvulsants, timing of exposure, and various psychosocial factors which were not controlled for in studies examining anticonvulsants in pregnancy (Altshuler *et al.*, 1996). One small study showed that infants born to mothers on carbamazepine had small head circumference, and failed to demonstrate catch-up growth by 18 months (Hillesmaa *et al.*, 1981). Another prospective controlled trial demonstrated no adverse neurobehavioural outcome, as measured by IQ, and language development in exposed children (Scolnik *et al.*, 1994).

Antipsychotic agents

Teratogenicity

Low doses of antipsychotics are not infrequently used to treat hyperemesis gravidarum, generating a fairly large database pertaining to the safety of antipsychotic use during pregnancy. Although there are a few reports of congenital malformations in infants of mothers receiving phenothiazines in the first trimester (Rumeau-Roquette *et al.*, 1977), the general consensus among experts is that there is no convincing evidence linking the use of conventional antipsychotics during pregnancy to the development of congenital malformations in the fetus (Wisner and Perel, 1996; Cohen and Rosenbaum, 1998). Altshuler *et al.* (1996) suggest a 20% increase (from a baseline rate of 2.0% to 2.4% with phenothiazine exposure) in the occurrence of congenital anomalies with phenothiazine exposure, and Rumeau-Roquette *et al.* (1977) observed that phenothiazines with an aliphatic side-chain (e.g. chlorpromazine), but not those with a piperidine (e.g. thioridazine) or piperazine (e.g. trifluoperazine) side-chain were associated with this teratogenic risk. Since conventional antipsychotics have been widely used for four decades and there are very few reports describing their teratogenic effects, it is reasonable to assume that such effects are minimal, if that.

There are few reports of haloperidol use during pregnancy and these do not document any teratogenic effect. There are even fewer reports of atypical antipsychotic exposure during pregnancy; no suggestion of teratogenicity has been noted thus far. Consequently, all atypical antipsychotics other than clozapine are categorized as teratogenic risk category C denoting the absence of documented risk with the caveat of sparse data; there are a few case reports of clozapine use during pregnancy not being associated with congenital malformations and this is ostensibly the reason why it is assigned a category B risk.

Behavioural toxicity

Data regarding potential long-term neurobehavioural effects of antipsychotic exposure during pregnancy are limited. Animal studies document a wide array of neurobehavioural abnormalities following fetal exposure to conventional antipsychotics (Clark and Gorman,1970; Coyle et al., 1976); these effects include difficulties in learning and memory. Studies in humans, however, have failed to find any differences in intelligence in children exposed to antipsychotics during pregnancy when compared to children who were not thus exposed (Kris, 1965; Slone et al., 1977).

Antiparkinsonian medications (such as diphenhydramine and amantadine) have been linked with teratogenicity (Saxen, 1974; Miller, 1991) and the use of anticholinergic antiparkinsonian medications late in pregnancy is associated with neonatal intestinal obstruction (Falterman and Richardson, 1980) and other neonatal toxicity. Such medications should be avoided during pregnancy, if possible.

Neonatal effects

In contrast to the paucity of data suggesting antipsychotic teratogenicity, antipsychotic exposure has been linked to neonatal toxicity. Extrapyramidal side effects (Tamer et al., 1969; Auerbach et al., 1992), motor hyperreflexia, vasomotor instability, neonatal jaundice (Scokel and Jones, 1962), and bowel obstruction (Falterman and Richardson, 1980) have been related to pre-delivery phenothiazine exposure. These adverse effects have generally been time-limited. The prevalence of antipsychotic neonatal toxicity is not known. Similarly, whether there are differences between conventional and atypical antipsychotics with regard to the occurrence of these effects is not known, although one would conjecture that neonatal extrapyramidal and related adverse effects may be less likely if atypical rather than conventional antipsychotics were used during pregnancy (Jibson and Tandon, 1998).

Management of psychiatric disorders in pregnancy

All decisions about medications in pregnancy require balancing the health of the woman, the risk of untreated illness and risk of psychotropic exposure to the developing fetus. A decision to discontinue medications prior to or at conception are influenced by (1) severity and frequency of illness in prior episodes; (2) illness-free interval; (3) current symptoms and ability to meet nutritional and medical needs; and (4) nature of pharmacotherapy.

Non-pharmacological treatment of depression

For women with histories of mild to moderate illness particularly in the first trimester of pregnancy, a trial off medication should be considered. Patients on medication should be counselled as to the importance of pregnancy planning to allow time to make decisions about medication. Medications should be weaned, as precipitous discontinuation may predispose to relapse. Medications should be given adequate time for wash out prior to conception to avoid exposure during organogenesis. This is particularly important for medications with a long half-life such as fluoxetine. When a patient becomes pregnant while using psychotropic medications, they should be tapered at conception if there has been a long period of interepisode well-being in women with mild to moderate illness.

Women who are medication free should be carefully followed for recurrence or exacerbation of symptoms and their care must be coordinated with obstetrics staff who can alert psychiatric clinicians if concern arises. To prevent exacerbations of minor symptoms, clinicians should employ a variety of strategies, including an emphasis on a healthy diet free of alcohol, nicotine, and caffeine, maintaining circadian rhythms, and encouraging exercise as pregnancy permits. Stress management, and mobilizing support systems may also be helpful in preventing relapse. Individual therapies may assist in maintaining remission and conjoint treatment is indicated when significant marital tensions exist. Family and significant others should be included early in the treatment. It is critical to educate family members about the illness and use of medication, as their opinions may clearly influence a woman's decision about self-medication.

Pharmacological treatments of major depression

Women who have moderate to severe illness which impedes their ability to get adequate rest, care for themselves nutritionally or medically, or who are predisposed to risk-taking behaviours or suicidal ideation are candidates for pharmacotherapy in pregnancy. Women who are in remission and conceive while on antidepressant therapy, but have had severe episodes of depression that have recurred promptly with prior attempts at medication discontinuation should also continue pharmacotherapy.

All decisions to continue or begin pharmacotherapy in pregnancy should be made in collaboration with a woman, her family and her obstetric team. Women are understandably very concerned about the medication risks to their infants, and they may have extreme difficulty in balancing decisions about their own health and exposing their infants to psychotropic agents. They should be assisted with this dilemma by thoughtful treatment planning with a compassionate clinician. Careful attention to documentation and written medication consents with full discussion of available research, treatment options, risks and benefits of medication is paramount in pregnancy. Medications should be used at the lowest dose and minimum time necessary to ameliorate symptoms. Increased hepatic metabolism, renal clearance and decreased serum albumin and protein binding may necessitate increased dosing relative to prepregnancy. Levels should be monitored when tricyclic agents are used and quickly adjusted at delivery (Mortola, 1989; Altshuler *et al.*, 1996).

The selective serotonin reuptake inhibitor fluoxetine has been studied in pregnancy and appears safe for use even in the first trimester. Preliminary studies on sertraline and paroxetine are similarly encouraging without evidence of teratogenicity or adverse pregnancy outcomes, and should be considered in those women who have had a previous good response. The tricyclic agents also appear safe, and nortriptyline and desipramine are good candidates for use in pregnancy because they tend to cause less orthostasis and constipation. Use of the tricyclic agents near the time of labour and delivery may require the assistance of specialized paediatric care due to possible neonatal difficulties and should be planned for in advance. Weaning of tricyclic antidepressants prior to the time of delivery is not advised because fetal withdrawal syndromes may pose greater risk to the fetus than extrauterine withdrawal. MAOIs are contraindicated in pregnancy due to potential interaction with tocolytics which may be necessary to forestall premature labour. There is limited information about pregnancy risks of bupropion, nefazodone, and venlafaxine. Similarly herbal remedies are not studied in pregnancy.

Women who have had prior postpartum depression may wish to consider reintroduction of their antidepressant in the third trimester, even if they remain healthy through the pregnancy so that they will have adequate blood levels upon delivery to prevent relapse. Others choose to begin their antidepressants 'on the delivery table'. In any event, all women at risk for postpartum exacerbation of their illness require close monitoring in the puerperium.

Management of bipolar illness in pregnancy

Bipolar illness is less common, but its management is complicated by the fact that the mood stabilizers all cause increased risk of congenital anomalies in the first trimester. When women have had long periods of quiescence in their illness prior to conception, a medication wean should be considered. Medications should be tapered gradually, over a 4-week period to avoid relapse. In such cases, kits which predict ovulation may be helpful to minimize medication-free period and concurrent risk of recurrence. When a woman's clinical situation warrants it, medication should be continued. Coordination of care with obstetricians and appropriate counselling of the woman and her family about risks of medications including cardiac and neural tube defects, as well as more substantial risks of untreated illness, are paramount to assist women in acceptance and encourage compliance with medications. Relapses of bipolar illness should be treated aggressively with mood stabilizers and neuroleptics when clinically indicated. ECT is indicated if rapid reconstitution is essential. Psychosis with delusions and command hallucinations present a psychiatric emergency, and it is this clinical situation which may predispose to the disastrous consequence of infanticide. Hospitalization is always required if the woman and her infant are at risk.

Lithium should be prescribed in multiple daily dosing to avoid exposing the infant to large variations in blood levels. Lithium levels need to be monitored closely, and lithium dosage requirements are increased (30–40%) in the second/third trimesters due to increased maternal fluid volumes and increased renal clearance of lithium. Likewise lithium should be reduced by as much as 30% a few weeks prior to delivery to avoid postpartum maternal lithium toxicity (Wisner and Perel, 1996). Lithium should not be discontinued within the immediate postpartum period because of the extreme risk of exacerbation of bipolar illness (Cohen et al., 1995). Ultrasound with full fetal survey should be obtained at 16–18 weeks to assess for congenital anomalies. Prenatal syndromes have been reported and paediatric teams should be arranged at the time of delivery to optimize neonatal outcomes (Wisner and Perel, 1996; Altshuler et al., 1996; Burt and Hendrick, 1997).

Exposure to the anticonvulsants in the first trimester are associated with an increased risk of neural tube defects (0.5–1% with carbamazepine and 1–5% with valproic acid); therefore, lithium is preferred in the first trimester as its risk for Ebstein's anomaly is relatively remote (0.1%). Women who are treatment refractory to lithium, and have severe bipolar illness are candidates for the anticonvulsants (Altshuler et al., 1996). Valproic acid should be used in the lowest dose which is effective as the risk for spina bifida appears to be dose related (Wisner and Perel, 1996). When valproic acid or carbamazepine are used, an amniotic alpha-fetoprotein analysis at 16 gestational weeks followed by ultrasound is recommended to screen for neural tube defects. Folate (4 mg/day) is also recommended for all women 4 weeks prior to conception and throughout the first trimester when the anticonvulsants are used (MRC Vitamin Study Research Group 1991). Medications should be continued postpartum to prevent relapse of bipolar illness after delivery.

Management of schizophrenia during pregnancy

Untreated or inadequately treated schizophrenic illness is associated with substantial risks to the mother and the fetus. Inadequate maintenance antipsychotic treatment of schizophrenic illness during pregnancy substantially increases the risk of a relapse, which in turn has adverse short- and long-term effects on the mother. In the long term, relapses substantially increase the risk of chronicity and treatment resistance in schizophrenia (DeQuardo, 1998). In the short term, psychosis increases the likelihood of impulsive and risky behaviours (Miller, 1991) and is associated with impaired self-care and nutrition. Poor maternal state (poor nutrition, infection or other negative consequences of poor self-care, etc.) obviously increases fetal morbidity and untreated schizophrenia in the mother has been found to result in an increase in perinatal mortality (Rieder *et al.*, 1975). Psychotic symptomatology clearly interferes with the mother's ability to access and accept necessary prenatal care.

In contrast to the significant maternal and fetal risks of antipsychotic discontinuation, the risks of fetal exposure to antipsychotics are less well-defined. While there is minimal evidence for teratogenicity and long-term neurobehavioural effects of antipsychotic exposure during pregnancy, neonatal toxicity is better documented. In a patient with chronic schizophrenia receiving maintenance antipsychotic medication, prevention of relapse by continuing the antipsychotic at the minimal effective dose should generally take precedence over the small risk to the fetus from *in utero* exposure to the antipsychotic. Although discontinuation of antipsychotic 2 weeks before the expected date of delivery to minimize neonatal toxicity was recommended earlier, this practice is not now recommended in view of the substantial risk of relapse (Cohen and Rosenbaum, 1998). Obviously the patient and her family unit need to be intimately involved in this decision-making process. Antiparkinsonian medications are best avoided.

In a patient receiving antipsychotics for non-psychotic illness or unclear reasons, discontinuation of antipsychotic is appropriate. If a patient develops a psychotic illness during pregnancy, its effective treatment is appropriate after a careful assessment for a possible organic aetiology. In terms of choice of antipsychotic, chlorpromazine is best avoided despite the fact that data indicating its teratogenicity appear spurious. Atypical antipsychotics are generally preferable to conventional antipsychotics (Jibson and Tandon, 1998), although information about their use in pregnancy is sparse.

Conclusions

All psychotropic agents freely cross the placental barrier, and expose the fetus to medication; therefore the risks of untreated psychiatric illness must always be balanced with the risk of fetal exposure. While some agents may increase the absolute risk for teratogenicity, that risk should be considered in the entire context of the woman's illness and the adverse consequences which may be incurred if the illness is left untreated. A decision to use medication in pregnancy should be informed by: (1) past history and severity of illness; (2) illness-free interval; (3) current symptoms, their risk to mother and fetus; and (4) nature of pharmacotherapy. When psychiatric illness poses substantial risk to the pregnancy, psychotropic agents are recommended. Choice of agent should be guided by those with least risk for teratogenicity. Treatment should always be coordinated with the obstetric team. Thoughtful treatment planning also requires much discussion with a woman and her family, for discussion of the risks both of medication and of undertreatment of psychiatric illness. These discussions serve to engage the family as allies in the treatment, enhance adherence, and recruit support systems for secondary prevention of depression and schizophrenia.

Further study is essential to elucidate risk factors which predispose women to relapse during pregnancy with discontinuation of medication. Additional information and long-term studies examining behavioural effects in children who are accidentally or intentionally exposed to these agents in pregnancy and lactation are also essential. Additional study on newer agents (nefazodone, venlafaxine, mitrazepine and atypical antipsychotics) is also critical. Finally, information relative to herbal treatments which many women self-prescribe with the belief that these agents are natural and therefore 'safe' is necessary in pregnancy.

In summary, while more study is necessary for newer agents the absolute risk of medication in pregnancy is frequently outweighed by the risk of undertreating psychiatric illness itself. Balancing that risk, and assisting a woman and her family with these delicate decisions is one of the most important jobs of the clinician who treats pregnant women.

References

Altshuler, L.L., Hendrick, V. and Cohen, L.S. (1998). Course of mood and anxiety disorders during pregnancy and the postpartum period. *J. Clin. Psychiatry*, **59**, 9–33.

Altshuler, L.L., Cohen, L., Szuba, M.P., *et al.* (1996). Pharmacologic management of psychiatric illness during pregnancy: dilemmas and guidelines. *Am. J. Psychiatry*, **153**, 592–606.

Auerbach, J.G., Hans, S.L., Marcus, J., *et al.* (1992). Maternal psychotropic medication and neonatal behavior. *Neurotoxicol. Teratol.*, **14**, 399–406.

Burt, V.K. and Hendrick, V.C. (1997). *Concise Guide to Women's Mental Health*, Washington, DC, AP Press, Inc.

Carroll, B.J., Feinberg, M., Greden, J.F., *et al.* (1980). Diagnosis of endogenous depression. Comparison of clinical, research and neuroendocrine criteria. *J. Affect. Dis.*, **2**, 177–194.

Clark, C.V.H., Gorman, D. and Vernadakis, A. (1970). Effects of prenatal administration of psychotropic drugs on behavior of developing rats. *Develop. Psychobiol.*, **3**, 225–235.

Cohen, L.S., Friedman, J.M., Jefferson, J.W., *et al.* (1994). A reevaluation of risk of in utero exposure to lithium. *J. Am. Med. Assoc.*, **271**, 146–150.

Cohen, L.S., Heller, V.L. and Rosenbaum, J.F. (1989). Treatment guidelines for psychotropic drug use in pregnancy. *Psychosomatic*, **30**, 25–33.

Cohen, L.S. and Rosenbaum, J.F. (1988). Psychotropic drug use during pregnancy: weighing the risks. *J. Clin. Psychiatry*, **59**, 18–28.

Cohen, L.S., Sichel, D.A., Robertson, L.M., *et al.* (1995). Postpartum prophylaxis for women with bipolar disorder. *Am. J. Psychiatry*, **152**, 1641–1645.

Compendium of Drug Therapy (The Obstetrician and Gynecologist's.) (1984). New York, Biomedical Information Corp.

Cowe, L., Lloyd, D.J. and Dawling, S. (1982). Neonatal convulsions caused by withdrawal from maternal clomipramine. *Br. Med. J.*, **284**, 1837–1838.

Coyle, I., Wayner, M.J. and Singer, G. (1976). Behavioral teratogenesis: a critical evaluation. *Pharmacol. Biochem. Behav.*, **4**, 191–200.

DeQuardo, J.R. (1998). Pharmacologic treatment of first episode schizophrenia: early intervention is key to outcome. *J. Clin. Psych.* **59** (Suppl. 19), 9–17.

DeQuardo, J.R. and Tandon, R. (1998). Do atypical antipsychotic medications favorably alter the long-term course of schizophrenia? *J. Psychiatric. Res.*, **32**, 229–242.

Elia, J., Katz, I.R. and Simpson, G.M. (1987). Teratogenicity of psychotherapeutic medications. *Psychopharmacol. Bull.*, **23**, 531–586.

Faedda, G.L., Tondo, L., Baldessarini, R.J., *et al.* (1993). Outcome after rapid vs. gradual discontinuation of lithium treatment in bipolar disorders. *Arch. Gen. Psychiatry*, **50**, 448–455.

Falterman, C.G. and Richardson, C.J. (1980). Small left colon syndrome associated with maternal ingestion of psychotropic drugs. *J. Pediatr.*, **97**, 308–310.

Fisher, J.B., Edgren, B.E., Mammel, M.C., *et al.* (1985). Neonatal apnea association with maternal clonazepam therapy: a case report. *Obstet. Gynecol*, **66** (Suppl.), 34S–35S.

Frank, K., Kupfer, D.J., Perel, J.M., *et al.* (1990). Three-year outcome for maintenance therapies in recurrent depression. *Arch. Gen. Psychiatry*, **47**, 1093–1099.

Gilbert, P.L., Harris, M.J., McAdams, L.A., *et al.* (1995). Neuroleptic withdrawal in schizophrenic patients: a review of the literature. *Arch. Gen. Psychiatry*, **52**, 173–188.

Gotlib, I.H., Whiffen, V.E., Mount, J.H., *et al.* (1989). Prevalence rates and demographic characteristics associated with depression in pregnancy and the postpartum. *J. Consult. Clin. Psychol.*, **57**, 269–274.

Greden, J. and Tandon, R. (1995). Long-term treatment for lifetime disorders. *Arch. Gen. Psychiatry*, **52**, 197–200.

Hillesmaa, V.K., Teramo, K., Granstrom, M.L., et al. (1981). Fetal heart growth retardation associated with maternal antiepileptic drugs. *Lancet*, **2**, 165–167.

Istvan, J. (1986). Stress anxiety, and birth outcomes: a critical review of the evidence. *Psychol. Bull.*, **100**, 331–348.

Jacobson, S.J., Jones, K., Johnson, K., *et al.* (1992). Prospective multicenter study of pregnancy outcome after lithium exposure during first trimester. *Lancet*, **1**, 530–533.

Jibson, M.D. and Tandon, R. (1998). New atypical antipsychotic medications. *J. Psych. Res.*, **32**, 215–228.

Jones, K.L., Lacro, R.V., Johnson, K.A., *et al.* (1989). Pattern of malformations in the children of women treated with carbamazepine during pregnancy. *N. Engl. J. Med.*, **320**, 1661–1666.

Kallen, B. and Tandberg, A. (1983). Lithium and pregnancy: a cohort study on manic-depressive women. *Acta Psychiatr. Scand.*, **68**, 134–139.

Karlsson, K., Lindstedt, G., Lundberg, P.A., *et al.* (1975). Transplacental lithium poisoning: Reversible inhibition of fetal thyroid. *Lancet*, **1**, 1295.

Kendell, R.E., Chalmers, J.C. and Platz, C. (1987). Epidemiology of puerpereal psychoses. *Br. J. Psychiatry*, **150**, 662–673.

Kerns, L.L. (1986). Treatment of mental disorders in pregnancy: a review of psychotropic drug risks and benefits. *J. Nerv. Ment. Dis.*, **174**, 652–659.

Kessler, R.C., McGonagle, K.A., Nelson, C.B., *et al.* (1993). Sex and depression in the National Comorbidity Survey. II: Cohort effects. *J. Affect. Dis*, **30**, 15–26.

Kris, E.B. (1965). Children of mothers maintained on pharmacotherapy during pregnancy and postpartum. *Curr. Therapeut. Res.*, **7**, 785–789.

Kulin, N.A., Pastuszak, A., Sage, S.R., *et al.* (1998). Pregnancy outcome following maternal use of the new selective serotonin reuptake inhibitors: A prospective controlled multicenter study. *J. Am. Med. Assoc.*, **279**, 609–610.

Kupfer, D.J., Frank, E., Perek, J.M., *et al.* (1992). Five-year outcome for maintenance therapies in recurrent depression. *Arch. Gen. Psychiatry*, **49**, 769–773.

Lammer, E.J., Sever, L.E. and Oakley, G.P. (1987). Teratogen update: valproic acid. *Teratology*, **35**, 465–473.

Lindhout, D., Meinardi, H., Meijer, J.W., *et al.* (1992). Antiepileptic drugs and teratogenesis in two consecutive cohorts: changes in prescription policy paralleled by changes in pattern of malformations. *Neurology*, **43** (Suppl. 5), 94–110.

McNeil, T.F., Kaij, L. and Malmquist-Larsson, A. (1984). Women with nonorganic psychosis: pregnancy's effect on mental health during pregnancy. *Acta Psychiatr. Scand.*, **70**, 140–148.

Miller, L.J. (1991). Clinical strategies for the use of psychotropic drugs during pregnancy. *Psychiatr. Med.*, **9**, 275–298.

Mortola, J.F. (1989). The use of psychotropic agents in pregnancy and lactation. *Psychiatr. Clin. N. Am.*, **12**, 69–87.

MRC Vitamin Study Research Group (1991). Prevention of neural-tube defects: results of the Medical Research Council Vitamin Study. *Lancet*, **2**, 131–137.

Nelson, K. and Holmes, L.B. (1989). Malformations due to presumed spontaneous mutations in newborn infants. *N. Eng. J. Med.*, **320**: 19–23.

Nulman, I., Rovet, J., Stewart, D.E., *et al.* (1997). Neurodevelopment of children exposed in utero to antidepressant drugs. *N. Eng. J. Med.*, **336**, 258.

O'Hara, M.W. (1986). Social support, life events, and depression during pregnancy and the puerperium. *Arch. Gen. Psychiatry*, **43**, 569–573.

O'Hara, M.W. and Swain, A.M. (1996). Rates and risk of postpartum depression – a meta-analysis. *Int. Rev. Psychiatry*, **8**, 37–54.

Omtzigt, J.G.C., Los, F.J., Grobbee, D.E., *et al.* (1992). The risk of spina bifida aperta after first-trimester exposure to valproate in a prenatal cohort. *Neurology*, **42** (Suppl. 5), 119–125.

Patuszak, A., Shick-Boschetto, B., Zuber, C., *et al.* (1993). Pregnancy outcome following first-trimester. *JAMA*, **269** (17), 2246–8.

Rane, A., Bertilsson, L. and Palmer, L. (1975). Disposition of placentally transferred carbamazepine in the newborn. *Eur. J. Clin. Pharmacol.*, **8**, 283.

Rieder, R.O., Rosenthal, D., Wender, P., *et al.* (1975). The off-spring of schizophrenics: fetal and neonatal deaths. *Arch. Gen. Psychiatry*, **32**, 220–211.

Rumeau-Roquette, C., Goujard, J. and Huel, G. (1977). Possible teratogenic effects of phenothiazines in human beings. *Teratology*, **15**, 57–64.

Saxen, I. (1974). Cleft palate and maternal diphenhydramine intake. *Lancet*, **1**, 407–408.

Schearer, W.T., Schreiner, R.L. and Marshall, R.E. (1972). Urinary retention in a neonate secondary to maternal ingestion of nortriptyline. *J. Pediatr.*, **81**, 570–572.

Schou, M., Amdisen, A. and Steenstrup, O.H. (1973). Lithium and pregnancy, II: hazards to women given lithium during pregnancy and deliver. *Br. Med. J.*, **2**, 137–138.

Schou, M. (1976). What happened later to the lithium babies? A follow-up study of children born without malformations. *Acta Psychiatr. Scand.*, **54**, 193–197.

Scokel, P.W. and Jones, W.D. (1962). Infant jaundice after phenothiazine drugs for labour: an enigma. *Obstet. Gynecol.*, **20**, 124–127.

Scolnik, D., Nulman, I., Rovet, J., *et al.* (1994). Neurodevelopment of children exposed in utero to phenytoin and carbamazepine monotherapy. *J. Am. Med. Assoc.*, **271**, 767–770.

Slone, D., Siskind, V., Heinonen, O., *et al.* (1977). Antenatal exposure to the phenothiazines in relation to congenital malformations, perinatal mortality rate, birth weight, and intelligence quotient score. *Am. J. Obstet. Gynecol.*, **128**, 486–488.

Steer, R.A., Scholl, T.O., Hediger, M.L., *et al.* (1992). Self-reported depression and negative pregnancy outcomes. *J. Clin. Epidemiol*, **45**, 1093–1099.

Suppes, T., Baldessarini, R.J., Faedda, G.L. and Tohen, M. (1991). Risk of recurrence following discontinuation of lithium treatment in bipolar disorder. *Arch. Gen. Psychiatry*, **48**, 1082–1088.

Tamer, A., McKey, R., Arias, D., *et al.* (1969). Phenothiazine-induced extrapyramidal dysfunction in the neonate. *J. Pediatr.*, **75**, 479–480.

Tandon, R., Greden, J.F., Shirley, J.E., *et al.* (1991). Muscarinic/cholinergic hyperactivity in schizophrenia: relationship to positive and negative symptoms. *Schizophrenia Res.*, **4**, 23–30.

Tandon, R. (1995). The pathophysiology of increase and decrease symptoms in schizophrenia: contemporary issues in treatment of schizophrenia. *APA Press*, 109–124.

Wiebyl, J.R., Blake, D.A., Freeman, J.M., *et al.* (1979). Carbamazepine levels in pregnancy and lactation. *Obstet Gynecol.*, **53**, 139–140.

Wheatley, D. (1997). LI 160, an extract of St. John's Wort, versus amitriptyline in mildly to moderately depressed outpatients – a controlled 6-week clinical trial. *Pharmacopsychiatry*, **30** (Suppl.), 77–80.

Wilson, N., Forfar, J.C. and Godman, M.J. (1983). Atrial flutter in the newborn resulting from maternal lithium ingestion. *Arch. Dis. Child*, **58**, 538–549.

Wisner, K.L. and Perel, J.M. (1996). Psychopharmacological treatment during pregnancy and lactation. In: *Psychopharmacology and Women: Sex, Gender and Hormones* (M.F. Jensvold, U. Halbreich and J.A. Hamilton, eds) Washington DC, AP Press, Inc., pp. 191–224.

Woody, J.N., London, W.L. and Wilbanks, G.D. (1971). Lithium toxicity in a newborn. *Pediatrics*, **47**, 94–96.

Wyatt, R.J. (1991). Neuroleptics and the natural course of schizophrenia. *Schizophrenia Bull.*, **17**, 325–351.

Yoder, M.C., Belik, J., Lannon, R.A., *et al.* (1984). Infants of mothers treated with lithium during pregnancy have an increased incidence of prematurity, mactrosomia and perinatal mortality. *Pediatr. Res.*, **18**, 163A.

20

Psychopharmacology in the young

Sophia Frangou and Sanjiv Kumra

Key points

- The diagnosis of severe mental illness in children and adolescents carries specific treatment and prognostic implications and therefore diagnostic accuracy is important. Differential diagnosis is often challenging because of low prevalence rates, variability and atypicality of presentation and phenomenological overlap with other disorders.
- Early Onset Schizophrenia: Treatment with atypical antipsychotics may be preferable because of their favourable risk–benefit profile. The optimal length of maintenance treatment has not been established but early discontinuation is not advisable.
- Early Onset Major Depression: Selective Serotonin Re-uptake inhibitors may be more effective. Close monitoring is paramount because of the risk of treatment induced mania.
- Early Onset Bipolar Disorder: Lithium is effective but may be associated with more side effects in this age group. Little is known about its safety in long-term use in this population.

Introduction

Severe mental illness in children and adolescents is associated with significant functional impairment, loss of productivity, promise and fulfilment, frequent hospitalization and prolonged outpatient treatment. The emotional and financial burden imposed on the families of affected young people is enormous. This chapter provides a brief summary of the clinical features of schizophrenia and affective disorders beginning in childhood and adolescence and then focuses on diagnostic issues and drug treatment principles.

Clinical features

Early onset schizophrenia (EOS)

Schizophrenia is rare in very young children but its incidence rises sharply and steadily at about 12–14 years of age (Galdos *et al.*, 1993; Remschmidt, 1993; Hafner and Nowotny, 1995). Follow-back studies suggest that prodromal symptoms of the disorder may include developmental delays, disruptive behaviour disorders, expressive and receptive language deficits, impaired gross motor functioning, learning and academic problems, borderline to low average full-scale IQ, and transient symptoms of pervasive developmental disorder (Watkins *et al.*, 1988; Werry *et al.*, 1991; Russell, 1994; Alaghband-Rad *et al.*, 1995). Although similar premorbid abnormalities have been observed in patients with adult-onset schizophrenia (Parnas *et al.*, 1982; Walker and Levine, 1990), the rate of non-specific and transient autistic-like symptoms and language impairment appears higher in EOS (Hafner and Nowotny, 1995; Hollis, 1995).

The few studies to examine the phenomenology in EOS using DSM-III criteria (Cantor *et al.*, 1982; Green *et al.*, 1992; Russell, 1994) support continuity with the adult onset form. EOS is frequently insidious rather than acute in onset, and the most commonly reported psychotic features are auditory hallucinations and delusions (Kolvin, 1971; Kolvin *et al.*, 1971; Green *et al.*, 1992; Russell, 1994). The presence of formal thought disorder is more variable across studies and depends on the sample and definition (Caplan, 1994).

The outcome of EOS patients is generally thought to be poor and possibly worse than that of adult onset cases. Three studies that examined outcome after an average interval of about 5 years, have reported rates of improvement ranging from 3% (Werry *et al.* 1991) up to 56% (Asarnow *et al.*, 1994a; Russell, 1994). Schmidt *et al.* (1995) examined the clinical and social outcome of EOS patients compared to that of adult onset ones after a mean follow-up period of 7.4 years. They found that over two-thirds of the 118 cases in their sample had had at least one further schizophrenic episode and were in need of continuing psychiatric treatment. Social impairment was greater for the EOS patients particularly in the areas of self-care and social contacts. In two studies with longer follow-up periods (average between 15 and 16 years), the reported rates of full remission were 5% and 20% respectively with the majority of patients experiencing continuing symptoms (Eggers, 1978; Maziade *et al.*, 1996). Eggers and Bunk (1997) have reported the longest follow-up data (42 years) on a small sample ($n = 44$) of EOS cases. They found that 50% of the patients had continuous symptoms and 25% were in partial remission. Premorbid function, mode and age of onset appear to be the best predictors of clinical outcome (Werry and McClellan, 1992; Amminger *et al.*, 1997; Eggers and Bunk, 1997).

Early onset major depression

The risk of major depression (MD) is low in childhood (between 0.6 and 2%) (Fleming and Offord, 1990) and increases substantially in mid-adolescence (Cohen *et al.*, 1993; Giaconia *et al.*, 1994; Lewinsohn *et al.*, 1994). Childhood rates of depression are similar between the two genders with a female excess (about 2:1) becoming evident in the adolescent years (Fleming and Offord, 1990; Lewinsohn *et al.*, 1994).

The signs and symptoms of MD in children and adolescents are broadly similar to those for adult cases. However, there are some important differences. Irritability, rather than overt sadness, is a prominent symptom of depression in this age group and psychomotor agitation in children often takes the form of aggressive or oppositional behaviour (Emslie *et al.*, 1995). Multiple somatic complaints, symptoms of anxiety and phobias and school refusal are also age-specific expressions of depression (Berney *et al.*, 1991; Emslie *et al.*, 1995; Birmaher *et al.*, 1996).

Early onset of MD is associated with continued impairment in behavioural and emotional functioning. Recovery from an initial episode of depression appears quite high, the actual percentage depending on the length of the follow-up period, ranging from 6.9% at 12 weeks to 66% at 1 year and nearly 90% at 2 years (Strober *et al.*, 1993; Sanford *et al.*, 1995). The presence of anxiety or psychotic symptoms as well as family discord were associated with poor short-term prognosis (Warner *et al.*, 1992; Strober *et al.*, 1993; Sanford *et al.*, 1995). Early onset MD is a recurrent disorder and the probability of recurrence increases with the length of follow-up period. In a community-based study of MD in adolescents, a third of the sample had at least a second episode within 4 years (Lewinsohn *et al.*, 1994). Children with MD may have a higher rate of relapse than adolescents with more than one-third having a second episode within 2 years (Kovacs *et al.*, 1984; Asarnow *et al.*, 1988). Studies on adult patients, whose initial clinical diagnoses as children or adolescents were retrospectively assessed based on clinical records, suggest that adult recurrence of early onset MD may be as high as 70% (Garber *et al.*, 1988; Harrington *et al.*, 1990).

MD carries a significant risk of suicide or attempted suicide. Kessler and Walters (1998) examined the prevalence of MD and suicidal behaviour in a representative American cohort of 1769 young people. The lifetime prevalence of MD in the sample was 15.3% and 21.9% of the young people with MD had attempted suicide. The lifetime prevalence rate of completed adolescent suicides range from 3%–7% (Birmaher *et al.*, 1996a,b). Factors that increase suicide risk in early onset depression include comorbid anxiety, conduct and personality disorders as well as the presence of substance abuse and disruptive family environment (Birmaher *et al.*, 1996a,b).

Early onset bipolar disorder

As with MD, information about the prevalence of bipolar disorder (BD) in children and adolescents is very limited. The diagnosis is often missed either because clinicians do not consider the possibility of BD in this age group or fail to recognize it because of its often atypical presentation (Gammon *et al.*, 1983). The prevalence of BD in mid-adolescence is similar to that seen in adult populations (Sibisi,1990; Lewinsohn *et al.*, 1995). The prevalence of childhood onset BD appears to be less but remains considerable as 20–40% of adult bipolar patients report first becoming ill when children (Joyce, 1984; Lish *et al.*, 1994).

Bipolar disorder is characterized by symptoms of mania or depression occurring separately or together in mixed affective states. In children and adolescents, BD tends to be less episodic and the different affective states are less clearly demarcated (Carlson, 1984; Geller and Luby, 1997). The early signs of the disorder can be very non-specific, characterized by emotional lability, impulsivity, irritability and low tolerance of frustration, explosive outbursts and destructive behaviour (Carlson, 1984; Emslie *et al.*, 1995). Psychotic symptoms may also be present. These may be transient or may dominate the clinical picture (Ballenger et al., 1982; Strober and Carlson, 1982).

Onset of BD in childhood is a predictor of poor outcome and poor response to treatment (Delong and Aldershof, 1987; Strober et al., 1988). However, BD with adolescent onset may have a similar prognosis to the adult onset form (Carlson et al., 1977). In general, cycle duration and length of remission may become longer with increasing age (Kimura et al., 1980). A 5-year follow-up study of adolescents with BD suggested that premorbid adjustment and IQ were the best predictors of outcome (Werry et al., 1991).

Diagnostic assessment

Since the diagnosis of schizophrenia or affective disorder carries specific treatment and prognostic implications, diagnostic accuracy is of considerable importance. A detailed clinical evaluation is the key to diagnosis and may help overcome the difficulties associated with the low base rates of these disorders, their often variable and atypical presentation and their considerable phenomenological overlap with other disorders.

The clinical evaluation of a child or adolescent involves obtaining a careful history and assessment of mental state over multiple sessions. The history should focus on the onset of the condition, clarification of the type of signs and symptoms and their evolution over time and on changes in academic and social functioning. A developmental history is an important part of this evaluation (McClellan and Werry, 1994). It is important that both parents and patients are interviewed as there appears to be little concordance on diagnosis based either on parental or child interviews alone (Puura et al., 1998).

Collateral data should be collected from other sources (e.g. school reports, previous neuropsychological assessments, speech and language evaluations, neurological and genetics consultation). In diagnostically complex cases, a drug-free evaluation period in an inpatient unit may be of value.

Differential diagnosis

In many aspects, the differential diagnosis of early onset schizophrenia and affective disorders is similar to that of the adult onset forms. There is a substantial number of neurological and medical conditions that may lead to affective or psychotic symptoms. These include epilepsy, CNS neoplasms, infections, traumas, demyelinating diseases, disorders affecting neuronal metabolism as well as systemic and endocrine disorders (Coffey and Brumback, 1998). Substance abuse should always be considered in differential diagnosis as its presence carries significant therapeutic and prognostic implications (Alpert et al., 1994; Geller and Luby, 1997; Mueser et al., 1999).

In this section, we will focus on the differential diagnosis with psychiatric disorders that are particularly relevant to early onset schizophrenia and affective disorders.

Early onset schizophrenia (EOS)

Affective disorders

The differential diagnosis between patients presenting with a manic episode and those presenting with schizophrenia is often difficult. The younger the age at onset the more likely it is for manic patients to receive the diagnosis of schizophrenia (Joyce, 1984). A major factor contributing to these diagnostic difficulties is that the prevalence of psychotic symptoms is negatively associated with age of onset in bipolar patients (Stephens and McHugh, 1991; Werry et al., 1991).

Pervasive developmental disorders

As mentioned earlier developmental delays, expressive and receptive language deficits, impaired gross motor functioning, learning and academic difficulties as well as transient symptoms of pervasive developmental disorder (PDD) are often seen in patients with schizophrenia giving rise to diagnostic difficulties especially in very early onset cases. However, PDDs, of which autism is the prototype, arise during infancy as opposed to schizophrenia that is rare before middle childhood. Furthermore, the presence of family history of schizophrenia or of psychotic features is rare in PDDs (Rutter, 1978).

Anxiety and conduct disorders

Compared to adult onset cases, patients with EOS present with an excess of non-specific neurotic symptoms (social anxiety, panic attacks and obsessional ideas) particularly during the prodromal phase and at first presentation (Hafner and Nowotny, 1995). Increased rates of antisocial behaviour leading to contact with the legal system and/or a diagnosis of conduct disorder are also seen in young patients with schizophrenia (Lewis et al., 1984; Hafner and Nowotny, 1995). In a study on hospitalized adolescents, the most common discharge misdiagnosis of those finally diagnosed as having schizophrenia was conduct disorder (Lewis et al., 1984). Similarly, in a study of adolescents with schizophrenia referred to a tertiary centre, 55% of the sample had been in contact with psychiatric services for behavioural problems that predated the onset of any psychotic symptoms by a mean of about 29 months (Frangou, unpublished data). Young people presenting with emotional and/or behavioural problems but without clear psychotic symptoms, pose significant diagnostic difficulties (McKenna et al., 1994a; Kumra et al., 1998a). A positive family history of schizophrenia, when present, is helpful in identifying high risk individuals but, in most cases, only longitudinal psychiatric follow-up is of any diagnostic value.

Early onset major depression

Bipolar disorder

Depression is often the initial presentation of young people with early onset BD (Lish *et al.*, 1994) and the rate of early onset depression switching to mania is high, ranging between 20–30% (Strober and Carlson, 1982; Geller and Luby, 1997). Although longitudinal follow-up is the only means of clarifying the diagnosis, it has been suggested some cross-sectional characteristics of a depressive episode may point to BD. These are rapid onset, the presence of psychotic features, family history of BD and antidepressant induced hypomania (Strober and Carlson, 1982; Geller *et al.*, 1993; Birmaher *et al.*, 1996a).

Anxiety disorders

Several studies have reported premorbid anxiety symptoms or disorders in children and adolescents with MD (Berney *et al.*, 1991; McCauley *et al.*, 1993; Birmaher *et al.*, 1996) and the rate of comorbidity has been reported to be between 30% and 80% (Lewinsohn *et al.*, 1994; Birmaher *et al.*, 1996). As anxiety disorders seem to have an earlier onset than mood disorders it is possible that they may represent a variant of the expression of depression in children or a risk factor for the development of mood disorders. Lewinsohn *et al.* (1994) examined possible determinants of the age of onset of MD in a randomly selected sample of community adolescents. They reported that comorbid anxiety disorders increased the risk of developing MD, but were not specifically predictive of an early onset. In the same study the presence of anxiety disorders did not appear to influence outcome measures such as length of episode or inter-episode interval.

Conduct disorder

The relationship of conduct and other disruptive disorders with MD in childhood and adolescence is quite complex. Angold and Costello (1993) reviewed the relevant epidemiological studies and found that the comorbidity of depression with conduct and oppositional/defiant disorder ranged from 21% to 83%. However, a study on large American (*n* = 500) and Australian (*n* = 2093) clinical cohorts of adolescents found that the comorbidity of conduct disorder and depression was not higher than that expected for any psychiatric disorder (Rey, 1994). Cohen *et al.* (1993), who examined general population samples of ages 10–20, reported that the association between conduct disorder and MD may be more significant for girls.

Warner *et al.* (1992) conducted a 2-year follow-up study of 174 children at high or low risk of MD. Within the follow-up period the incidence of MD was 8.5%, with all cases occurring exclusively among the high risk offspring. Preceding diagnosis of conduct disorder or subclinical depression were predictors of incidence suggesting that at the very early stages disruptive behaviour dominates the clinical picture or that conduct disorder is an independent risk factor for the development of MD. Kovacs *et al.* (1988), however, in a longitudinal observation of the evolution of MD in school aged children, found that in the majority of the cases conduct disorder developed after the onset of depression and persisted after the resolution of the depressive symptoms. Meller and Borchardt (1996) reported that, on a cross-sectional basis, the presence of anxiety was the variable best discriminating, between childhood depression and conduct disorder.

Early onset bipolar disorder

The issues of differential diagnosis of BD patients presenting with an initial depressive or psychotic episode have already been covered in the previous sections. Here we will concentrate on two other relevant conditions:

Attention Deficit Hyperactivity Disorder (ADHD)

Diagnostic problems between BD and ADHD usually arise in the early phase of BD or at the beginning of a manic episode. In these cases, as previously discussed, the affective component may be less clear and the clinical symptoms may be dominated by ADHD-like symptoms such as poor concentration, impulsivity, and hyperactivity. During a manic episode approximately 90% of children and 30% of adolescents will also fulfil criteria for ADHD (Geller and Luby, 1997). However, a chronic nature of such symptoms as opposed to an episodic one should point more towards a diagnosis of ADHD (Coll and Bland, 1979; Delong and Nieman, 1983). The onset of ADHD is early in childhood, often before the age of 6, while BD is rare in this age range (Bowring and Kovacs, 1992). Rates of depression, psychosis, conduct disorder and the degree of psychosocial impairment appear to be higher in BD than ADHD children (Wozniak *et al.*, 1995). However, one has to keep in mind that the comorbidity of ADHD and BD is high and in some patients both diagnoses may be warranted (Wozniak *et al.*, 1995; Biederman *et al.*, 1996).

Conduct disorder

Mania may lead to reckless and risk taking behaviour or to aggressive and destructive outbursts. These behaviours can also be seen in conduct disorder, which also often starts in adolescence. Kovacs and Pollock (1995) suggest that nearly half of the children and adolescents with mania may fulfil diagnostic criteria for conduct disorder while in episode. However, young people with conduct disorder appear to have more antisocial motives and general behavioural style (Bowring and Kovacs, 1992). The presence of psychotic symptoms, thought disorder and episodic nature of antisocial-like behaviour is more suggestive of BD rather than conduct disorder (Delong, 1978).

Special investigations

These should include:

1 detailed medical history as well as family history of psychiatric and hereditary neurological disorders
2 thorough physical examination with measurement of height and weight, neurological examination for tics, stereotypies, or drug induced movement disorder and attention to dysmorphic features

3 baseline laboratory evaluations (e.g. thyroid function tests, screen for toxic substances, pregnancy test, serum ceruloplasmin, erythrocyte sedimentation rate, antinuclear factor, complete blood count, urinalysis, renal function tests, liver function tests)
4 magnetic resonance scan of the brain
5 encephalogram
6 karyotype, molecular fragile X analysis
7 cerebrospinal fluid analysis may be clinically indicated but this is rare.

Treatment principles and options

The development of a treatment plan for a child/adolescent with schizophrenia or affective disorder requires the consideration of many issues, including current clinical status, cognitive level, developmental stage, and severity of illness. Ideally, treatment should be provided within the context of a multidisciplinary team consisting of a psychiatrist, a primary nurse, school teacher, social worker, occupational therapist and neuropsychologist. Having access to various specialist consultants (e.g. neurologist, geneticist, speech and language therapist) is also important. The foundation of treatment is the establishment and maintenance of a supportive therapeutic alliance with both the patient and family. It is important to involve families at the outset in the decision to initiate medication and to inform them about possible side effects and limitations of the treatment.

Very little information is available regarding appropriate pharmacological treatment in children and adolescents with schizophrenia or affective disorders. In this chapter we concentrate on double-blind controlled studies and open clinical trials are only mentioned when no other information is available. Most of the studies published to date concentrate on short-term (6–8 weeks) efficacy and safety of drug treatment. Even then, study samples are universally small with questionable statistical power. Studies on the pharmacokinetics and pharmacodynamics of psychotropic medication in children and adolescents are also few and the question of effective dosage and titration of these drugs in this age group is open. Finally, there is a dearth of information on long-term efficacy and tolerability of psychotropic medication in children and adolescents.

Pharmacological treatment for early onset schizophrenia

Conventional antipsychotic medications

There have been two controlled trials, one in children (Spencer *et al.*, 1992) and one in adolescents (Pool *et al.*, 1976) which support the use of typical antipsychotics for the treatment of schizophrenia in this age group. Spencer *et al.* (1992) examined the clinical efficacy of haloperidol in 16 children with schizophrenia, aged 5.5 to 11.75 years, who participated in a 10-week randomized double-blind placebo-controlled trial. Haloperidol was clinically and statistically superior to placebo as measured by reduction in the total pathology scores and scores for positive symptoms such as ideas of reference, persecution, hallucinations and thought disorder. Therapeutic doses ranged from 0.5 to 3.5 mg/day; most common untoward effects were excessive sedation and extrapyramidal symptoms (EPS). Good clinical response to haloperidol was inversely related to duration of illness and positively related to age and level of intellectual functioning (Spencer and Campbell, 1994). Pool *et al.* (1976) conducted a double-blind placebo controlled trial comparing haloperidol to loxapine employing a parallel groups design in 75 adolescents with acute schizophrenia, aged 13–18 years. At daily doses ranging from 2 to 16 mg (mean 9.8) haloperidol and 10–200 mg/day (mean 87.5) loxapine, there was no statistical difference between drugs and placebo with significant reduction of symptoms being present in all three treatment conditions. However, severely or very severely ill patients tended to show greater improvement on active drugs than on placebo. Untoward effects, mainly EPS and sedation, were common with both haloperidol and loxapine.

The major limitations of conventional antipsychotic drugs in EOS, as in older patients, include EPS, tardive dyskinesia, galactorrhoea, gynaecomastia, excessive weight gain and sedation (Kumra *et al.*, 1996). As most of the EOS cases will probably require antipsychotic treatment for many years, it is important to monitor closely the development of movement disorders and particularly emergent tardive dyskinesia. For abnormal movements, the Abnormal Involuntary Movement Scale (AIMS) should be used following a schedule recommended for children (Campbell and Palij, 1985).

Atypical antipsychotics
Recently, an increasing number of atypical antipsychotics, of which clozapine is the prototype, have been introduced and are being prescribed in the treatment of children and adolescents with schizophrenia (Siefen and Remschmidt, 1986; Birmaher *et al.*, 1991; Mozes *et al.*, 1994; Remschmidt *et al.*, 1994). Most reports in EOS patients are open clinical trials conducted in small samples. Armenteros *et al.* (1997) conducted an open pilot study of risperidone in 10 adolescents with acute schizophrenia, aged 11–18 years. At daily doses ranging from 4 to 10 mg (mean 6.6) there was a statistically significant clinical improvement without major adverse reactions. EPS were minimal to mild at low doses, but increased at doses above 6 mg/day. Grcevich *et al.* (1996) conducted a retrospective study of risperidone in 16 children and adolescents with psychotic disorders, aged 9–20 years. Good clinical improvement was seen at daily doses ranging from 2 to 10 mg (mean, 5.9). The major adverse effects reported were mild sedation and EPS (in 31% and 19% of the patients respectively). Although olanzapine is fast becoming the most widely prescribed atypical antipsychotic the only available clinical data on its efficacy and side effects in EOS come from a NIMH study on treatment resistant cases (see Treatment-non-responsive childhood onset schizophrenia). To date there has been only one controlled clinical trial on the use of clozapine in treatment-resistant EOS cases that is described in detail below (see Treatment-non-responsive childhood onset schizophrenia).

There are no systematic data to provide guidance for the comprehensive treatment of EOS during the maintenance phase. The biggest therapeutic dilemma in this phase is whether to continue medication or not in the case of patients who are in remission after their initial episode. As discussed above outcome studies suggest that the majority of EOS patients (up to 70%) will have a second psychotic episode within 5–7 years. Variables to be considered in deciding on discontinuation of medication are: the mental state of the patient at the time, the number and frequency of previous relapses; the risks associated with relapse (with emphasis on dangerous or suicidal behaviour exhibited by the patient during previous acute episodes); the degree of disruption to the patient's life caused by a further relapse; the level of side effects experienced by the patient and the extent to which they hinder daily living; and the presence of an adequate supportive social network. The balance of probability suggests that clinicians should consider long-term maintenance treatment and avoid early discontinuation. However, if discontinuation is attempted, additional precautions should be instituted such as gradual dose reduction over several months, frequent monitoring and contingency plans in case of relapse.

As in adults, pharmacokinetic processes vary from individual to individual, and may be variable within the same individual. Children eliminate psychoactive agents more rapidly than do adults and may require a greater dose (mg/kg) than adults and may be more sensitive to the extrapyramidal side effects of neuroleptic drugs (Baldessarini and Teicher, 1995). The half-life of psychotropic drugs in children and adolescents is often unknown. Plasma drug levels can be used to identify patients with low levels who are non-compliant, non-responders, or rapid metabolizers and/or to aid in the differential diagnosis of patients with high plasma levels and drug toxicity.

Neuroleptic-non-responsive early onset schizophrenia

Thirty children and adolescents with treatment-refractory schizophrenia (all with onset of psychotic symptoms before age 12; mean age 14.0 years) have been studied at the National Institute of Mental Health (NIMH) in either open or double-blind protocols. A double-blind parallel comparison of haloperidol and clozapine in 21 of these patient found clozapine superior to haloperidol for both positive and negative symptoms and for measures of overall improvement (Kumra et al., 1996). Clozapine doses began at 6.25–25 mg/day, depending on the patient's weight and could be increased every 3–4 days by one to two times the starting dose (Kumra et al., 1996). The mean dose of clozapine at the sixth week of treatment was 149 mg/day (range 25–525 mg/day). Medical monitoring included: weekly complete blood cell counts with differential liver function tests, an encephalogram, and an electrocardiogram prior to drug initiation and at week 6 of treatment. Thirteen of 21 patients who participated in the double-blind trial continued on clozapine for an additional 30–45 months after completion of the study, and continued benefits in overall functioning have been seen at 2-year follow-up (S. Kumra and L.K. Jacobsen, unpublished data). In the NIMH sample, seven out of 27 patients had to stop otherwise effective clozapine therapy due to serious adverse events: two because of neutropenia which recurred with drug re-challenge; three because of persistent seizure activity despite anticonvulsant treatment; one because of excessive weight gain; one because of a threefold elevation in liver enzymes. There were no permanent or long-lasting negative consequences after drug withdrawal.

Similar findings were reported by Turetz *et al.* (1997) in 11 treatment-resistant schizophrenic children treated with clozapine in an open label study. Treatment response was monitored over a period of 16 weeks. Clinical condition showed an overall improvement, mostly within the first 6–8 weeks, that was greater for positive symptoms. Somnolence and hyper-salivation were the most serious side effects and there were no incidents of agranulocytosis.

Ten treatment-refractory schizophrenic children from the NIMH cohort were also treated with olanzapine in either open or double-blind trials (Kumra *et al.*, 1998b). In general, olanzapine was well tolerated in this group using doses up to 20 mg/day. For this protocol, olanzapine doses were initiated at 2.5 mg every day or every other day depending on the child's weight. The doses were doubled on day 3 and afterwards were adjusted upward to a maximum of 20 mg/day by 2.5 mg to 5 mg increments every 5–9 days. The mean dose of medication at the sixth week of treatment for olanzapine was 17.5 mg/day (range, 12.5–20 mg). After 8 weeks, of the 10 patients who participated in this trial, three were rated much improved, four minimally improved, one no change, one minimally worse and one much worse (Kumra *et al.*, 1998b). The most frequent side effects included increased appetite, constipation, nausea/vomiting, headache, somnolence, insomnia, difficulty concentrating, sustained tachycardia, increased ner-vousness and transient elevation of liver transaminases. No cases of neutro-penia or seizures have occurred with olanzapine.

Preliminary data based on a comparison of 23 patients who received 6-week open trials of clozapine and/or olanzapine at the NIMH, show that clozapine has superior efficacy for both positive and negative symptoms for this group of severely ill children (Kumra *et al.*, 1998b). In addition, four patients who were clozapine responsive but who could not continue on the drug due to serious adverse events received an open trial of olanzapine. For this group, each patient was less symptomatic at week 6 of treatment while on clozapine compared to olanzapine ($P = 0.03$) (Kumra *et al.*, 1998b). The results of this comparison should be considered preliminary due to the small number of patients studied, lack of randomization, open-label design, fixed order of drug trials (most patients received a trial of clozapine first) and the limitations of comparing open-label with double-blind data. To evaluate directly the relative safety and efficacy of these treatments, an 8-week dou-ble-blind comparison trial of clozapine and olanzapine has been initiated at NIMH.

Pharmacological treatments for early onset major depression

Antidepressants

Controlled double-blind studies that have examined the clinical efficacy of tricyclic antidepressants (imipramine, amitriptyline, desipramine and nor-triptyline) in children and adolescents with MD over a 4–8-week period have failed to find any advantage of active treatment over placebo (Kramer and

Feiguine, 1981; Petti and Law, 1982; Kashani *et al.*, 1984; Puig-Antich *et al.*, 1987; Geller *et al.*, 1989; Hughes *et al.*, 1990; Kutcher *et al.*, 1994; Kye *et al.*, 1996; Klein *et al.*, 1998).

Two double-blind placebo controlled studies have examined the clinical efficacy of the selective serotonin reuptake inhibitor (SSRI), fluoxetine. In the earlier study (Simeon *et al.*, 1990), 30 adolescents with depression received either fluoxetine or placebo for a period of 8 weeks. Patients in both treatment groups improved, but although fluoxetine showed some superiority to placebo this did not reach statistical significance. Emslie *et al.* (1997, 1998) reported a more clear therapeutic advantage of fluoxetine in the acute treatment of depression in a group of 96 children and adolescents who were randomly assigned to treatment with fluoxetine or placebo for a period of 8 weeks. Both study groups, however, were in agreement regarding the lack of a differential effect of initial treatment (fluoxetine or placebo) on subsequent recurrences.

Dugas *et al.* (1985) conducted a 15-week open clinical trial of mianserin on 110 children and adolescents with depression and reported significant clinical improvement that was noticeable after the first week.

Lithium

Two open label studies suggest a possible role for lithium augmentation of tricyclic treatment (Ryan *et al.*, 1988; Strober *et al.*, 1992). Lithium was combined with imipramine in the treatment of 24 adolescents who remained symptomatic on imipramine monotherapy. Ten of the patients appeared to have benefited from lithium augmentation (Strober *et al.*, 1992).

Pharmacological treatments for early onset bipolar disorder

Lithium

To date, lithium carbonate has been the most commonly used pharmacological intervention. Three open lithium treatment studies have examined the clinical efficacy of lithium in acute mania. Varanka *et al.* (1988) examined the effect of lithium treatment in pre-pubertal children with mania and associated psychotic features and reported that the psychotic symptoms resolved without the addition of other medication within 2 weeks of lithium initiation. DeLong and Aldershof (1987) examined a group of 59 bipolar children and adolescents and reported that over two-thirds of the sample showed a favourable response. Strober *et al.* (1988), who studied the efficacy of lithium in acute mania in a group of 50 bipolar adolescents, also reported similar rates of response to lithium after 6 weeks of treatment. The two studies differ however with regards to their findings on the effect of age at onset and response to lithium. In the first study children and adolescents responded equally well, while in the second, onset in childhood (before the age of 12) was associated with decreased response rate. Other investigators have suggested that predictors of poor response to lithium also include mixed affective states (Himmelhoch and Garfinkel, 1986), rapid-cycling (Jones and Berney, 1987) and the presence of comorbid personality disorders (Kutcher *et al.*, 1990). In contrast, one may especially expect a positive reaction to lithium when there is a family history of positive response to this medication (DeLong and Aldershof, 1987).

A single study has examined the merits of lithium prophylaxis in bipolar adolescents. Strober *et al.* (1990) in a naturalistic follow-up of 37 adolescents who had responded to acute treatment with lithium reported that the rate of relapse was nearly three times higher for those who did not take lithium prophylactically.

Side effects of lithium, such as weight gain, vomiting, headaches and tremor may be more frequent in children than in adults (Campbell *et al.*, 1991). Caroll *et al.* (1987) also reported inactivity, sedation, and irritability in children and adolescents treated with lithium. Khandelwal *et al.* (1984) examined the long-term (3–5 years) effects of lithium treatment in four adolescents who did not appear to experience any side effects. However, in the absence of reliable safety data on long-term lithium use in this age group one has to be particularly aware of the possibility of lithium having a negative impact on kidney, thyroid and bone growth (Reisberg and Gershon, 1979).

In spite of the higher clearance rate in children no dose adjustment for lithium appears necessary and effective drug levels are the same as those required for the treatment of adult cases of BD (McKnew *et al.*, 1981; Geller *et al.*, 1992).

Anticonvulsants

Papatheodorou *et al.* (1995) conducted a 7-week open clinical trial of divalproex sodium on 15 acutely manic patients aged 12–20. All but one showed significant improvements in all ratings of psychopathology. Patients were allowed concomitant medication, mostly chlorpromazine or benzodiazepines. Three patients developed clinically significant side effects (elevation of liver enzymes, sedation and dizziness and low thyroid and cortisol blood levels) leading to withdrawal from the trial in one case. Deltito *et al.* (1998) examined the use of divalproex sodium in ordinary clinical practice by examining the clinical records of patients admitted to an adolescent unit over a 1-year period. They found that divalproex sodium was most commonly prescribed in manic or mixed affective presentations and its use was associated with reduction in the symptoms of mania, psychosis, agitation, affective lability, aggression and anxiety in the majority of patients.

Antipsychotics

Schreier (1998) conducted an open label study of low dose risperidone (0.75–2.5 mg daily) in a group of 11 children and adolescents with manic-like symptoms and aggressive behaviour. They were also receiving a variety of concomitant medication. A marked to moderate improvement in behaviour was noted for seven of the patients in the sample. However, a recent systematic review of medical records to assess the efficacy of prescribed treatments to young manic patients found that the use of antipsychotics was of no significant benefit and only lithium appeared to produce a significant decrease in manic symptoms (Biederman *et al.*, 1998).

Antidepressants

Particular caution is needed in the treatment of depressive episodes in early onset BD. Tricyclic antidepressants can precipitate the onset of a manic episode, especially in the presence of a family history of BD (Geller *et al.*, 1993). Depressive episodes with biological or other episodic symptoms may respond favourably to treatment with lithium (DeLong and Aldershof, 1987).

Psychosocial interventions

In addition to medication, specific psychosocial treatment strategies can be introduced as the patients' clinical status stabilizes. The main aim of psychosocial interventions is to address the many psychological and social problems that afflict young patients and their families.

Educational and vocational support

Academic performance can be severely impaired even during the prodromal and residual phase of a psychotic or affective episode and in most cases school attendance becomes unattainable in acute phases. Even for patients in full remission re-integration into academic life may be very difficult. It is therefore important that clinical teams forge close working relationships with educational authorities. Providing information to school teachers about the nature of disorders and the likely impairments that it can cause is an essential first step. It may be possible for some patients to return to mainstream education, but they would need additional support (e.g. dedicated classroom assistant). For others, more specialized arrangements may be necessary in the form of home tuition or specialized school setting.

Family interventions

It has long been recognized that the quality of the family environment has a significant impact on the course of schizophrenia and affective disorders (Warner *et al.*, 1992; Bebbington and Kuipers, 1994; Sanford *et al.*, 1995). Most child and adolescent patients have regular contact with their families and the quality of family relationships is more important for this age group than it is for older patients. Some form of family intervention is therefore recommended and there are several models to choose from. Regardless of the model adopted, successful family intervention aims to increase understanding of the disorder and the limitations that it imposes on the individual. Other goals include education about treatment options and limitations, improvement of communication within the family, encouraging respect for and acceptance of the patient and help with solving daily living problems as well as discrete events.

Cognitive behavioural therapy

Harrington *et al.* (1998) critically reviewed all randomized trials comparing the efficacy of cognitive behaviour therapy (CBT) with inactive treatment in children and adolescents (aged 8 to 19) with depression. They found that patients receiving active treatment were three times more likely to recover from depression compared to the control group. They comment, however, that, although encouraging, these results should be viewed with caution as most studies of CBT in children and adolescents focused on cases with mild to moderate depression and had other significant methodological limitations.

References

Alaghband-Rad, J., McKenna, K., Gordon, C.T., et al. (1995). Childhood-onset schizophrenia: the severity of premorbid course. J. Am. Acad. Child. Adolesc. Psychiatry, **34**, 1273–1283.

Alpert, J.E., Maddocks, A., Rosenbaum, J.F. (1994). Childhood psychopathology retrospectively assessed among adults with early onset major depression. J. Affect. Dis. **31**, 165–171.

Amminger, G.P., Resch, F., Mutschlechner, R., et al. (1997). Premorbid adjustment and remission of positive symptoms in first-episode psychosis. Eur. Child. Adolesc. Psychiatry, **6**, 212–218.

Angold, A. and Costello, E.J. (1993). Depressive comorbidity in children and adolescents: empirical, theoretical, and methodological issues. Am. J. Psychiatry, **150**, 1779–1791.

Armenteros, J.L., Whitaker, A.H., Welikson, M., et al. (1997). Risperidone in adolescents with schizophrenia: an open pilot study. J. Am. Acad. Child. Adolesc. Psychiatry, **36**, 694–700.

Asarnow, J.R., Goldstein, M.J., Carlson, G.A., et al. (1988). Childhood onset depressive disorders. A follow-up study of rates of rehospitalization and out-of-home placement among child psychiatric inpatients. J. Affect. Dis. **15**, 245–253.

Asarnow, J.R., Tompson, M.C. and Goldstein, M.J. (1994a). Childhood-onset schizophrenia: a follow-up study. Schizophr. Bull., **20**, 599–617.

Asarnow, R.F., Asamen, J., Granholm, E., et al. (1994b). Cognitive/neuropsychological studies of children with a schizophrenic disorder. Schizophr. Bull., **20**, 647–669.

Baldessarini, R.J. and Teicher, M.H. (1995). Dosing of antipsychotic agents in pediatric populations. J. Child. Adolesc. Psychopharmacol., **5**, 1–4.

Ballenger, J.C., Reus, V.I. and Post, R.M. (1982). The atypical clinical picture of adolescent mania. Am. J. Psychiatry, **139**, 602–606.

Bebbington, P. and Kuipers, L. (1994). The predictive utility of expressed emotion in schizophrenia: an aggregate analysis. Psychol. Med., **24**, 707–718.

Berney, T.P., Bhate, S.R., Kolvin, I., et al. (1991). The context of childhood depression. The Newcastle Childhood Depression Project. Br. J. Psychiatry, **11** (Suppl.), S28–S35.

Biederman, J., Faraone, S., Mick, E., et al. (1996). Attention-deficit hyperactivity disorder and juvenile mania: an overlooked comorbidity? J. Am. Acad. Child. Adolesc. Psychiatry, **35**, 997–1008.

Birmaher, B., Baker, R., Kapur, S., et al. (1991). Clozapine for the treatment of adolescents with schizophrenia. J. Am., Acad. Child. Adolesc. Psychiatry, **3**, 160–164.

Birmaher, B., Ryan, N.D., Williamson, D.E., et al. (1996a). Childhood and adolescent depression: a review of the past 10 years. Part I. J. Am. Acad. Child. Adolesc. Psychiatry, **35**, 1427–1439.

Birmaher, B., Ryan, N.D., Williamson, D.E., et al. (1996b). Childhood and adolescent depression: a review of the past 10 years. Part II. J. Am. Acad. Child. Adolesc. Psychiatry, **35**, 1575–1583.

Bowring, M.A. and Kovacs, M. (1992). Difficulties in diagnosing manic disorders among children and adolescents. J. Am. Acad. Child. Adolesc. Psychiatry, **31**, 611–614.

Campbell, M. and Palij, M. (1985). Measurement of side effects including tardive dyskinesia. Psychopharmacol. Bull., **21**, 1063–1082.

Campbell, M., Silva, R., Kafantaris, V., et al. (1991). Predictors of side-effects associated with lithium administration in children. Psychopharmacol. Bull., **27**, 373–380.

Cantor, S., Evans, J., Pearce, J. (1982). Childhood schizophrenia: present but not accounted for. Am. J. Psychiatry, **139**, 758–762.

Caplan, R. (1994). Thought disorder in childhood. *J. Am. Acad. Child Psychiatry*, **33**, 605–615.

Carlson, G.A. (1984). Classification issues of bipolar disorders in Childhood. *Psychiatric Development*, **4**, 273–285.

Carlson, G.A., Davenport, Y.B. and Jamison, K. (1977). A comparison of outcome in adolescent- and later-onset bipolar manic-depressive illness. *Am. J. Psychiatry*, **134**, 919–922.

Caroll, J.A., Jefferson, J.W. and Greisl, J.H. (1987). Psychiatric use of lithium for children and adolescents. *Hosp. Com. Psychiatry*, **38**, 927–928.

Coffey, C.E. and Brumback, R.A. (1998). *Textbook of Pediatric Neuropsychiatry*, Washington, American Psychiatric Press, pp. 359–1274.

Cohen, P., Cohen, J., Kasen, S., *et al.* (1993). An apidemiological study of disorders in late childhood and adolescence – I. Age- and gender-specific prevalence. *J. Child. Psychol. Psychiatry*, **34**, 851–867.

Coll, P.G. and Bland, R. (1979). Manic-depressive illness in adolescence and childhood. *Can. J. Psychiatry*, **24**, 255–263.

DeLong, G.R. (1978). Lithium carbonate treatment of select behavior disorders in children suggesting manic-depressive illness. *J. Pediatr.*, **93**, 689–694.

DeLong, G.R. and Nieman, M.A. (1983). Lithium induced behavior changes in children with symptoms suggesting manic-depressive illness. *Psychopharmacol. Bull.*, **19**, 258–263.

DeLong, G.R. and Aldershof, A.L. (1987). Long-term experience with lithium treatment in childhood: correlation with clinical diagnosis. *J. Am. Acad. Child. Adolesc. Psychiatry*, **26**, 389–394.

Deltito, J.A., Levitan, J., Damore, J., *et al.* (1998). Naturalistic experience with the use of divalproex sodium on an in-patient unit for adolescent psychiatric patients. *Acta Psychiatr. Scand.*, **97**, 236–240.

Dugas, M., Mouren, M.C., Halfon, O., *et al.* (1985). Treatment of childhood and adolescent depression with mianserin. *Acta. Psychiatr. Scand. Suppl.*, **320**, S48–S53.

Eggers, C. (1978). Course and prognosis of childhood schizophrenia. *J. Austism Child. Schizophr.*, **8**, 21–36.

Eggers, C. and Bunk, D. (1997). The long-term course of childhood-onset schizophrenia: a 42-year follow up. *Schizophr. Bull.*, **23**, 105–117.

Emslie, G.J., Kennard, B.D. and Kowatch, R.A. (1995). Affective disorders in children: diagnosis and management. *J. Child. Neurol.*, **10** (Suppl. 1), S42–S49.

Emslie, G.J., Rush, A.J., Weinberg, W.A., *et al.* (1997). A double-blind, randomized, placebo-controlled trial of fluoxetine in children and adolescents with depression. *Arch. Gen. Psychiatry*, **54**, 1031–1037.

Emslie, G.J., Rush, A.J., Weinberg, W.A., *et al.* (1998). Fluoxetine in child and adolescent depression: acute and maintenance treatment. *Depress. Anxiety*, **7**, 32–39.

Fleming, J.E. and Offord, D.R. (1990). Epidemiology of childhood depressive disorders: a critical review. *J. Am. Acad. Child. Adolesc. Psychiatry*, **29**, 571–580.

Galdos, P.M., Van Os, J.J. and Murray, R.M. (1993). Puberty and the onset of psychosis. *Schizophr. Res.*, **10**, 7–14.

Gammon, G.D., Karen John, M.S., Rothblum, E.D., *et al.* (1983). Use of a structured diagnostic interview to identify bipolar disorder in adolescent inpatients: frequency and manifestations of the disorder. *Am. J. Psychiatry*, **140**, 543–547.

Garber, J., Kriss, M.R., Koch, M., *et al.* (1988). Recurrent depression in adolescents: a follow-up study. *J. Am. Acad. Child. Adolesc. Psychiatry*, **27**, 49–54.

Geller, B., Cooper, T.B., McCombs, H.G., *et al.* (1989). Double-blind, placebo-controlled study of nortriptyline in depressed children using a 'fixed plasma level' design. *Psychopharmacol. Bull.*, **25**, 101–108.

Geller, B., Cooper, T.B., Watts, H.E., *et al.* (1992). Early findings from a pharmacokinetically designed doubleblind and placebo-controlled study of lithium for adolescents comorbid with bipolar and substance dependency disorders. *Progres. Neurol.*, **16**, 281–289.

Geller, B., Fox, L.W. and Fletcher, M. (1993). Effect of tricyclic antidepressants on switching on mania and on the onset of bipolarity in depressed 6- to 12-year-olds. *J. Am. Acad. Child Adolesc. Psychiatry*, **32**, 43–50.

Geller, B. and Luby, J. (1997). Child and adolescent bipolar disorder: a review of the past 10 years. *J. Am. Acad. Child. Adolesc. Psychiatry*, **36**, 1168–1176.

Giaconia, R.M., Reinherz, H.Z., Silverman, A.B., *et al.* (1994). Ages of onset of psychiatric disorders in a community population of older adolescents. *J. Am. Acad. Child. Adolesc. Psychiatry*, **33**, 706–717.

Grcevich, S.J., Findling, R.L., Rowane, W.A., *et al.* (1996). Risperidone in the treatment of children and adolescents with schizophrenia: a retrospective study. *J. Child Adolesc. Psychopharmacol.*, **6**, 251–257.

Green, W.H., Padron-Gayol, M., Hardesty, A.S., *et al.* (1992). Schizophrenia with childhood-onset: a phenomenological study of 38 cases. *J. Am. Acad. Child. Adolesc. Psychiatry*, **31**, 968–976.

Hafner, H.B. and Nowotny, B. (1995). Epidemiology of early-onset schizophrenia. *Eur. Arch. Psychiatry Clin. Neurosci.*, **245**, 80–92.

Harrington, R., Fudge, H., Rutter, M., *et al.* (1990). Adult outcomes of childhood and adolescent depression. I. Psychiatric status. *Arch. Gen. Psychiatry*, **47**, 465–473.

Harrington, R., Whittaker, J., Shoebridge, P., *et al.* (1998). Systematic review of efficacy of cognitive behaviour therapies in childhood and adolescent depressive disorder. *Br. Med. J.*, **316**, 1559–1563.

Himmelhoch, J.M. and Garfinkel, M.E. (1986). Sources of lithium resistance in mixed mania. *Psychopharmacol. Bull.*, **22**, 613–620.

Hollis, C. (1995). Child and adolescent (juvenile onset) schizophrenia: a case control study of premorbid development impairments. *Br. J. Psychiatry*, **166**, 489–495.

Hughes, C.W., Preskorn, S.H., Weller, E., *et al.* (1990). The effect of concomitant disorders in childhood depression on predicting treatment response. *Psychopharmacol. Bull.*, **26**, 235–238.

Jones, P.M. and Berney, T.P. (1987). Early onset rapid cycling bipolar affective disorder. *J. Child. Psychol. Psychiatry*, **28**, 731–738.

Joyce, P.R. (1984). Age of onset in bipolar affective disorder and misdiagnosis as schizophrenia. *Psychol. Med.*, **14**, 145–149.

Kashani, J.H., Shekim, W.O. and Reid, J.C. (1984). Amitriptyline in children with major depressive disorder: a double-blind crossover pilot study. *J. Am. Acad. Child Psychiatry*, **23**, 348–351.

Kessler, R.C. and Walters, E.E. (1998). Epidemiology of DSM-III-R major depression and minor depression among adolescents and young adults in the National Comorbidity Survey. *Depress. Anxiety*, **7**, 3–14.

Khandelwal, S.K., Varma, V.K. and Srinivasa-Murthy, R. (1984). Renal function in children receiving long-term lithium prophylaxis. *Am. J. Psychiatry*, **141**, 278–279.

Kimura, S., Fujito, T. and Wakabayashi, T. (1980). On adolescent manic-depressive psychosis. Long-term observation and follow-up study. *Folia Psychiatr. Neurol. Jpn*, **34**, 433–450.

Klein, R.G., Mannuzza, S., Koplewicz, H.S., *et al.* (1998). Adolescent depression: controlled desipramine treatment and atypical features. *Depress. Anxiety*, **7**, 15–31.

Kolvin, I. (1971). Studies in the childhood psychoses: I. Diagnostic criteria and classification. *Br. J. Psychiatr.*, **118**, 381–384.

Kolvin, I., Ounsted, C., Humphrey, M., *et al.* (1971). Studies in childhood psychoses: II. The phenomenology of childhood psychoses. *Br. J. Psychiatr.*, **118**, 385–395.

Kovacs, M., Feinberg, T.L., Crouse-Novak, M.A., *et al.* (1984). Depressive disorders in childhood. I.A longitudinal prospective study of characteristics and recovery. *Arch. Gen. Psychiatry*, **41**, 229–237.

Kovacs, M., Paulauskas, S., Gatsonis, C., *et al.* (1988). Depressive disorders in childhood. III. A longitudinal study of comorbidity with and risk for conduct disorders. *J. Affect. Dis.*, **15**, 205–217.

Kovacs, M. and Pollock, M. (1995). Bipolar disorder and comorbid conduct disorder in children and adolescents. *J. Am. Acad. Child. Adolesc. Psychiatry*, **34**, 715–723.

Kramer, A. and Feiguine, R. (1981). Clinical effects of amitriptyline in adolescent depression. *J. Am. Acad. Child. Adolesc. Psychiatry*, **20**, 636–644.

Kumra, S., Frazier, J.A., Jacobsen, L.K., *et al.* (1996). Childhood-onset schizophrenia: a double-blind clozapine-haloperidol comparison. *Arch. Gen. Psychiatr.*, **53**, 1090–1097.

Kumra, S., Jacobsen, L.K., Lenane, M., *et al.* (1998a). 'Multidimensionally impaired disorder', Is it a variant of very early-onset schizophrenia? *J. Am. Acad. Child. Adolesc. Psychiatry*, **37**, 91–99.

Kumra, S., Jacobsen, L.K., Lenane, M., *et al.* (1998b). Childhood-onset schizophrenia: an open-label study of olanzapine in adolescents. *J. Am. Acad. Child. Adolesc. Psychiatry*, **37**, 377–385.

Kutcher, S.P., Marton, P. and Korenblum, M. (1990). Adolescent bipolar disorder and personality disorder. *J. Am. Acad. Child. Adolesc. Psychiatry*, **29**, 355–358.

Kutcher, S., Boulos, C., Ward, B., *et al.* (1994). Response to desipramine treatment in adolescent depression: a fixed-dose, placebo-controlled trial. *J. Am, Acad. Child. Adolesc. Psychiatry*, **33**, 686–694.

Kye, C.H., Waterman, G.S., Ryan, N.D., *et al.* (1996). A randomized, controlled trial of amitriptyline in the acute treatment of adolescent major depression. *J. Am. Acad. Child. Adolesc. Psychiatry*, **35**, 1139–1144.

Lewinsohn, P.M., Clarke, G.N., Seeley, J.R., *et al.* (1994). Major depression in community adolescents: age at onset, episode duration, and time to recurrence. *J. Am. Acad. Child. Adolesc. Psychiatry*, **33**, 809–818.

Lewinsohn, P.M., Klein, D.N., and Seeley, J.R. (1995). Bipolar disorders in a community sample of older adolescents: prevalence, phenomenology, comorbidity, and course. *J. Am. Acad. Child. Adolesc. Psychiatry*, **34**, 454–463.

Lewis, D.O., Lewis, M., Unger, L., *et al.* (1984). Conduct disorder and its synonyms: diagnoses of dubious validity and usefulness. *Am. J. Psychiatry*, **141**, 514–519.

Lish, J.D., Dime-Meenan, S., Whybrow, P.C., *et al.* (1994). The National Depressive and Manic-Depressive Association survey of bipolar members. *J. Affect. Dis.*, **31**, 281–294.

Maziade, M., Gingras, N., Rodrigue, C., *et al.* (1996). Long-term stability of diagnosis and symptom dimensions in asystematic sample of patients with onset of schizophrenia in childhood and early adolescence. I: nosology, sex and age of onset. *Br. J. Psychiatr.*, **169**, 361–370.

McCauley, E., Myers, K., Mitchell, J., *et al.* (1993). Depression in young people: initial presentation and clinical course. *J. Am. Child. Adolesc., Psychiatry*, **32**, 714–722.

McClellan, J. and Werry, J. (1994). Practice parameters for the assessment and treatment of children and adolescents with schizophrenia. *J. Am. Child. Adolesc. Psychiatry*, **33**, 616–635.

McKenna, K., Gordon, C.T., Lenane, M., *et al.* (1994). Looking for childhood-onset schizophrenia. The first 71 cases screened. *J. Am. Acad. Child. Adolesc. Psychiatry*, **33**, 636–644.

McKnew, D.H., Cytryn, Z., Buchsbaum, M.S., *et al.* (1981). Lithium in children of lithium responsive parents. *Psychiatry Res.*, **4**, 171–180.

Meller, W.H. and Borchardt, C.M. (1996). Comorbidity of major depression and conduct disorder. *J. Affect. Dis.*, **39**, 123–126.

Mozes, T., Toren, P. and Chernauzan, N. (1994). Case study: clopazine treatment in very early onset schizophrenia. *J. Am. Acad. Child. Adolesc. Psychiatry*, **33**, 65–70.

Mueser, K.T., Rosenberg, S.D., Drake, R.E., *et al.* (1999). Conduct disorder, antisocial personality disorder and substance use disorders in schizophrenia and major affective disorders. *J. Stud. Alcohol.*, **60**, 278-2–84.

Papatheodorou, G., Kutcher, S.P., Katic, M., *et al.* (1995). The efficacy and safety of divalproex sodium in the treatment of acute mania in adolescents and young adults: an open clinical trial. *J. Clin. Psychopharmacol.*, **15**, 110–116.

Parnas, J., Schulsinger, F., Schulsinger, H., *et al.* (1982). Behavioral precursors of schizophrenia spectrum: a prospective study. *Arch. Gen. Psychiatry*, **39**, 658–664.

Petti, T. and Law, W. (1982). Imipramine treatment of depressed children: a double blind pilot study. *J. Clin. Psychopharmacol.*, **2**, 107–110.

Pool, D., Bloom, W., Mielke, D., *et al.* (1976). A controlled evaluation of loxitane in seventy-five adolescent schizophrenic patients. *Curr. Ther. Res.*, **19**, 99–104.

Puig-Antich, J., Perel, J.M., Lupatkin, W., *et al.* (1987). Imipramine in prepubertal major depressive disorders. *Arch. Gen. Psychiatry*, **44**, 81–89.

Puura, K., Almqvist, F., Tamminen, T., *et al.* (1998). Psychiatric disturbances among prepubertal children in southern Finland. *Soc. Psychiatry Psychiatr. Epidemiol.*, **33**, 310–318.

Reisberg, B. and Gershon, S. (1979). Side effects associated with lithium therapy. *Arch. Gen. Psychiatry*, **36**, 879–887.

Remschmidt, H. (1993). Childhood and adolescent schizophrenia. *Curr. Opinion Psychiatry*, **6**, 470–479.

Remschmidt, H., Schulz, E. and Martin, M. (1994). An open trial of clopazine in thirty-six adolescents with schizophrenia. *J. Child. Adolesc. Psychiatry*, **4**, 31–41.

Rey, J.M. (1994). Comorbidity between disruptive disorders and depression in referred adolescents. *Aust. NZ J. Psychiatry*, **28**, 106–113.

Russel, A.T. (1994). The clinical presentation of childhood-onset schizophrenia. *Schizophr. Bull.*, **20**, 631–646.

Rutter, M. (1978). Diagnosis and definition of childhood autism. *J. Autism Childh. Schizophrenia*, **8**, 139–161.

Ryan, N.D., Meyer, V., Dachille, S., *et al.* (1988). Lithium antidepressant augmentation in TCA-refractory depression in adolescents. *J.Am. Acad. Child. Adolesc. Psychiatry*, **27**, 371–376.

Sanford, M., Szatmari, P., Spinner, M., *et al.* (1995). Predicting the one-year course of adolescent major depression. *J. Am. Acad. Child. Adolesc. Psychiatry*, **34**, 1618–1628.

Schmidt, M., Blanz, B., Dippe, A., *et al.* (1995). Course of patients diagnosed as having schizophrenia during first episode occurring under age 18 years. *Eur. Arch. Psychiatry Clin. Neurosci.*, **245**, 93–100.

Schreier, H.A. (1998). Risperidone for young children with mood disorders and aggressive behavior. *J. Child. Adolesc. Psychopharmacol.*, **8**, 49–59.

Sibisi, C.D. (1990). Sex differences in the age of onset of bipolar affective illness. *Br. J. Psychiatry*, **156**, 842–845.

Siefen, G. and Remschmidt, H. (1986). Treatment results with clopazine in schizophrenic adolescents. *Z. Kinder, Jugenpsychiatr*, **14**, 245–257.

Simeon, J.G., Dinicola, V.F., Ferguson, H.B., *et al.* (1990). Adolescent depression: a placebo-controlled fluoxetine treatment study and follow-up. *Prog. Neuropsychopharmacol. Biol. Psychiatry*, **14**, 791–795.

Spencer, E.K., Kafantaris, V., Padron-Gayol, M.V., *et al.* (1992). Haloperidol in schizophrenic children: early findings from a study in progress. *Psychopharmacol. Bull.*, **28**, 183–186.

Spencer, E.K. and Campbell, M. (1994). Children with schizophrenia: diagnosis, phenomenology, and pharmacotherapy. *Schizophr. Bull.*, **20**, 713–725.

Stephens, J.H. and McHugh, P.R. (1991). Characteristics and long-term follow-up of patients hospitalized for mood disorders in the Phipps Clinic. *J. Nerv. Men. Dis.*, **179**, 64–73.

Strober, M. and Carlson, G. (1982). Bipolar illness in adolescents with major depression. *Arch. Gen. Psychiatry*, **39**, 549–555.

Strober, M., Morell, W., Burroughs, J., *et al.* (1988). Family study of bipolar I disorder in adolescence. Early onset of symptoms linked to increased familial loading and lithium resistance. *J. Affect. Dis.*, **15**, 255–268.

Strober, M., Morrell, W., Lampert, C., *et al.* (1990). Relapse following discontinuation of lithium maintenance therapy in adolescents with bipolar I illness: a naturalistic study. *Am. J. Psychiatry*, **147**, 457–461.

Strober, M., Freeman, R., Rigali, J., *et al.* (1992). The pharmacotherapy of depressive illness in adolescence: II. Effects of lithium augmentation in nonresponders to imipramine. *J. Am. Acad. Child. Adolesc. Psychiatry*, **31**, 16–20.

Strober, M., Lampert, C., Schmidt, S., *et al.* (1993). The course of major depressive disorder in adolescents: I. Recovery and risk of manic switching in a follow-up of psychotic and non-psychotic subtypes. *J. Am. Acad. Child. Adolesc. Psychiatry*, **32**, 34–42.

Turetz, M., Mozes, T., Toren, P., *et al.* (1997). An open trial of clozapine in neuroleptic-resistant childhood-onset schizophrenia. *Br. J. Psychiatry*, **170**, 507–510.

Varanka, T.M., Weller, R.A., Weller, E.B., *et al.* (1988). Lithium treatment of manic episodes with psychotic features in prepubertal children. *Am. J. Psychiatry*, **145** (12), 1557–1559.

Walker, E. and Levine, R.J. (1990). Prediction of adult-onset schizophrenia from childhood home movies of the patients. *Am. J. Psychiatry*, **147**, 1052–1056.

Warner, V., Weissman, M.M., Fendrich, M., *et al.* (1992). The course of major depression in the offspring of depressed parents. Incidence, recurrence, and recovery. *Arch. Gen. Psychiatry*, **49**, 795–801.

Watkins, J.M., Asarnow, R.F. and Tanguay, P.E. (1988). Symptom development in childhood onset schizophrenia. *J. Child. Psychol. Psychiatry*, **29**, 865–878.

Werry, J.S., McClellan, J.M. and Chard, L. (1991). Childhood and adolescent schizophrenic, bipolar, and schizoaffective disorders: a clinical and outcome study. *J. Am. Acad. Child. Adolesc. Psychiatry*, **30**, 457–465.

Werry, J.S. and McClellan, J.M. (1992). Predicting outcome in child and adolescent (early onset) schizophrenia and bipolar disorder. *J. Am. Acad. Child. Adolesc. Psychiatry*, **31**, 147–150.

Wozniak, J., Biederman, J., Kiely, K., *et al.* (1995). Mania-like symptoms suggestive of childhood-onset bipolar disorder in clinically referred children. *J. Am. Acad. Child. Adolesc. Psychiatry*, **34**, 867–876.

21

Drug treatment of schizophrenia and mood disorders in older people

Ruth Allen, Barbora Richardson, Tim Stevens and Cornelius Katona

---

Key points

- Medication only one element of management.
- Inform patient and caregiver of:
  (a) typical side effects
  (b) delay in onset of therapeutic action
  (c) need for continued treatment after onset of response.
- Begin with low dose (subtherapeutic if necessary) and titrate upwards against response and tolerability.
- Aim for single daily dose regimen to improve compliance.
- Reassess for response and side effects, weekly if possible.
- Allow sufficient time for response.

Introduction

Elderly people suffer from the same range of functional psychiatric illnesses as younger patients. These can often be successfully treated and there is no excuse for therapeutic nihilism among clinicians working with patients in the older age group. When prescribing in the elderly, doctors need to be aware of the general principles of pharmacokinetics and pharmacodynamics and the effect on them of ageing.

The World Health Organisation (1970) has suggested that an adverse drug reaction (ADR) is any response to a drug which is noxious and unintended and occurs at usual doses. The risk of adverse drug reactions increases with age (Castleden and Pickles, 1988) and is two to three times more common in the elderly than in the young and middle aged (Grahame-Smith and Aronson, 1984). It has been estimated from geriatric admissions that 11–16% of elderly patients prescribed medication experience ADRs (Anon, 1988). This is likely to be an underestimate as not all will result in hospital admission. The increased incidence of ADRs in older age groups may be due to a number of reasons – increased prescribing, altered pharmacokinetics, altered pharmacodynamics and compliance issues.

Increased prescribing rates

As might be expected, the elderly consume the greatest amounts of medication and utilize around 25–30% of health service expenditure on drugs.

Polypharmacy is common; one survey showed 34% of over 75-year-olds were taking three or four different drugs daily (Gillies *et al.*, 1986). The number of ADRs increases with the number of drugs prescribed (Williamson and Chopin, 1980). In addition, elderly people purchase 70% of over-the-counter medicines and it is important to enquire about all drug usage prior to prescribing. Multiple drug prescribing increases the risk of drug–drug interactions and as few drugs as possible should be used.

Pharmacokinetics

Pharmacokinetics includes drug absorption, metabolism and excretion. Knowledge of age effects on these factors influences choice of dose, frequency and route of administration.

Absorption

Most drugs are given orally and absorption mainly takes place in the upper small intestine while some occurs in the stomach depending on the pKa of the drug and the pH of the stomach. Absorption does not appear to decline with age provided that gastrointestinal function is normal (Gillies *et al.*, 1986; Kinirons and Wood, 1998).

Distribution

Ageing is associated with an increase in the ratio of fat to muscle and water. This increases the volume of distribution of lipophilic drugs such as diazepam and tricyclic antidepressants. An increase in volume of distribution leads to an increased half-life of these drugs and hence the need for dose reduction in older patients.

Only unbound drugs are free to cross plasma membranes. Drugs that are highly protein bound (> 90%) will be affected by changes in concentration of such proteins. In such cases, small decreases in albumin may lead to a clinically relevant increase in the free drug. Evidence for a decrease in serum albumin with age is mixed. However, levels are consistently lower in frail elderly people (Woodhouse *et al.*, 1988) and those with chronic disease (Pickart, 1983).

Metabolism

The principal organ for drug metabolism is the liver. The liver's ability to metabolize a drug is determined by intrinsic enzyme capacity, liver size and blood flow. The most important phase 1 enzyme systems are the cytochrome P450 dependent microsomal mono-oxygenases. There appears to be no decline in the amount or activity of cytochrome P450 with age and age-related decreases in the body's ability to eliminate a drug reflects fall in liver volume and blood supply (Kinirons *et al.*, 1994). A suggestion has been made that the induction of cytochrome P450 enzymes is decreased with age, but data are conflicting (Woodhouse, 1998). There is no evidence of age-related decline in the esterase or alcohol dehydrogenase enzymes that are used in phase 1 reactions. However, physical frailty may have more effect than the ageing process *per se* on these drug metabolizing enzymes (Williams *et al.*, 1989), although the impact on cytochrome P450 is unclear (Wynne *et al.*, 1989).

Excretion

The final elimination of drugs predominantly involves the kidneys and the liver. There is no simple way to predict the decline in hepatic excretion with age, in contrast with the kidneys, where drug elimination is correlated with creatinine clearance. Creatinine clearance decreases by 1% per year after the age of 20 (Kinirons and Wood, 1998) and dosing should be decreased in proportion to the fall in clearance. Serum creatinine levels alone are not a good indicator of drug elimination as creatinine production decreases with age. Estimating creatinine clearance at the bedside can be done using the Cockcroft formula (Cockcroft and Gault, 1976).

Pharmacodynamics

Evidence that the elderly are intrinsically more sensitive to drugs is scarce. Most studies use highly selected samples of fit elderly people; their findings cannot always be generalized to the majority of elderly patients. Greater heterogeneity in pharmacological responses occurs in the elderly compared with younger people. Ford *et al.* (1998) suggest the following mechanisms for age-related pharmacodynamic change: altered receptor density, decreased affinity of receptors to second messenger systems, altered post-receptor mechanisms and non-receptor functional alterations of cells or organs.

Compliance

Non-compliance is reported to occur in 30–50% of elderly patients (Morrow *et al.*, 1988). It is important to keep the drug regimen simple and explain it carefully. Cognitive problems in the elderly may also be a barrier to understanding how their drugs should be taken. Involvement of carers and use of a dosette box may help. Formulations such as syrup may be easier for elderly patients to swallow. When prescribing for an elderly patient, it is generally advisable to consider their general physical state and intercurrent medical problems, start with a low dose, monitor carefully and increase the dose only if necessary. General issues relating to compliance are considered in Chapter 24.

Consideration will now be given to specific functional mental disorders and to advances in their treatment in older people.

Mood disorders in the elderly

Mood disorders are the most commonly occurring psychiatric conditions in people over the age of 65, with reported prevalence rates ranging from 11.5% (Copeland *et al.*, 1987) to 26% (Kay *et al.*, 1964). As in younger patients, demographic, social and biological factors have been implicated in the aetiology of the illness. Depression is more common in physically ill than in healthy older people and this is of particular significance when considering pharmacological therapy with potential side effects. The clinical features and drug treatment of mania are similar to those in younger patients but first onset mania in old age is frequently associated with an underlying organic cause.

Treatment of depression

Controlled trials of tricyclic and newer antidepressant drugs have consistently demonstrated response rates of 50–60% in older patients (Anstey and Brodaty, 1995; Katona and Judge, 1996), compared with 25% for placebo (Rockwell *et al.*, 1988). Nonetheless, and surprisingly, antidepressant medication is seldom used in this age group, particularly in primary care; for example, less than 10% of a sample of elderly subjects with depression identified in a recent community survey were receiving antidepressants (Manela *et al.*, 1996). There are several possible reasons for this underprescribing. Depression in older patients may be missed owing to its frequent manifestation as symptoms not immediately identifiable as depressive, such as anxiety or somatic complaints. It may also not be diagnosed if the symptoms displayed are viewed as a 'normal' response to ageing, physical impairment or living alone. Doctors may be reluctant to prescribe medication to elderly patients because of concerns about adverse effects and lack of knowledge about the different side effects of the various agents; this may account for the common prescription of medication at subtherapeutic doses (Donoghue *et al.*, 1998).

The pharmacotherapy of depression may be considered in regard first to the acute phase of the illness, and secondly to the prevention of relapse and recurrence.

Acute phase

The categories of antidepressant available are the tricyclic antidepressants (TCAs), the selective serotonin reuptake inhibitors (SSRIs), the monoamine oxidase inhibitors (MAOIs), the reversible inhibitors of MAO-A (RIMAs), and atypical antidepressants such as the serotonin and noradrenaline reuptake inhibitor venlafaxine, the noradrenaline reuptake inhibitor reboxetine, the noradrenaline and specific serotonin antidepressant mirtazapine, and others such as mianserin and trazodone. The recommended starting and maintenance doses and the most significant adverse effects are shown in Table 21.1.

Table 21.1 Classes of antidepressants, recommended doses and significant side effects in older patients

Antidepressant class	Examples	Starting dose (mg/day)	Maintenance dose (mg/day)	Adverse effects
TCA	Amitriptyline	25	100–150	Confusion, blurred vision, constipation, urinary retention, orthostatic hypotension, cardiac effects, sedation (less with lofepramine)
	Imipramine	10	30–50	
	Lofepramine	70	140–210	
SSRI	Fluoxetine	10–20	20–40	Nausea, diarrhoea, headache, agitation, sedation
	Citalopram	10–20	20–40	
MAOI	Phenelzine	15	15–45	Confusion, constipation, urinary retention, sedation, hypertensive crisis
RIMA	Moclobemide	150	150–600	Agitation
Atypical	Mianserin	30	30–90	Sedation, aplastic anaemia
	Trazodone	100	300	Sedation, priapism
	Venlafaxine	37.5	75–150	Agitation, insomnia, somnolence, nausea

Efficacy of antidepressants

The overall superiority of antidepressants over placebo has been mentioned earlier. A recent meta-analysis of published studies (Mittman *et al.*, 1997) suggests that there is little difference in efficacy between classes of antidepressant, though mianserin and trazodone may be less effective. There is however a dearth of placebo-controlled trials of the newer drugs in particular, with the exception of citalopram (Nyth *et al.*, 1992), fluoxetine (Tollefson and Holman, 1993) and moclobemide (Amrein *et al.*, 1997). Conclusions from meta-analyses such as this should, however, be tempered by awareness that clinical trial samples are somewhat unrepresentative of clinical populations. Reboxetine is currently not recommended for use in the elderly because of lack of published efficacy data.

Tolerability and safety

The reduced creatinine clearance, hepatic blood flow and plasma protein levels in older patients typically result in higher plasma levels of TCAs than of other agents. The elimination half-life of citalopram and paroxetine (but not fluoxetine or fluvoxamine) is significantly increased in older subjects. However, it should be borne in mind that considerable variability exists in drug absorption, distribution, metabolism and excretion between individuals of different chronological and biological ages.

Both TCAs and MAOIs have a propensity to produce adverse effects likely to be more hazardous in older patients. These include anticholinergic, antihistaminic and antiadrenergic effects. In addition, MAOIs require dietary restriction, and TCAs may have a quinidine-like effect and cause tachycardia and prolongation of the Q–T interval. An increase in falls and consequent fractures is perhaps the most hazardous consequence of these effects (Ray *et al.*, 1992). Nortriptyline (Miller *et al.*, 1991) and lofepramine (Ghose and Sedman, 1987) are less likely to produce these effects and are hence better tolerated.

The SSRIs may cause sedation in the elderly; however, their chief side effects of gastrointestinal disturbance, headache and agitation appear less troublesome to older patients. The Mittman *et al.* (1997) meta-analysis concluded that, in the context of controlled clinical trials, there was little difference in tolerability between the different classes. In naturalistic clinical practice, however, a higher proportion of the elderly may be suitable for treatment with SSRIs than with TCAs (Mullan *et al.*, 1994). 'Real-life' compliance may also be better with SSRIs because of their simpler dosage regimen.

Ancillary medication

This is sometimes necessary for symptoms of depression such as sleep disturbance and anxiety, before antidepressant medication has begun to take effect. The former may be treated with hypnotics such as benzodiazepines, zopiclone or zolpidem, the latter by benzodiazepines or low-dose antipsychotics. Important principles to consider are avoiding polypharmacy as far as possible, and slowly withdrawing the ancillary medication as core depressive symptoms resolve following antidepressant treatment.

Psychotic (delusional) depression usually responds poorly to antidepressants alone, and electroconvulsive therapy (ECT) is usually regarded as the treatment of first choice. Patients may, however, respond well to a combination of an antidepressant and an antipsychotic drug; this combination may be particularly useful in older people unfit for, or unwilling to receive, ECT. The use of antipsychotic medication in older patients is considered later in this chapter.

Refractory depression

Older patients who have failed to respond to treatment, and in whom other factors such as inadequacy of dose, duration of treatment or compliance, or significant social or physical maintaining factors, have been ruled out, may be considered for augmentation with lithium, which is as effective in the elderly as in younger patients (Abou-Saleh and Coppen, 1983). Lithium levels are dependent on renal excretion and, as clearance decreases, lower doses are needed but there is much inter-patient variation. Careful dose titration is advisable, starting at 100–200 mg/day, and the aim is for lower levels than in younger adult patients, usually 0.4–0.6 mmol/l (Wood and Castledon, 1991). Lithium may cause neurotoxic symptoms at relatively low serum concentrations in older patients (Mirchandani and Young, 1993). Patients with cognitive impairment or diffuse neurological disease are particularly vulnerable to lithium neurotoxicity. Lithium also interacts with diuretics, ACE inhibitors and most non-steroidal anti-inflammatory drugs which are often prescribed in the elderly. Coadministration of these agents leads to increased lithium levels and therefore increases the risk of toxicity. Great care should be taken in these patients; a decrease in the dose of lithium may be required. Aspirin does not affect serum lithium concentration.

Other 'refractory depression' drug regimens which may be useful in older people include monoamine oxidase inhibitors and the psychostimulant methylphenidate. These regimes are succinctly reviewed by Flint (1995).

Continuation and maintenance treatment

Most relapses of depressive illness occur within the first year of an episode, and older patients may be at high risk of relapse for up to 2 years (Flint, 1995). Treatment should therefore be continued for at least 2 years, at a dose as close to the initial effective therapeutic one as possible, and for life in patients with a particularly severe index episode, two or more episodes in the previous 2 years, chronic physical illness or significant social stressors (Baldwin, 1997).

There is good evidence for the prophylactic efficacy of the tricyclic antidepressant dothiepin in long-term treatment in older people. The Old Age Depression Interest Group (1993) study reported that the relative rate of risk of relapse over 2 years was two and a half times greater in a placebo group than in patients receiving the TCA dothiepin at 75 mg/day. There is less evidence for the efficacy of the newer agents such as SSRIs though open trial data suggest a similar prophylactic effect. Lithium may also be used prophylactically, though precautions must be taken as noted above.

Mood stabilizers

In older, just as in younger patients, lithium is often used in the prophylaxis of bipolar affective disorder (BPD). As noted earlier, the low therapeutic index and changes in lithium handling in the elderly mandates careful monitoring.

Carbamazepine is also used but there are few studies in the elderly. It is often favoured in rapid-cycling affective disorder, which is defined as more than four mood episodes in 1 year. Conlon (1989) describes successfully using carbamazepine 100 mg bid in a 67-year-old man with a rapid-cycling disorder. The elimination half-life of carbamazepine increases linearly with age, so a dose reduction is needed in the elderly.

Sodium valproate has been shown to be effective in acute and maintenance treatment of BPD and a few studies have looked at its use in the elderly (Eastham et al., 1998). It is well absorbed, largely protein bound and metabolized by the liver. Dosage requirements for patients with affective disorder have not been adequately characterized, but elderly patients may need lower doses than younger patients. Valproate seems well tolerated in the elderly; its main side effects are nausea and sedation.

Lamotrigine is a new anticonvulsant used for resistant partial seizures. It is well absorbed, metabolized in the liver and eliminated by the kidney.

Toxic effects have not been reported at less than 90 times the therapeutic dose. Kotler and Matar (1998) describe its use in an 81-year-old man with a long history of bipolar affective disorder to treat successfully a resistant depressive episode. The drug was given in combination with fluoxetine and lithium and there were no adverse effects.

The use of verapamil as an antimanic drug has been described, but there are no specific data from the elderly. Verapamil is well absorbed orally, is extensively protein bound and metabolized by the liver. The increased adiposity and decreased hepatic metabolism with age lead to a prolonged half-life. Doses should be lower and less frequent in the elderly (Wei, 1989).

Schizophrenia and its treatment in the elderly

Patients aged 65 and over with schizophrenia include the so-called 'graduate' population as well as late onset cases. Although there have been several studies (Pearlson et al., 1989; Howard et al., 1993; Watkin and Katona, 1998) outlining the differences between early and late onset schizophrenia, significant similarities remain allowing for common treatment strategies.

Pearlson et al. (1989) carried out a comparative review of symptoms in patients with schizophrenia with early and late onset of psychosis. They found a similar prevalence of core positive (Schneiderian first rank) symptoms. Late onset patients however presented with significantly less affective flattening and other negative features, as well as less thought disorder. Late onset patients tended to have more delusions and experience hallucinations in many different modalities, compared to the early onset patients. The modalities of sensory delusions were not related to modalities of sensory impairment.

Drug treatment of schizophrenia in elderly patients

Although pharmacotherapy is an important part of treatment of elderly patients with schizophrenia, it must be remembered that drugs are only one part of the treatment plan which should also comprise good medical, nursing and social care.

Conventional antipsychotics (chlorpromazine, thioridazine, haloperidol, etc.) are undoubtedly effective in the treatment of schizophrenia and related psychoses in older people. They carry a considerable side-effect burden, however, and there has been increasing interest in the use of newer 'atypical' antipsychotics in this population. Some recent studies of these newer agents have focused on age-related pharmacokinetic and pharmacodynamic aspects. The effects of ageing on the liver and kidneys generally lengthen the half-life of these primarily lipophilic agents with a high hepatic first pass effect and metabolism, resulting in susceptibility to adverse effects even at recommended therapeutic doses. Added multisystem disease resulting in polypharmacy, nutritional deficiencies and dehydration in an individual with paranoid delusions, all predispose to the possible development of adverse events. Substantially lower doses (Table 21.2) and smaller dose increments are therefore advised in the population aged over 65 to decrease

Table 21.2 Summary of clinical information on antipsychotics in people aged over 65

	Recommended dose	*Clinical features*
Amisulpride	Low doses (50–300 mg) less likely to result in EPSE	Studies suggest that positive and negative symptoms are affected. Additional interest in treatment of dysthymia and depression
Clozapine	Doses of 50 mg may be effective, above 300 mg autonomic side effects are more likely	Beneficial for treatment of tardive dyskinesia and negative symptoms. Incidence of agranulocytosis increased in elderly
Olanzapine	Lower starting doses in elderly with smaller increases	Somnolence. Some anticholinergic effects. 'Patch' preparation being developed
Quetiapine	Generally tolerated well in elderly in doses from 12.5 mg to 200 mg. Clearance is reduced in elderly	Orthostatic hypotension is more common
Risperidone	0.5 mg bd. starting dose with slower titration in increments of 0.5 mg is advised, above 4 mg a day EPSE more likely	Possible cognitive improvement in elderly patients with schizophrenia, compared to haloperidol. Orthostatic hypotension. Parenteral preparation being developed
Sertindole	Once daily dose, lower maintenance dose and slower titration advised	ECG and initial BP monitoring recommended, Q–T prolongation reported. Rhinitis
Sulpiride	Initially 50–100 mg bd	Generally well tolerated but can result in EPSE at relatively low doses
Thioridazine	Usually 30–100 mg daily	Orthostatic hypotension, urinary retention, balance, low EPSE
Ziprasidone	Pharmacokinetics in elderly not fully evaluated	Antidepressant and anxiolytic properties

the likelihood of adverse events and ensure greater compliance. Patients who have been clinically stable while receiving neuroleptic medication, particularly 'graduates' from the adult service who may be continuing on depot preparations, should be reviewed regularly with a view to reduction in dosage of neuroleptics to reduce risk of emerging side effects (particularly tardive dyskinesia, see below). Monitoring of possible psychotic relapse is also important, however. Long-acting injectable or skin-patch preparations of some of the newer antipsychotic drugs such as risperidone and olanzapine (see below) will further increase treatment options and should contribute to improving patient compliance.

Efficacy

The overall efficacy of new atypical antipsychotics in the treatment of schizophrenia is based on double-blind placebo-controlled trials and comparisons with conventional antipsychotics in adult populations. In the elderly the pharmacological studies focus on the effects of ageing on frequency of adverse drug reactions and may include patients with additional diagnoses, such as psychotic symptoms as a result of dementia associated with Alzheimer's and Parkinson's disease. The outcomes of such studies are summarized in Table 21.2.

Adverse drug reactions

While the adverse reactions of conventional antipsychotics are well documented in the elderly, the number of patients treated with atypical antipsychotics has been comparatively low and their side-effect profile continues to be evaluated.

Extrapyramidal side effects (EPSEs)

These occur commonly with older antipsychotic agents (Casey and Keepers, 1988) as a result of non-selective dopaminergic antagonism in nigrostriatal pathways. In an elderly population, EPSEs are not only troublesome in themselves but can also lead to falls; drugs with fewer EPSEs are therefore to be welcomed. In the adult group the reports of EPSE and clozapine are much lower (Lieberman and Safferman, 1992) at 3% compared to conventional neuroleptics. Clozapine has been successfully used in patients with Parkinson's disease (PD) with starting doses of 6.25 mg every other day (Wolters et al., 1990). There are reports of good tolerability of low dose risperidone (starting at 0.25 mg) in patients with PD, but, as in younger patients, good EPSE profile is lost in the elderly treated with higher doses (Marder and Meibach, 1994). Amisulpride has also been shown to produce EPSEs at higher doses. In adult trials the other atypical neuroleptics have similar EPSE rates to placebo.

Tardive dyskinesia (TD)

Several risk factors for the development of TD are recognized. These include length and quantity of exposure to antipsychotics, diagnoses of schizophrenia or of affective disorders, age, organicity and female sex (Woerner et al., 1998). TD-like abnormal movements may occur in the absence of treatment with antipsychotics. A significant proportion of patients prescribed atypical antipsychotics would have also been exposed to older agents, and reports of new cases of TD in patients treated with the newer agents are therefore difficult to evaluate. Data available so far suggest that clozapine is effective in ameliorating TD movements as well as in treating psychotic symptoms in patients with TD (Lieberman et al., 1991).

Cardiovascular

Orthostatic hypotension occurs more commonly in the elderly as a result of several organic factors such as arteriosclerosis and can lead to serious consequences. This group of patients is thus highly susceptible to alpha-adrenergic blockade. While information on the effect of atypical antipsychotics on blood pressure is incomplete, monitoring is advisable with clozapine, risperidone and sertindole. Prolongation of Q–T interval has been noted with sertindole and a pretreatment ECG is advised.

Central nervous system effects

Cognitive decline in patients with schizophrenia has been reported (Berman *et al.*, 1995) and this can be exacerbated further by medication with centrally acting anticholinergic properties. Compared to older antipsychotic agents, there have been reports of beneficial effect on cognitive function in patients with schizophrenia treated with risperidone (Berman *et al.*, 1995) and quetiapine (Stip *et al.*, 1996). Sedation, which may impair cognitive functioning and mobility, can arise as a result of treatment with atypical antipsychotic agents and has been noted with clozapine, olanzapine and quetiapine.

Atypical antipsychotics given in adjusted doses present a more acceptable side-effect profile to the elderly patient with schizophrenia compared to the conventional neuroleptic agents. The more novel of these preparations continue to be evaluated and may have wider psychiatric application.

References

Abou-Saleh, M.T. and Coppen, A. (1983). The prognosis of depression in old age: the case for lithium therapy. *Br. J. Psychiatry*, **143**, 527–528.

Amrein, R., Stabl, M., Henauer, S., *et al.* (1997). Efficacy and tolerability of moclobemide in comparison with placebo, tricyclic antidepressants and selective serotonin reuptake inhibitors in elderly depressed patients: a clinical overview. *Can. J. Psychiatry*, **42**, 1043–1050.

Anon (1988). Need we poison the elderly so often? *Lancet*, **2**, 20–22.

Anstey, K. and Brodaty, H. (1995). Antidepressants and the elderly: double-blind trials 1987–1992. *Int. J. Geriatr. Psychiatry*, **10**, 265–279.

Baldwin, R. (1997). The prognosis of depression in later life. In: *Advances in Old Age Psychiatry* (C. Holmes and R. Howard, eds), Petersfield, Wrightson, pp. 194–224.

Berman, I., Marson, A., Allan, E., *et al.* (1995). Effect of risperidone on cognitive performance in elderly schizophrenic patients: a double blind comparison study with haloperidol. *Psychopharmacol. Bull.*, **31**, 552.

Casey, D.E. and Keepers, G.A. (1988). Neuroleptic side effects: acute extrapyramidal syndromes and tardive dyskinesia. *Psychopharmacol. Series*, **5**, 74–93.

Castleden, C.M. and Pickles, H. (1988). Suspected adverse drug reactions in elderly patients reported to the CSM. *Br. J. Clin. Pharmacol.*, **26**, 347–353.

Cockcroft, D.W. and Gault, M.H. (1976). Prediction of creatinine clearance from serum creatinine. *Nephron*, **16**, 31–41.

Conlon, P. (1989). Rapidly cycling mood disorder in the elderly. *J. Geriartr. Psychiatry Neurol.*, **2**, 109–112.

Copeland, J.R.M., Dewey, M.E., Wood, N., *et al.* (1987). Range of mental illness among the elderly in the community: prevalence in Liverpool using the GMS-AGECAT package. *Br. J. Psychiatry*, **150**, 815–823.

Donoghue, J., Katona, C. and Tylee, A. (1998). The treatment of depression: antidepressant prescribing for elderly patients in primary care. *Pharmaceutical J.*, **260**, 500–502.

Eastham, J.H., Jeste, D.V. and Young, R.C. (1998). Assessment and treatment of bipolar disorder in the elderly. *Drugs and Aging*, **12**, 205–224.

Flint, A.J. (1995). Augmentation strategies in geriatric depression. *Int. J Geriatr. Psychiatry*, **10**, 137–146.

Ford, G.A., Hoffman, B.B. and Blaschke, T.F. (1998). Pharmacodynamics. In: *Drug Therapy In Old Age* (C.F. George, K.W. Woodhouse, M.J. Denham, *et al.*, eds), Chichester, John Wiley & Sons Ltd, pp. 59–72.

Ghose, K. and Sedman, E. (1987). A double-blind comparison of the pharmacodynamic effects of single doses of lofepramine, amitriptyline and placebo in elderly subjects. *Eur. J. Clin. Pharmacol.*, **33**, 505–509.

Gillies, H.C., Rogers, H.J., Spector, R.G., *et al.* (1986). Drugs in pregnancy and at the extremes of age. In: *A Textbook Of Clinical Pharmacology*, London, Edward Arnold, pp. 145–167.

Grahame-Smith, D.G. and Aronson, J.K. (1984). Drug therapy in the young, in the elderly and in pregnancy. In: *Oxford Textbook Of Clinical Pharmacology and Drug Therapy*, Oxford, Oxford University Press, pp. 172–187.

Howard, R., Castle, D., Wessely, S., *et al.* (1993). A comparative study of 470 cases of early-onset and late-onset schizophrenia. *Br. J. Psychiatry*, **163**, 325–357.

Katona, C.L.E. and Judge, R. (1996). Antidepressants for elderly people: should selective serotonin reuptake inhibitors be the first-line choice? *Primary Care Psychiatry*, **2**, 123–128.

Kay, D.W.K., Beamish, P. and Roth, M. (1964). Old age mental disorders in Newcastle upon Tyne. Part I: a study of prevalence. *Br. J. Psychiatry*, **110**, 146–158.

Kinirons, M.T., Morike, K., Shay, S., *et al.* (1994). Does selective inhibition of cytochrome P450s occur? *Clin. Res.*, **42**, 215A.

Kinirons, M.T. and Wood, A.J.J. (1998). Pharmacokinetics. In: *Drug Therapy In Old Age* (C.F. George, K.W. Woodhouse, M.J. Denham, *et al.*, eds), Chichester, John Wiley & Sons Ltd, pp. 39–46.

Kotler, M. and Matar, M.A. (1998). Lamotrigine in the treatment of resistant bipolar disorder. *Clin. Neuropharmacol.*, **21**, 65–67.

Lieberman, J.A. and Safferman, A.Z. (1992). Clinical profile of clozapine: adverse reactions and agranulocytosis. *Psychiatric Q.*, **63**, 51–70.

Lieberman, J.A., Saltz, B.L., Johns, C.A., *et al.* (1991). The effects of clozapine on tardive dyskinesia. *Br. J. Psychiatry*, **158**, 503–510.

Manela, M., Katona, C.L.E. and Livingston, G. (1996). How common are the anxiety disorders in old age? *Int. J. Geriatr. Psychiatry*, **11**, 65–70.

Marder, R. and Meibach, R.C. (1994). Risperidone in the treatment of schizophrenia. *Am. J. Psychiatry*, **151**, 825–835.

Miller, M., Pollock, B.G., Rifai, A.H., *et al.* (1991). Longitudinal analysis of nortriptyline side effects in elderly depressed patients. *J. Geriatr. Psychiatry Neurol.*, **4**, 226–230.

Mirchandani, I. and Young, R.C. (1993). Management of mania in the elderly: an update. *Ann. Clin. Psychiatry*, **5**, 67–77.

Mittman, N., Hermann, N., Einarson, T.R., *et al.* (1997). The efficacy, safety and tolerability of antidepressants in late-life depression: a meta-analysis. *J. Affect. Dis.*, **46**, 191–217.

Morrow, D., Leirer, V. and Sheikh, J. (1988). Adherence and medication instructions: review and recommendations. *J. Am. Geriatr. Soc.*, **36**, 1147–1160.

Mullan, M., D'Ath, P., Katona, P., *et al.* (1994). Screening, detection and management of depression in elderly primary care attenders. 2. Detection and fitness for treatment: a case record study. *Fam. Pract.*, **11**, 267–270.

Nyth, A.L., Gottfries, C.G., Lyby, K., *et al.* (1992). A controlled multicentre clinical study of citalopram and placebo in elderly depressed patients with and without concomitant dementia. *Acta Psychiatrica Scand.*, **86**, 138–145.

Old Age Depression Interest Group (1993). How long should the elderly take antidepressants? A double-blind placebo-controlled study of continuation/prophylaxis therapy with dothiepin. *Br. J. Psychiatry*, **162**, 175–182.

Pearlson, G.D., Kreger, L., Rabins, P.V., *et al.* (1989). A chart review study of late-onset and early-onset schizophrenia. *Am. J. Psychiatry*, **146**, 1568–1574.

Pickard, L. (1983). Increased ratio of free fatty acids to albumin during normal ageing and in patients with cardiovascular disease. *Atherosclerosis*, **46**, 21–28.

Ray, W.A., Fought, R.L. and Decker, M.D. (1992). Psychoactive drugs and the risk of injurious motor vehicle crashes in elderly drivers. *Am. J. Epidemiol.*, **136**, 873–883.

Rockwell, E., Lam, R.W. and Zisook, S. (1988). Antidepressant drug studies in the elderly. *Psychiatr. Clin. N. Am.*, **11**, 215–233.

Stip, E., Lusser, I., Babai, M., *et al.* (1996). Seroquel and cognitive improvement in patients with schizophrenia. *Biol. Psychiatry*, **40**, 434–435.

Tollefson, G.D. and Holman, S.L. (1993). Analysis of the Hamilton Depression Rating Scale factors from a double-blind, placebo-controlled trial of fluoxetine in geriatric major depression. *Int. Clin. Pharmacol.*, **8**, 253–259.

Watkin, M. and Katona, C. (1998). Functional psychiatric illness in old age. In: *Brocklehurst's Textbook of Geriatric Medicine and Gerontology* (R. Tallis, H. Fillit and J.C. Brocklehurst, eds), Edinburgh, Churchill Livingstone, pp. 741–755.

Wei, J.Y. (1989). Use of calcium entry blockers in elderly patients. Special considerations. *Circulation*, **80** (Suppl. IV), 171–177.

Williams, F.M., Wynne, H., Woodhouse, K.W., *et al.* (1989). Plasma aspirin esterase: the influence of old age and frailty. *Age and Ageing*, **18**, 39–42.

Williamson, J. and Chopin, J.M. (1980). Adverse reactions to prescribed drugs in the elderly: a multicentre investigation. *Age and Ageing*, **9**, 73–80.

Woemer, M.G., Alvir, J.M.J., Salts, B.L., *et al.* (1998). Prospective study of tardive dyskinesia in the elderly: rates and risk factors. *Am. J. Psychiatry*, **155**, 1521–1528.

Wolters, E.C., Hurwitz, T.A., Mak, E., *et al.* (1990). Clozapine in the treatment of parkinsonian patients with dopaminomimetic psychosis. *Neurology*, **40**, 832–834.

Wood, P. and Castledon, C.M. (1991). Psychopharmacology in the elderly. In: *Psychiatry in the Elderly* (R. Jacoby and C. Oppenheimer, eds), Oxford, Oxford University Press, pp. 339–372.

Woodhouse, K.W. (1998). Biochemical pharmacology of ageing: In: *Drug Therapy in Old Age* (C.F. George, K.W. Woodhouse, M.J. Denham, *et al.*, eds), Chichester, John Wiley & Sons Ltd., pp. 47–58.

Woodhouse, K.W., Wynne, H., Baille, S., *et al.* (1988). Who are the frail elderly? *Queensland J. Med.*, **68**, 505–506.

World Health Organisation (1970). International drug monitoring – the role of hospital. *Drug Intelligence Clin. Pharmacol.*, **4**, 101.

Wynne, H., Cope, L.H., James, O.F.W., *et al.* (1989). The effect of age and frailty upon acetanilide clearance. *Age and Ageing*, **18**, 415–418.

22

Treatment of substance misuse in schizophrenia

Kim Mueser and Shôn Lewis

Key points

- 25%–40% of people with schizophrenia have a substance misuse problem.
- Comorbid substance misuse is a risk factor for relapse and other adverse outcomes.
- Comprehensive, assertive outreach with a substance misuse engagement model is most successful.
- Effective antipsychotic drug treatment is central.
- Clozapine may have a particular place in some patients.

Introduction

The use of alcohol and street drugs among people with a diagnosis of schizophrenia appears to be widespread and increasing (Cuffel, 1996). Estimates of the prevalence of alcohol and drug misuse in schizophrenia vary, but studies typically report life-time comorbidity rates ranging between 40% and 60%, and recent substance misuse (e.g., past 6 months) in the 25–40% range (Mueser *et al.*, 1995). At issue is whether individuals with a diagnosis of schizophrenia and other psychotic disorders are at increased risk of substance misuse, compared to the general population. Difficulties facing epidemiological research in this area include the geographical and temporal variations in alcohol and street drug use in the general population; the challenge in identifying a representative control group; and the difficulty inherent in obtaining reliable estimates of substance misuse, particularly in a patient population where disclosure of such information may result in withdrawal of certain privileges (Galanter *et al.*, 1988; Drake *et al.*, 1996). Despite these problems, evidence from community surveys indicates that patients with schizophrenia are at substantially increased risk for substance misuse compared to either non-psychiatric patients or persons with less severe psychiatric disorders, such as major depression and anxiety disorders (Regier *et al.*, 1990).

Substance misuse comorbidity in schizophrenia is important for several reasons. First, substance misuse, particularly of stimulant drugs, can trigger a first psychotic episode (Breakey *et al.*, 1974; Mueser *et al.*, 1990). The nosological status of such episodes has long been debated. With schizophrenia, the consensus is that drugs such as amphetamines, by virtue of their functional dopaminergic activity, can trigger a first episode of schizophrenia in individuals who are predisposed and would likely have developed the disorder anyway (Tsuang *et al.*, 1982). Thus, drug misuse can determine the timing of the onset of schizophrenia but not its presence. Secondly, the evidence concerning drug misuse precipitating relapse in individuals with established schizophrenia is clearer. The best evidence for this comes from first episode studies, such as that by Linszen *et al.* (1994). This study followed up a cohort of people with first episode schizophrenia and showed that those with moderate or heavy misuse of cannabis showed a worse 2-year outcome on variables such as relapse rates than those patients with no or mild use, after controlling for other factors. Similar prospective research has documented that alcohol misuse is associated with increased relapses and rehospitalizatons in mixed cohorts of schizophrenic patients (Drake *et al.*, 1989). A revolving door pattern of emergency hospital admissions can result (Shaner *et al.*, 1993).

Models of comorbidity

Various hypotheses have been proposed about the apparently increased risk of people with schizophrenia developing substance misuse disorders (Mueser *et al.*, 1998b). One of the most popular is the self-medication hypothesis, where substance misuse is seen as an understandable strategy adopted on behalf of the patient to reduce the distress associated with psychotic symptoms, or the dysphoric effects of conventional antipsychotic drugs (Kosten and Ziedonis, 1997). This may take the form of use of stimulant drugs to offset subjective experiences of negative symptoms such as anhedonia, or through the use of alcohol or drugs such as opiates to suppress positive symptoms. There is some evidence for this, in that several studies have shown an inverse relationship between substance misuse and total symptoms (Dixon *et al.*, 1991), and between amphetamine or cocaine misuse and negative symptoms (Serper *et al.*, 1995). However, most studies fail to report associations between symptom severity and substance misuse, nor is there evidence that specific symptoms tend to be correlated with a predilection to misuse specific types of substances, as might be predicted by the self-medication hypothesis (Mueser *et al.*, 1998b).

Alternatively to this hypothesis, or in addition, it is plausible that the cognitive deficits which are part of the schizophrenia syndrome impair the person's ability to shift attention away from substance-related environmental cues which seem to be important in mechanisms of craving. Both these formulations allow potentially for specific therapeutic pharmacological intervention. Mesolimbic dopamine transmission is involved both in positive psychotic symptoms and the reinforcement of adaptive, and maladaptive, behaviours.

Another hypothesis accounting for the high rate of substance use disorders in schizophrenia is that the biological vulnerability which characterizes the illness renders patients highly susceptible to the effects of very low quantities of alcohol and drugs (Mueser *et al.*, 1998b). In line with this hypothesis, patients with schizophrenia and substance use problems tend to use lower quantities of substances and are less vulnerable to developing physical dependence on substances than persons with primary substance use disorders (Test *et al.*, 1989; Lehman *et al.*, 1994; Corse *et al.*, 1995). Furthermore, they are less capable of sustaining a pattern of moderate drinking without negative consequences over time (Drake and Wallach, 1993), and they are prone to experiencing exacerbations of symptoms following the administration of low doses of drugs, especially psychostimulants (Lieberman *et al.*, 1987). This hypothesis suggests that the misuse of substances in patients with schizophrenia is largely due to their heightened sensitivity to psychoactive substances, rather than to increased use of substances *per se*.

One final hypothesis concerning the excessive comorbidity of substance misuse in schizophrenia is that antisocial personality is a common factor that increases the risk of both disorders. Antisocial personality disorder, and its precursor conduct disorder, is over-represented in both primary substance use disorders (Regier *et al.*, 1990; Kessler *et al.*, 1997) and schizophrenia (Asarnow, 1988). Furthermore, patients with schizophrenia with a history of conduct disorder, adult antisocial personality disorder, or both are at increased risk of comorbid substance misuse (Mueser *et al.*, 1999). Finally, among patients with schizophrenia and substance misuse, antisocial personality disorder is related to a more severe history of substance misuse, including earlier age of onset of substance misuse, more treatment episodes, and more severe consequences of substance use (Mueser *et al.*, 1997). Thus, antisocial personality disorder may account for some of the increased comorbidity of substance misuse in schizophrenia. Other factors may account for comorbidity in some cases of substance misuse in schizophrenia, such as family history of substance misuse, but probably do not explain increased comorbidity (Mueser *et al.*, 1998b). Of course, no single hypothesis can explain all comorbidity of substance misuse in schizophrenia, and multiple models may apply for a given individual.

Assessment of comorbid substance misuse

Reliable assessment of recent substance misuse is important in both clinical practice and research. In clinical practice, both self-report measures, urine analysis, and clinician ratings have been the usual methods of assessment. Recently, self-report screening instruments for substance misuse have been developed and validated specifically for the psychiatric population. For example, the Dartmouth Assessment of Lifestyle Inventory (DALI; Rosenberg *et al.*, 1998) was developed for psychiatric patients with severe mental illness and has been found to be 85–90% accurate in detecting substance misuse in this population, significantly more accurate than other instruments designed for detecting substance misuse in the general population.

Explicit regular monitoring by urinalysis and/or breathalyser tests is an important part of many treatment programmes. More recently, analysis of hair has been proposed as a method that is both more informative and more acceptable. Street drugs and therapeutic drugs become bound within growing hair in a way that is resistant to washing and cosmetic hair preparations (McPhillips *et al.*, 1998). In practice, with the patient's consent, a lock of hair is cut from the head, arm pit, or pubic region. The hair sample can then be kept for a relatively long period of time if necessary before analysis takes place. The preferred analysis process consists of gas chromatography with mass spectrometry (GCMS). Unlike urine analysis, not only is this process potentially quantitative, such that the quantities of individual drugs taken can be specified, but it also allows for the dating of drug use over previous weeks and months, depending on the length of the hair sample obtained. Furthermore all drugs of misuse (except alcohol) can be tested for individually, even when different drugs come from the same chemical class, as in the case of dexamphetamine and ecstasy. Both false positives and false negatives are less with hair analysis than with urine analysis. Preliminary studies using hair analysis as a gold standard to validate self-report have given important pointers in dual diagnosis patients. McPhillips *et al.* (1997) showed in an epidemiologically defined sample of schizophrenic patients that both self-reported and hair analysis results confirmed widespread comorbid substance misuse. Importantly, wide divergence was found between self-report and hair analysis for particular drugs. Although the use of cannabis was widely volunteered by patients, the use of drugs such as opiates proved to be common on hair analysis although usually denied on self-report.

A further important aspect of hair analysis is its acceptability. Although, at first glance the procedure might seem intrusive, in fact it seems to be at least as acceptable as urine analysis in patients with schizophrenia. Haddock *et al.* (in press) used hair analysis in a randomized controlled trial of a specific psychological intervention incorporating motivational interviewing in a sample of 36 young patients with clinical problems arising out of comorbid substance misuse in schizophrenia. Hair analysis, used as a repeated measure in this study, proved to be acceptable to over 95% of participants.

Hair analysis and urine analysis both provide valuable, quantitative estimates of drug use, although they are less useful in detecting the most commonly used substance, alcohol. In addition, while detection of substance use is vital to effective treatment of substance misuse, laboratory tests are not informative as to the consequences of substance use. Information on the consequences of substance use is necessary in order to determine whether the use truly constitutes misuse in the form of substance abuse (i.e. negative social, health, or psychological consequences) or substance dependence (i.e. tolerance, physical withdrawal symptoms indicating physical dependence, or excessive involvement in substance use and inability to cut down despite attempts indicating psychological dependence). Self-reports using structured interviews can be helpful in evaluating the consequences of substance use, but such reports are prone to under-detection due to patient minimization and denial (Drake *et al.*, 1996).

A valuable method for obtaining reliable diagnostic information concerning the consequences of substance use is to obtain reports from trained clinicians (Carey *et al.*, 1996). Clinicians need to be trained to recognize the most common consequences of substance misuse in patients with schizophrenia, including symptom exacerbations, family conflict, money problems, aggression, depression and suicidality, and legal problems. Once trained, clinicians are ideally suited to collect information concerning patients' substance use and its consequences from a variety of sources, including patients themselves, collaterals, laboratory measure, medical records, their own observation, and the observations of other treatment providers. This information can be combined to produce reliable and valid ratings of substance misuse that are useful in both determining who needs treatment and monitoring the effects of intervention.

For example, the Clinician Rating Scales for Alcohol and Drugs (Mueser et al., 1995b) yields scores on two five-point scales corresponding to substance use over the past 6 months: 1 = no substance use; 2 = substance use without impairment; 3 = substance abuse (or misuse) characterized by a pattern of negative consequences resulting from substance use; 4 = substance dependence, characterized by both negative consequences and either physical or psychological dependence; and 5 = severe dependence, including both negative consequences, physical or psychological dependence, and frequent (or extended) institutionalization.

Service frameworks and psychological interventions

Intervention for patients with comorbid substance misuse (or dually diagnosed patients) needs to comprise several components. Interventions must be coordinated and preferably integrated as part of a targeted service that treats both disorders simultaneously in a seamless fashion. This has often been difficult in the USA and the UK because of the historical separation of services for persons with mental illness and those with substance misuse problems. In order to be successful, any potentially effective drug treatment needs to be set within a service framework which includes elements of assertive outreach and follow-up, as well as specific social support mechanisms and psychological interventions.

Drake et al. (1993) and Mueser et al. (1998a) have articulated a number of features of effective integrated dual diagnosis treatment programmes, including assertiveness, comprehensiveness, stage-wise treatment, shared decision-making, and long-term perspective. These overarching programme components guide the development of specific dual diagnosis treatment modalities, including case management and individual treatment, as well as group and family interventions. A wide range of therapeutic interventions are provided within these different modalities, such as education, cognitive-behavioural counselling, social skills training, problem solving with social network members, and motivational strategies designed to help clients understand how substance misuse has affected their lives.

Assertiveness, which refers to the process of outreach and work with patients in their natural living environments as opposed to strictly clinic or hospital-based work, is needed to engage dually diagnosed patients who otherwise fall between the cracks of the mental health and substance misuse service systems, and is also helpful in monitoring the effects of dual diagnosis treatment. Without assertiveness, many patients fail to receive the services needed to help them overcome their substance misuse.

Comprehensiveness refers to the recognition that effective dual diagnosis programmes must target a broad range of different outcomes in addition to substance misuse if they are to be successful in reducing problems related to substance use. Dually diagnosed patients have multiple needs in the areas of social skill deficits, family strife, unsafe and unstable living environments, unemployment, and distress from symptoms. Problems in any and all of these areas may compound substance misuse and therefore need to be addressed if progress is to be made.

Stage-wise treatment is based on the recognition that patients with a dual disorder progress through a series of stages in response to treatment, and that recognition of the different stages can help clinicians identify interventions that are matched to patients' motivational level at each stage. Osher and Kofoed (1989) identified four stages, including *engagement* (in which the goal is to establish a working relationship with the patient), *persuasion* (in which the goal is to convince the patient that substance use is disadvantageous and he or she should attempt to cut down), *active treatment* (in which the goal is to assist the patient in reducing substance use), and *relapse prevention* (in which the goal is to maintain awareness that relapse could happen and to expand recovery to other areas of functioning). By matching interventions to patients' current motivational levels, treatment outcomes can be optimized.

Shared decision-making is based on the importance of working collaboratively with patients and their families in order to ensure the involvement of all stakeholders, and to maximize the chances that treatment plans will be followed through. Finally, a *long-term perspective* is needed in the treatment of dually diagnosed patients. For at least some individuals, both substance misuse and severe mental illness are chronic disorders, characterized by multiple relapses and slow progress. At the same time, research suggests that treatment of dual disorders is frequently effective over the long-run. For this reason, mental health and substance misuse services need to be configured so that long-term and individualized treatment is available.

Research on psychological interventions

Over the past several years 10 studies have been completed examining the effects of comprehensive and integrated outpatient programmes for dually diagnosed patients assessed over 1–3 years (Drake *et al.*, 1998b). Most of these studies have included mixed samples of psychiatric patients and have not employed experimental research designs. Nevertheless, the findings have been encouraging by demonstrating high rates of retention of dually diagnosed patients in more integrated treatments, and higher rates of substance misuse remission as compared to traditional services.

For example, one experimental study (Godley *et al.*, 1994) and one quasi-experimental study (Drake *et al.*, 1997) have compared integrated and traditional dual diagnosis treatment for dually diagnosed patients, with both studies reporting higher rates of substance misuse remission in the integrated treatment groups. In a quasi-experimental study, Jerrell and Ridgley (1995) compared the effects of behavioural skills training, case management and 12-step programmes for dually diagnosed patients. The first two groups represented more integrated treatments since the same clinicians assumed responsibility for treating both disorders. Although outcomes varied depending on specific domain, in general the behavioural skills training group fared the best, including substance misuse outcomes, and the 12-step group did the worst over the 2-year follow-up. In a 3-year experimental study conducted at seven different community mental health centres, Drake *et al.* (1998a) compared the effects of two integrated treatment programmes for dually diagnosed patients (77% schizophrenia), an assertive community treatment model (ACT) and a standard case management model. Overall, the outcomes for both groups were excellent, with the more intensive ACT group having better outcomes for alcohol misuse, but not drug misuse. These studies provide modest support that the integration of mental health and substance misuse services improves the outcomes of dually diagnosed patients with schizophrenia.

Drug treatments for primary substance misuse

Specific serotonin reuptake inhibitors such as citalopram have been shown to reduce craving in alcohol and drug dependence. There is no pharmacological reason not to use these in schizophrenic patients, but formal evaluations have not been published. Cocaine is known to exert its powerful reinforcing effects at least partly through the dopaminergic system, by inhibiting presynaptic reuptake of dopamine. Desipramine, a tricyclic which blocks presynaptic catecholamine reuptake, has been shown in one randomized controlled trial of 80 patients with cocaine misuse and schizophrenia, in combination with standard antipsychotic drug treatment, to reduce rates of misuse at 12 weeks (Wilkins, 1997).

No data exist for the use in schizophrenia of acamprosate, a drug with a GABA-like chemical structure which probably blocks glutamatergic transmission and has been shown to reduce craving and relapse in abstinent alcohol-dependent subjects. Naltrexone also reduces relapse rates during abstinence from alcohol. One older treatment, disulfiram, was used successfully in one small trial of patients with schizophrenia and alcohol misuse (Kofoed *et al.*, 1987), although low doses are recommended because of interactions with antipsychotic drugs.

Lofexidine is an alpha$_2$ adrenergic agonist like clonidine which has been shown to reduce withdrawal symptoms from opiates. It has not been evaluated in schizophrenia.

Antipsychotic drug treatment

The efficacy of conventional and new atypical antipsychotic drugs in schizophrenic patients with comorbid substance misuse is poorly understood. The main reason for this is the widespread identification of substance use as a principal exclusion criterion in phase three drug efficacy studies. Thus, the protocol for randomized controlled trials of new antipsychotic agents in clinical populations specifically excludes patients who are known to be misusing drugs. In recent years, this practice has become an increasing anomaly in view of the steady rise of substance use as a comorbid problem in people with schizophrenia. Nonetheless, the formal evidence in the form of randomized controlled trials concerning the effectiveness of these drugs in improving outcomes in patients with dual diagnosis, is sparse.

The self-medication hypothesis would predict that substance misuse will be less likely if primary positive and negative symptoms are well-controlled, with a minimum of adverse effects. The hypothesis that the cognitive deficits found in schizophrenia predispose to substance misuse by impairing ability to resist environmental cues would predict that antipsychotic drug treatment will help if it reverses these deficits. Optimal symptom treatment with an effective antipsychotic drug would therefore seem to be an appropriate goal. The use of depot antipsychotic drugs is anecdotally successful in the subpopulation of substance misusers whose lifestyle is chaotic. Their use in the schizophrenia population generally is considerably higher in the UK than in the USA. The new atypical antipsychotic drugs such as risperidone and olanzapine, by virtue of their reduced neurological side effects and apparent action on negative symptoms presumably through $5\text{-}HT_2$ blockade in ascending dopaminergic systems, are likely to be useful (Buckley, 1998).

The next question is whether some or all antipsychotic drugs have a direct effect on the substance misuse, rather than just controlling psychotic symptoms. Berger et al. (1996) showed that haloperidol reduced cue-elicited craving in (non-schizophrenic) cocaine-dependent subjects. However, the effect of chronic haloperidol administration may be paradoxically to increase the reinforcing properties of dopamine agonist stimulants such as cocaine, as suggested by animal studies (Kosten, 1997), presumably as a result of eventual upregulation of post-synaptic dopamine receptors. It may be that long-term treatment with conventional antipsychotic drugs is itself a risk factor for the development and maintenance of stimulant drug misuse (Buckley, 1998).

Haloperidol primarily antagonizes dopamine D_2 activity. There is strong evidence that the reinforcing effects of cocaine and other stimulant drugs of misuse are mediated particularly through dopamine D_1 systems (Kosten, 1997). Clozapine binds to postsynaptic D_1 receptors with an affinity equal or greater than for D_2 receptors and anecdotal evidence suggests it may be particularly useful in substance-misusing schizophrenic patients. Animal studies have produced some evidence that it does not lead to the paradoxical supersensitivity to cocaine over the long-term shown by haloperidol (Kosten, 1997). Buckley et al. (1994) showed that substance-misusing patients improved in symptoms and social functioning on clozapine treatment over 6 months to the same degree as non-misusing patients. Furthermore, Drake et al. (in press) found in a naturalistic study that clozapine was associated with significant reductions in alcohol misuse, but not drug misuse in schizophrenic patients, and that these remissions of alcohol misuse could not be explained by either improvements in positive or negative symptoms. Clozapine has been shown to improve engagement in a range of psychosocial interventions in schizophrenia (Rosenheck et al., 1998) and this effect might be particularly valuable in patients with comorbid substance misuse, where such non-drug interventions are a crucial part of a successful treatment programme (Table 22.1).

Table 22.1 Issues in substance misuse and approaches to management in schizophrenia

Issues	Approaches
Assessment of substance use is important	Use a combination of objective measures such as urine screening and validated rating scales
Service interventions need to be integrated	Intervention programmes need to involve both substance misuse and psychiatric services. Comprehensive, assertive outreach models are best
Engagement is often difficult	Stage-wise approaches are most likely to succeed
Patients may abuse substances to minimize negative symptoms or adverse drug effects	Effective drug therapy with low rates of adverse effects is important

References

Asarnow, J.R. (1988). Children at risk for schizophrenia: converging lines of evidence. *Schizophrenia Bull.*, **14**, 613–631.

Berger, S.P., Hall, S., Mickhalian, J., *et al.* (1996). Haloperidol antagonism of cue-elicited cocaine craving. *Lancet*, **347**, 504–8.

Breakey, W.R., Goodell, H., Lorenz, P.C., *et al.* (1974). Hallucinogenic drugs as precipitants of schizophrenia. *Psychol. Med.*, **4**, 255–261.

Buckley, P., Thompson, P., Way, L. and Meltzer, H.Y. (1994). Substance abuse among patients with treatment-resistant schizophrenia: Characteristics and implications for clozapine therapy. *Am. J. Psychiatry*, **151**, 385–389.

Buckley, P.F. (1998). Substance abuse and schizophrenia – a review. *J. Clin. Psychiatry*, **59**, 26–30.

Carey, K.B., Cocco, K.M. and Simons, J.S. (1996). Concurrent validity of substance abuse ratings by outpatient clinicians. *Psychiatric Serv.*, **47**, 842–847.

Corse, S.J., Hirschinger, N.B. and Zanis, D. (1995). The use of the Addiction Severity Index with people with severe mental illness. *Psychiatric Rehab. J.*, **19**, 9–18.

Cuffel, B.J. (1996). Comorbid substance use disorder: prevalence, patterns of use, and course. In: *Dual Diagnosis of Major Mental Illness and Substance Abuse Disorder II: Recent Research and Clinical Implications. New Directions for Mental Health Services* (R.E. Drake and K.T. Mueser, eds), **70**, San Francisco, Jossey-Bass, pp. 65–77.

Dixon, L., Haas, G., Weiden, P.J.., *et al.* (1991). Drug abuse in schizophrenic patients: clinical correlates and reasons for use. *Am. J. Psychiatry*, **148**, 224–230.

Drake, R.E., Bartels, S.B., Teague, G.B., *et al.* (1993). Treatment of substance abuse in severely mentally ill patients. *J. Nerv. Ment. Dis.*, **181**, 606–611.

Drake, R.E., McHugo, G.J., Clark, R.E., *et al.* (1998a). Assertive community treatment for patients with co-occurring severe mental illness and substance use disorder: a clinical trial. *Am. J. Orthopsychiatry*, **68**, 201–215.

Drake, R.E., Mercer-McFadden, C., Mueser, K.T., *et al.* (1998b). A review of integrated mental health and substance abuse treatment for patients with dual disorders. *Schizophrenia Bull.*, **24**, 589–608.

Drake, R.E., Osher, F.C. and Wallach, M.A. (1989). Alcohol use and abuse in schizophrenia: a prospective community study. *J. Nerv. Ment. Dis.*, **177**, 408–414.

Drake, R.E., Rosenberg, S.D. and Mueser, K.T. (1996). Assessment of substance use disorder in persons with severe mental illness. In: *Dual Diagnosis of Major Mental Illness and*

Substance Abuse Disorder II: Recent Research and Clinical Implications. New Directions in Mental Health Services (R.E. Drake and K.T. Mueser, eds), **70**, San Francisco, Jossey-Bass, pp. 3–17.

Drake, R.E. and Wallach, M.A. (1993). Moderate drinking among people with severe mental illness. *Hosp. Comm. Psychiatry*, **44**, 780–782.

Drake, R.E., Xie, H., McHugo, G.J., *et al.* (in press). The effects of clozapine on alcohol and drug abuse among schizophrenic patients. *Schizophrenia Bull.*

Drake, R.E., Yovetich, N.A., Bebout, R.R., *et al.* (1997). Integrated treatment for dually diagnosed homeless adults. *J. Nerv. Ment. Dis.*, **185**, 298–305.

Galanter, M., Castaneda, R. and Ferman, J. (1988). Substance abuse among general pscychiatric patients: place of presentation, diagnosis and treatment. *Am. J. Drug Alcohol Abuse*, **142**, 211–235.

Godley, S.H., Hoewing-Roberon, R., Godley, M.D. (1994). *Final MISA report.* Bloomington, Lighthouse Institute.

Haddock, G., Barrowclough, C., Tarrier, N., *et al.* (in press). Hair analysis: acceptability in a clinical trial in dual diagnosis patients. *Br. J. Psychiatry.*

Jerrell, J. and Ridgely, M.S. (1995). Comparative effectiveness of three approaches to serving people with severe mental illness and substance abuse disorders. *J. Nerv. Ment.Dis.*, **183**, 566–576.

Kessler, R.C., Crum, R.M., Warner, L.A., *et al.* (1997). Lifetime co-occurrence of DSM-III-R alcohol abuse and dependence with other psychiatric disorders in the National Comorbidity Survey. *Arch. Gen. Psychiatry*, **54**, 313–321.

Kofoed, L., Tolson, R., Atkinson, R., *et al.* (1987). Treatment compliance of older alcoholics: An elder-specific approach is superior to "mainstreaming". *J. Studies Alcohol*, **48** (1), 47–51.

Kosten, T.A. (1997). Enhanced neurobehavioural effects of cocaine with chronic neuroleptic exposure in rats. *Schizophrenia Bull.*, **23**, 203–213.

Kosten, T.R. and Ziedonis, D.M. (1997). Substance abuse and schizophrenia: editors' introduction. *Schizophrenia Bull.*, **23**, 181–186.

Lehman, A.F., Myers, C.P., Dixon, L.B., *et al.* (1994). Defining subgroups of dual diagnosis patients for service planning. *Hosp. Comm. Psychiatry*, **45**, 556–561.

Lieberman, J.A., Kane, J.M., Alvir, J. (1987). Provocative tests with psychostimulant drugs in schizophrenia. *Psychopharmacology*, **91**, 415–433.

Linszen, D.H., Dingemans, P.M. and Lenior, M.E. (1994). Cannabis abuse and the course of recent onset schizophrenic disorders. *Arch. Gen. Psychiatry*, **51**, 237–279.

McPhillips, M.A., Kelly, F.J., Barnes, T.R.E., *et al.* (1997). Comorbid substance abuse among people with schizophrenia in the community: a study comparing self-report with analysis of hair and urine. *Schizophrenia Res.*, **25**, 141–148.

McPhillips, M., Strang, J., and Barnes, T.R.E. (1998). Hair analysis: a new laboratory ability to test for substance use. *Br. J. Psychiatry*, **173**, 287–290.

Mueser, K.T., Bennett, M. and Kushner, M.G. (1995). Epidemiology of substance abuse among persons with chronic mental disorders. In: *Double Jeopardy: Chronic Mental Illness and Substance Abuse* (A.F. Lehman and L. Dixon, eds), New York, Harwood Academic Publishers, pp. 9–25.

Mueser, K.T., Drake, R.E., Ackerson, T.H., *et al.* (1997). Antisocial personality disorder, conduct disorder, and substance abuse in schizophrenia. *J. Abnormal Psychol.*, **106**, 473–477.

Mueser, K.T., Drake, R.E., Clark, R.E., *et al.* (1995b). *Toolkit for Evaluating Substance Abuse in Persons with Severe Mental Illness.* Cambridge, MA: Evaluation Center at HSRI.

Mueser, K.T., Drake, R.E. and Noordsy, D.L. (1998a). Integrated mental health and substance abuse treatment for severe psychiatry disorders. *Practical Psychiatry Behav. Hlth.*, **4**, 129–139.

Mueser, K.T., Drake, R.E. and Wallach, M.A. (1998b). Dual diagnosis: a review of etiological theories. *Addictive Behaviors*, **23**, 717–734.

Mueser, K.T., Rosenberg, S.D., Drake, R.E., *et al.* (1999). Conduct disorder, antisocial personality disorder, substance use disorders in schizophrenia and major affective disorders. *J. Studies Alcohol*, **60**, 278–284.

Mueser, K.T., Yarnold, P.R., Levinson, D.F., *et al.* (1990). Prevalence of substance abuse in schizophrenia: demographic and clinical correlates. *Schizophrenia Bull.*, **16**, 31–56.

Osher, F.C. and Kofoed, L.L. (1989). Treatment of patients with psychiatric and psychoactive substance abuse disorders. *Hosp. Comm. Psychiatry*, **40**, 1025–1030.

Regier, D.A., Farmer, M.E., Rae, D.S., *et al.* (1990). Comorbidity of mental disorders with alcohol and other drug abuse: results from the Epidemiologic Catchment Area (ECA) study. *J. Am. Med. Assoc.*, **264**, 2511–2518.

Rosenheck, R., Tekell, J., Peters, J., *et al.* (1998). Does participation in psychosocial treatment augment the benefit of clozapine? *Arch. Gen. Psychiatry*, **55**, 618–625.

Rosenberg, S.D., Drake, R.E., Wolford, G.L., *et al.* (1998). The Dartmouth Assessment of Lifestyle Instrument (DALI): a substance use disorder screen for people with severe mental illness. *Am. J. Psychiatry*, **155**, 232–238.

Serper, M.R., Alpert, M., Richardson, N.A., *et al.* (1995). Clinical effects of recent cocaine use on patients with acute schizophrenia. *Am. J. Psychiatry*, **152**, 1464–1469.

Shaner, A., Khalsa, M.E., Roberts, L., *et al.* (1993). Unrecognized cocaine use among schizophrenia patients. *Am. J. Psychiatry*, **150**, 758–762.

Test, M.A., Wallisch, L.S., Allness, D.J., *et al.* (1989). Substance use in young adults with schizophrenic disorders. *Schizophrenia Bull.*, **15**, 465–476.

Tsuang, M.T., Simpson, J.C. and Kronfol, Z. (1982). Subtypes of drug abuse with psychosis. *Arch. Gen. Psychiatry*, **39**, 141–147.

Wilkins, J.N. (1997). Pharmacotherapy of schizophrenia patients with comorbid substance abuse. *Schizophrenia Bull.*, **23**, 215–228.

23

Treating violence in the context of psychosis

Pamela Taylor and Peter Buckley

Key points

- There is a small but significant association between violence and schizophrenia.
- There is considerable evidence for a relationship between symptoms of psychosis and violence among those with such illness.
- Comorbidity with substance misuse has been associated with multiplication of risk in the community.
- Clozapine may reduce both risk of repetition of violence and return to substance abuse among people with schizophrenia or similar psychotic illness.

The case for treatment

Psychiatrists are not agents of social control, so the concept of *treating* violence may, at first sight, seem wrong. Aggression – a rather broader term which tends to be applied to attacking behaviours of any kind, not necessarily resulting in physical injury – is very common in most human societies. The terms anger and hostility, which have different meanings again, are generally reserved for a relatively acute emotion and chronic state respectively; in the latter negative evaluations such as resentment, mistrust or hate of others predominate. There is mixed evidence as to the extent to which these correlate with the infliction of physical harm. Physical violence is the principal focus of attention in this chapter. It is fairly common in society as a whole – whether sanctioned, as in some sports or in declared war, or largely unsanctioned, as reported, for example by 2% of an interviewed community population (Swanson *et al.*, 1990) in the USA.

Although most violence in society is inflicted by people who have no detectable mental disorder, there is a small but significant statistical association between psychotic illnesses and violence. There is a widespread sense that this violence ought to be amenable to treatment. Its risk, however, is multiplied if such illnesses are accompanied by abuse of alcohol or other drugs (Swanson *et al.*, 1990). Such complication is probably an increasing problem (Mullen *et al.*, 1999). So, to what extent is violence in this context a direct result of features of the illness? Is it, rather, indirectly linked through the social decline or stresses that the more serious variants of such illnesses tend to create, or possibly increased proneness to substance misuse (Steadman *et al.*, 1998). In practice, there is evidence that occasional, serious violence may be mediated by a different route from more trivial but more repetitive violence, and that symptoms may take on differing import according to social context. Whichever way, how much can treatment really help?

Evidence that psychosis may increase the risk of violence

There is as yet no perfect epidemiological study which takes into account all forms of verified violence and mental disorder within a defined geographical area during any stated period of time, and tests for associations. The best evidence comes from three main sources – self-report by community residents of three USA cities (Swanson et al., 1990), case register work from Victoria, Australia (Wallace et al., 1998), and national homicide statistics (Taylor and Gunn, 1999).

The USA based work from the Epidemiologic Catchment Area Survey (Swanson et al., 1990) by definition excluded anyone resident in an institution at the time of the study and, therefore, it is likely, sicker and/or more violent people. Otherwise the sample was probably representative of these populations. In excess of 10 000 people were interviewed; 368 had been violent. Of the latter, 55.5% met criteria for a psychiatric disorder. Substance abuse formed by far the most prevalent cluster of diagnoses, and tended to magnify any risk posed by any other disorder. Schizophrenia alone increased the rate of self-reported violence for the year by fourfold over that among respondents without mental disorder. Tiihonen et al. (1997) emphasized the comorbidity from their findings.

The Australian work (Wallace et al., 1998) was a case linkage study between verified, if incomplete, estimates of antisocial behaviour in the form of official criminal records in the State of Victoria for 1993–5 and the Victorian Psychiatric Case Register which, given the system of health funding there, necessarily identified all contacts with psychiatric services for the State (not just admissions). A conviction for interpersonal violence was recorded for 0.5% of men and 0.05% of women with a diagnosis of schizophrenia, 2.5% of men and 0.4% of women with a personality disorder and 1.1% of men and 0.4% of women with a primary substance misuse disorder. Subsequent work (Mullen et al., 1999) has also incorporated controls from the register of voters matched for sex, age and district of residence. The rate of violent offending was five times higher among those with schizophrenia than the controls. There was no difference in violence by people with psychosis between two time periods – 1975, before the widespread introduction of community care in Victoria, and 1985, after it.

Homicide is an offence for which there is both a high reporting and clear up rate, and therefore for this subcategory of violence a near complete sample is available for several countries. The proportionate contribution of people with a mental disorder depends on national rates, being relatively low in countries of high homicide rates and relatively high where overall figures are low. In England and Wales and areas with similar overall rates, including other European countries, Contra Costa County in California, and Victoria in Australia, the representation of people with schizophrenia has been shown to be of the order of 10 times that in the general population. Nevertheless, this translates into low risk figures – of the order of nine in 10 000 men or one in 10 000 women with schizophrenia according to the

Victorian data (Wallace *et al.*, 1998). Figures for affective psychosis are generally recorded as much lower. In England and Wales, annual numbers of people with psychosis who have killed have remained more-or-less constant over time (1957–1995), but despite publicity around selected cases, which tends to alarm clinicians and the wider public alike, the proportionate contribution of people with a mental disorder to national homicide statistics has actually fallen as homicide rates have risen (Taylor and Gunn, 1999).

Evidence that the psychosis is relevant to violence

Lindqvist and Allebeck (1990), Hodgins (1992) and Wessely *et al.* (1994) each made some contribution to estimates of the frequency with which people with a psychosis become violent, but, in many ways, the principal interest of their work is in the illustration of differences in the violence career patterns of the subjects. Although each was wholly dependent on official criminal records, because each was a longitudinal study it is thus possible to begin to see the way in which psychosis may relate to violence. Taylor and Hodgins (1994) reviewed this evidence, from two Swedish cohorts and a south London (UK) psychiatric contact case register respectively. In effect, it confirmed earlier data (Walker and McCabe, 1973; Häfner and Böker, 1973) that violent offending, but probably not offending more generally, tended to occur late among men with psychosis compared with those without. A twin study (Coid *et al.*, 1993, as extended in Taylor and Hodgins, 1994), confirmed that violent offending specifically almost always post-dated the onset of a psychotic illness. In a study of pretrial prisoners (Taylor, 1993), among whom it was possible to explore histories of significant violence that had not necessarily led to a criminal conviction as well as that which had, nearly 90% had first acted violently only after the onset of their illness.

Management or treatment?

Psychosis, particularly when chronic, has a devastating effect on the lives of the people concerned; perhaps management in terms of ensuring care, reassurance and decent living conditions for the sufferers would be sufficient to ensure safety? These issues are important, but features of the illness seem to have a direct role in relation to serious violence as opposed to other sorts of antisocial behaviour for many, if not most, patients. Few studies have worked with symptoms of psychosis in relation to a particular event. Link and Stueve (1994) examined three acts – hitting, fighting and weapon use – and compared their occurrence over a 5-year period with report of symptoms using the Psychiatric Epidemiology Research Interview (PERI) applied to the last year of the five in about half the 521 respondents and to one month in the other half. They found that a cluster of symptoms – a sense of mind being dominated by external forces, thought insertion and persecutory beliefs – which they called threat/control-override symptoms correlated strongly with having been violent. These features accounted for the differences between patients and never-treated community controls. They were better predictors than other psychotic symptoms, and than popularly cited variables such as male sex, youth and ethnic minority status. Swanson *et al.* (1996) applied this symptom cluster to test the data from the Epidemiologic Catchment Area survey, and Link *et al.* (1998) in Israel with similar effect.

In the Brixton pretrial prisoner study (Taylor, 1985), extensive data were available from over 85% of subjects about mental state and an index offence just 3–6 weeks prior to interview; more time had elapsed between offending and interview for the remainder. In about half of cases, and nearly all of those where serious violence had been the issue, some independent data contemporaneous to the events were available from victims, other witnesses or the police. Over 90% of the 121 psychotic men had been symptomatic at the time of their offence and entry into custody. Although it would thus be hard to dismiss the illness as irrelevant, a direct relationship between symptoms and offending was established in only about 40% of these men. There was, however, a significant relationship between reported delusional drive and more serious violence. Delusions were the only symptoms to show a significant relationship, and, not unlike the Link and Stueve pattern, passivity delusions and the related religious and paranormal delusions were the most important in these terms. Their likely special importance in relation to serious violence was subsequently underscored in a study of high security hospital patients (Taylor *et al.*, 1998). Among the majority group with psychosis and no evidence of personality disorder, there was evidence from reports close in time to the index violence that over 75% at that time had been acting on delusions. The proportion was rather lower for those with evidence of pre-illness conduct, emotional and personality disorders.

An instrument developed for the assessment of the impact of delusions and, in turn, the likelihood of acting on them – the Maudsley Assessment of Delusions Schedule (MADS) (Taylor *et al.*, 1994), suggested that not only may delusions exert an effect by direct impact, for example depressing or frightening the affected individual, but also the nature of the social exchanges around the delusions may be important (Wessely *et al.*, 1993; Buchanan *et al.*, 1993). People who were inclined to modify their belief on challenge were more likely to act on it, and this may be a factor in an apparent interaction between symptoms and social context, with delusions in a community, commonly a family setting, more likely to lead to serious violence than in a specialist hospital setting. In the latter, poverty of communication seems to be a stronger correlate of violence (Heads *et al*; to be published).

Among seriously violent offenders, a number of researchers have explicitly explored the possibility that hallucinations, perhaps particularly command hallucinations may render a sufferer violence prone. There is some evidence that hallucinations may add to the effect of delusions (e.g. Juninger, 1990; Swanson *et al.*, 1996; Taylor *et al.*, 1998) but little to suggest that in themselves they pose more than an occasional threat in these circumstances. Rogers *et al.* (1988) found under 6% of 385 people under evaluation for an insanity defence in Canada had acted on their voices, a proportion in turn higher than in the slightly smaller Brixton (English) pretrial series (Taylor, 1985) and the special hospital serious offender study (Taylor *et al.*, 1998). In general psychiatric hospital inpatient samples, however, perhaps where less serious violence is involved but also perhaps more persistent, there is some suggestion that hallucinations may have a more important role. Werner *et al.* (1984) noted that the best predictor of violence among a small series of male inpatients was 'hallucinatory behaviour'. Depp (1983) found that 15% of 60 assaultive inpatients had acted on hallucinated commands. Hellerstein and colleagues (1987) noted a possible confounding factor against arriving at a true estimate in an inpatient setting. In a substantial series (789 patients, 151 hallucinating, of whom one-third had command hallucinations), there was no difference between hallucinating and non-hallucinating patients in terms of self- or other-directed violence, but the hallucinating patients had been more likely to have been specially treated by staff, including episodes of seclusion and/or one-to-one nursing.

The finding that patients with thought disorder or a predominantly negative symptom presentation were both more likely to have absent or smaller social networks than other patients and to be violent in the hospital setting (Heads *et al.*, to be published) raises the probability that, within such a context, these symptom clusters may be relatively neglected in research, partly because reliability of rating is more difficult to attain. Violence in the context of a mainly negative symptom presentation may be most likely to be of a reactive kind, in response to attempts on the part of professional staff or other carers to promote routine activities of daily living. Such a pattern was described by Nilsson *et al.* (1988), albeit mainly in a sample with dementia; Bartels *et al.* (1991) reported a relationship among outpatients. People with thought disorder were rated as at rather higher risk in this latter study, but still with a fraction of the problems of people with paranoid features. Janofsky *et al.* (1988), in a voluntary inpatient sample, found a slightly increased association with violence, but in the pretrial prisoner series (Taylor, 1985) thought disorder did not distinguish violent and non-violent psychotic men. Christison *et al.* (1991) raise the possibility that there is yet another relevant group of people, with treatment-resistant schizophrenia, and with refractory impulsive aggression that is relatively autonomous from their overtly psychotic symptoms. They suggest that such behaviour is particularly likely to respond to carbamazepine (e.g. Hakola and Laulumaa, 1982; Neppe, 1983; Luchins, 1984). Also consistent with hypotheses about the importance of serotinergic function to agression, they found a double-blind trial showing that L-tryptophan significantly reduced violent ward based incidents among people with schizophrenia hospitalized after violent crimes and persistently violent even when treated with neuroleptics (Morand *et al.*, 1983).

The relationship between violent and affective disorders or symptomatology is perhaps rather less clear than that with schizophrenia. It has already been noted that action on delusions may be more likely if they have first induced affective symptoms (Buchanan *et al.*, 1983), but primary affective disorders may also carry some risk. The rarity of serious harm to others in the course of a mania is generally agreed, but it can occur (Podolsky, 1964; Schipkowensky, 1968; Häfner and Böker, 1973; Craig, 1982). If it does, then it is most likely to follow from an act of omission – such as distractibility leading to dangerous driving – rather than an act of commission, although when paranoia attends grandiosity, perhaps especially when omnipotent delusions are resolving and doubts creep in, even the latter may be possible (Taylor *et al.*, 1983). The relative rarity of depression in conjunction with homicide has been emphasized (e.g. Häfner and Böker, 1973; Taylor and

Gunn, 1984), although several researchers have observed a relationship between depression and homicide among women who kill their children (e.g. West, 1965), and Häfner and Böker confirmed that the depressive homicide group was the only one in which women outnumbered men, by a ratio of 6:1. Nihilistic delusions and delusions of catastrophe are particularly blamed in what is, in these circumstances, commonly construed as an extended suicide. Swanson et al. (1990) cited major affective disorders as having a similar numerical relationship to schizophrenia with the forms of violence reported in the Epidemiologic Catchment Area Survey. Although it is undoubtedly the case that depression is a major problem among offender samples (e.g. Gunn et al., 1991; Maden et al., 1995), the direction of any relationship with violence to others is rather less clear. The risk of harm to self, including suicide is, however, certainly high in prisons, and in Scottish and English prisons it is rising at a rate of about 6% per year (Gunn, 1997).

The evidence that alcohol and illicit, self-chosen drugs increase the risk of violence among people with mental disorder as well as among those without is gaining ground (Tiihonen and Schwartz, in press), probably partly due to a real increase in use (Mullen et al., 1999), but the nature of the relationship is less clear. It is unlikely that there is a single, homogeneous route to increased risk, and mechanisms include the possibility that such drugs may: (1) constitute a direct precipitant, through a toxic or pharmacological disinhibiting effect; (2) facilitate violence through associated social context or relations; (3) precipitate psychiatric disorder, perhaps through organic brain damage, which in turn triggers the violence; (4) increases the occurrence of crime, inclusive of violence to support the habit; and (5) the substance abuse and the violence may be linked by a common aetiology. One or more of these situations may apply to people who have an established psychotic illness, but commonly the question also arises as to whether drug taking may be precipitated by a deterioration in condition, or experimentation brought about in part by the unpleasant side effects of conventional antipsychotic medications and/or to seek oblivion from the financial and social poverty trap in which so many patients with chronic, disabling illnesses find themselves. Thus substance misuse might be merely an indicator of growing risk of aggression or violence among people with psychosis, by one or more mechanisms a factor increasing it, or both. Either way, there are grounds for some optimism that appropriate treatment may reduce violence risks. One study of clozapine in such circumstances (Buckley et al., 1994), showed that such patients who were also substance abusers did at least as well as patients who were not, and that there was little tendency to return to substances of abuse while continuing to take clozapine. A further, potentially even more important finding in terms of countering the common clinical pessimism about such a group, however, lies in the community follow-up phase of the MacArthur risk study (Steadman et al., 1998). The occurrence of violent acts significantly decreased in both the treated psychotic and non-psychotic mental disorder groups who had abused substances prior to the index hospital admission, but not in the psychotic group who had not abused drugs. Tiihonen and Schwartz (in press) extend discussion of pharmacological treatment when violence may complicate comorbid psychosis and substance misuse disorders.

Non-pharmacological management of violence and risk of violence among people with psychosis

Clinical skills in engaging and maintaining engagement with difficult or aggressive patients

Neither assessment, management nor specific treatment will be maximally effective without engagement of the patient in the process, and this can be difficult when an individual is preoccupied with the distressing symptoms of psychosis alone. With the added burden of aggressive episodes, or pervasive hostility the challenge is even greater. It may be that one of the first things with which the clinician has to cope in order to be able to make effective contact with a prospective patient is this projected aggression, which can raise, in effect, and quite rapidly, a counter transference leading to failure to explore fully the individual's needs, or to reject him or her from services. Genuinely calm, warm and positive acceptance of the individual presenting may be a first step towards diffusing progression to actual violence. Reassurance together with clear guidance on what can be done to help and to avoid harm to anyone is commonly also useful and, given that all parties in a preliminary assessment may be in a state of high arousal and preoccupation, may need repeating more than once.

Such counsel generally requires that the person or people doing the assessment themselves feel safe, so it is important that as far as possible the environment for such assessment and subsequent management has been planned appropriately. In an inpatient setting this means attention both to the physical environment and the nature of staffing (e.g. Taylor *et al.*, 1993). For community assessment, the environment is hardly if at all in the control of the assessors, who are advised always to be scrupulous about scheduling appointments, regular communication and having the means of ready communication with their base. If there is thought to be any increased risk, it is sensible to take an accompanying colleague. It may even be wise to alert the police or security agencies to be on standby in situations agreed among clinicians to be particularly worrying. Stanko (1983) stresses, however, that for all planning for the foreseen, violence can still erupt as the dynamics in a relationship change – both in the course of a single exchange or over a longer period, and consequently safety remains a matter for negotiation. In chronically violent settings, for example within abusive families, such a process may in itself become pathological, but it is perhaps worth emphasizing that clinical risk assessment and management, which can look like a neat achievable package, should be a continuous process and that skills for negotiating with patients, for safety as well as for other valued goals, are important and are likely to need specific development.

Solo work is likely to leave practitioners most vulnerable to misinterpretation of a situation, or the development of counter-transference, while team work not only allows for the ready identification of such problems, but also offers the necessary support to foster maintenance of some kind of therapeutic alliance when appropriate. An invaluable asset to the longer-term assessment and management of a potentially violent patient is dynamic psychotherapeutic input, not necessarily as treatment *per se*, but most particularly to add understanding of the risky qualities in interpersonal relationships, and to assist in the monitoring of any progress (McGauley, 1997). Team work, however, demands clear communication, and designation of leadership and locus of responsibility is imperative.

Attaining an adequate information base

It is almost a truism that assessment is incomplete without some attempt to get independent reports of a patient's state, in effect to seek to verify information. Mulvey and colleagues (1994) provided evidence for this, although they never quite resolve the question of why and when uncorroborated positive reports should necessarily be accepted. About 45% of incidents were reported only by patients – perhaps they never happened? Twenty-seven per cent were reported only by carers, perhaps these too were an overestimate? Official records, including medical records, provided grossly inadequate data about the extent of violence. It is perhaps a pointer for clinicians to improve record keeping that medical records, if used as the only source, would have identified just 9% of the 779 violent incidents under study. If positive reports are accepted as true, the patient was by far the best source, reporting 58% of incidents, but family or carers reported a further 196.

In a larger, subsequent community study, adding informants to the subject provided relatively little gain in merely counting incidents (Steadman *et al.*, 1998), although that is only one aspect of information gain in these circumstances. Notwithstanding the desirability of attempting a broader picture of people taken on as long-term cases, these figures confirm that the value of taking a full history from the patient alone should not be disregarded.

Risk assessment and management

Clinical risk, including the risk of violence, cannot be eliminated. There is a high chance, however, that it can be limited by use of a systematic assessment process, a management strategy thus informed for the individual's needs or circumstances, and a continuing monitoring cycle which results in adjustments according to any change in circumstances. The Royal College of Psychiatrists (1996) (for Britain and Ireland) has offered potentially useful, pocket guidance for a clinical approach. The general principles are set out in Table 23.1. Monahan (1993) takes a notionally more defensive approach, but one which we would also commend as of practical value (Table 23.2).

There has been considerable debate about the advantages or otherwise of an actuarial, or statistically based, approach to risk assessment rather than a clinically determined approach, but it is difficult to extract strong messages from comparison of an approach that is at least well defined – the actuarial – with one that for research purposes has not been defined at all – the clinical – although that is not to say that it is not definable. Chaiken *et al.* (1994) and Gardner *et al.* (1986a,b) make the case in favour of an actuarial approach. *Chaiken et al.* also reviewed all true prediction studies to that date. The Gardner team, however, came to this conclusion on the same data used previously to demonstrate an advantage for clinicians' assessments of men

Table 23.1 Assessment and Clinical Management of Risk to Harm to Other People (Extracts from Royal College of Psychiatrists Council Report CR53, 1996)

General principles
- Risk cannot be eliminated; it can be rigorously assessed and managed, but outcomes cannot be guaranteed.
- Risk is dynamic and may depend on circumstances which can alter over often brief time periods. Therefore, risk assessment needs a predominantely short-term time perspective and must be subject to frequent review.
- Some risks are general while other risks are more specific, with identified potential victims.
- Interventions can increase risk as well as decrease it. The interaction between the clinician and the patient is crucial in the assessment and management of risk. Good relationships make assessment easier and more accurate and may reduce risk. Risk may be increased if doctor/patient relationships are poor.
- Among people with mental disorder, factors such as age, gender and ethnicity are, in general, unreliable predictors of risk of harm to others.
- Clinicians should always try to validate information gathered from a single source with other sources.
- An adequate risk assessment can rarely be done by the person alone. Wider information is needed and it is almost always helpful to discuss the assessment and the management plan with a peer or a supervisor.
- The outcome of the assessment and the management plan must be shared with others as appropriate. Information about a patient may be passed to someone else:
  - (a) with the patient's explicit consent; or
  - (b) on a 'need to know' basis when the recipient needs the information because he will be involved with the patient's care or treatment. Where staff from more than one agency are involved, the patient needs to be told that some sharing of information is likely to be necessary, *or*
  - (c) in some cases, if the need to protect the public outweighs the duty of confidence to the patient.
- Patients who present a risk to others are likely also to be vulnerable to other forms of risk, for example self-harm, self-neglect or exploitation by others.

The clinical management of risk
General principles
Two principles underlie the management of patients who present a risk of dangerous behaviour.
- A clinician, having identified the risk of dangerous behaviour, has a responsibility to take action with a view to ensuring that risk is reduced and managed effectively.
- The management plan should change the balance between risk and safety, following the principle of negotiating safety. When seeing a patient who presents a risk of dangerous behaviour, the clinician should aim to make the patient feel safer and less distressed as a result of the interview.

---

presenting to psychiatric emergency services (Lidz *et al.*, 1993). According to this last study the greatest problem for clinicians was in the under-prediction of violence by women. Therein may lie one of the explanations for any apparent discrepancy in approaches. Clinicians almost certainly incorporate some elements of statistical applications in their approach to patients, but it is important that their information for doing so is up-to-date. The assumption that risk factors largely generated from general criminal data will apply also to people with a mental disorder is not necessarily valid. Men tend to have been studied more than women in this field, but various studies have suggested that mental disorder tends to have an equalizing effect in this respect (e.g. Steadman *et al.*, 1993; McNeil and Binder, 1995). Another major source of over-prediction of violence has been in applying ethnic minority criteria (McNeil and Binder, 1993).

Table 23.2 Principles of risk containment (Monahan, 1993)

A. Risk assessment
1 Become educated in risk assessment, stay current with developments in the field, and be conversant with the law of the jurisdiction.
2 Obtain reasonably available records of recent prior treatment and carefully review current treatment records.
3 Directly question the patient and relevant others about violent acts and ideation.
4 Communicate information and concerns about violence to the person responsible for making decisions about the patient, and make important items salient.

B. Risk management
5 For cases that raise particular concerns about violence, consider intensified treatment, incapacitation, or target-hardening.
6 For especially difficult cases, seek consultation from an experienced colleague.
7 Follow-up on lack of compliance with treatment.

C. Documentation
8 Record the source, content, and date of significant information on risk and the content, rationale, and date of all actions to prevent violence.

D. Policy
9 Develop feasible guidelines for handling risk, and subject these guidelines to clinical and legal review.
10 Educate staff in the use of guidelines and audit compliance.
11 Revise forms to prompt and document the information and activities contemplated in the guidelines.

E. Damage control
12 Discourage public statements of responsibility and tampering with the record.

Perhaps the most important point, however, in relation to clinical prediction studies in a real clinical situation, is that management to reduce the risk of violence is almost invariably introduced as a result of the prediction, i.e. intervention in order to reduce the chance of the prediction coming true. A too high level of false positive predictions of violence is the commonest criticism of clinician predictions, which would tend to support the possibility that this point may explain some apparent deficiencies in prediction.

Management strategies

If attempts to defuse or prevent violence have failed, then the essence of general management of any violence is containment. Most national jurisdictions thus allow for the possibility of removal from the community situation, if indicated, on grounds of risk to others. In practice this commonly means compulsory admission to hospital. Other legal underpinning of clinical action for safety is more variable between jurisdictions, for example in terms of what may be permitted in enforcing specific treatments.

Within hospital, the general management of continued threat of violence can only mean intensification of care in some way. This may be achieved by increasing staff supervision, perhaps by a specified frequency of observations – say, documented at a minimum of every 15 minutes, perhaps moving to continuous, one-to-one nursing care, according to the perceived threat posed. Apart from the increased attention possible under these arrangements, the provision may allow for more active management of the patient within the space available – separating them from potential antagonists, possibly allowing for escorted, supervised and supported exits from the unit, or time out within the unit.

A behavioural plan should be negotiated by the team, preferably with guidance from an expert psychologist (Corrigan *et al.*, 1993; Ball, 1994). The behavioural plan should identify cues to aggression, alternative strategies, and modifying behaviours. It should have clear, measurable, and attainable treatment goals. These should be consistently applied by all team members and across all staff shifts. The plan should be reviewed and updated frequently.

Rarely, a patient may have to be restrained physically by staff, who should have received specific training in techniques for doing so with safety. Physical restraints are almost never used in the UK, but are used sparingly in state hospitals in the USA. Seclusion, the locked isolation of a patient from others on the unit, is another measure that may occasionally prove necessary. This is regarded as an exceptionally serious step and to require explicit policies which will incorporate specified times for various kinds of review (Royal College of Psychiatrists, 1990). Whenever such extreme measures have to be applied, the underlying principles must remain those of continuing to deliver the best care and treatment possible and discontinuing the more restraining and restrictive elements as soon as possible. Lion and Soloff's injunction remains as pertinent now as in 1984:

The staff restraining the patient today will be seeking a therapeutic alliance tomorrow. The patient remains a vulnerable human being and even when it appears that there is little rapport with the patient, every effort must be made to continue talking to him or her, explaining what is happening and why and reassuring.

Pharmacological management of aggression

The relative merits of commonly used drugs in treating violence in schizophrenic patients and their place in acute versus long-term management are highlighted in Table 23.3.

Benzodiazepines

In the USA benzodiazepines are frequently used for the acute treatment of violence in schizophrenia and other conditions (Fava, 1997). However, they are rarely used alone in England. Short and intermediate-acting agents are available in tablet, liquid, and intramuscular preparations. The main drawback to the use of benzodiazepines is that they are not helpful for persistent violence, wherein long-term use may result in pharmacological tolerance, delirium, cognitive impairments, respiratory depression, and even the potential for paradoxical aggression. The same is true for barbiturates which are still occasionally used in Europe and rarely used in the USA.

Typical antipsychotics

Typical antipsychotics, particularly mid- and high-potency agents, have been another mainstay of the treatment of violence in schizophrenia. Low

Table 23.3 Pharmacological management of violence in patients with psychosis

Drug class/agent	Advantages	Disadvantages	Therapeutic indication
Benzodiazepines	Effective; rapid onset; available in tablet, liquid, and I.M. forms; clinician experience with PRN use	Common side effects (excessive sedation, unsteadiness, respiratory depression); tolerance with prolonged use; abuse potential	Only for acute violent episodes; avoid in persistent violence
Mood stabilizers			
Lithium	Effective as adjunctive. Open trials have shown efficacy alone in non-psychotic patients	Requires monitoring; delayed onset; drug–drug interactions; not for PRN use	Limited benefit in persistent violence due to psychosis
Carbamazepine or valproic acid	Effective as adjunct	Requires monitoring; delayed onset; haematological adverse effects relatively common; drug–drug interactions; not for PRN[1] use	Used as combination therapy with neuroleptics, however carbamazepine cannot be used with clozapine
Typical antipsychotics Chlorpromazine (low potency) Loxapine (mid potency) Clopenthixol (mid potency) Haloperidol (high potency) Droperidol (high potency) Thioridazine (low potency)	Proven efficacy; rapid onset of action; available in tablet, liquid, and short-acting intramuscular forms; clinician experience with PRN use; best for short-term rather than long-term use	Low potency may cause postural hypotension; high potency causes EPS[2], especially acute dystonia. NMS[3] a risk with rapid titration in agitated patients	Currently still drugs of choice for acute situations; diminished efficacy in persistent violence; also, tardive dyskinesia a risk of long-term use. Long acting depot preparations are appropriate when medication compliance is inadequate but effectiveness established
Atypical antipsychotics Clozapine	Proven efficacy for treatment refractory psychosis; proposed selective antiaggressive action	Not used as PRN; not a first-line drug; no intramuscular preparation. Requires patient motivation	Indicated for persistent violence and accompanying psychosis; should be considered early in treatment. Measuring blood levels and manage treatment essential that blood count is monitored; blood levels of drug may assist accurate prescription
Risperidone	Efficacious; available in tablet and liquid form	No intramuscular preparation; limited experience with PRN use	May have acute use role, especially since also available in liquid form; more favourable side-effect profile over typical antipsychotics in long-term use
Olanzapine	Preliminary data suggest efficacy, once daily dose	Limited experience with PRN use, no liquid or I.M. preparation	May have acute use role, more favourable side-effect profile over typical antipsychotics in long-term use
Quetiapine	Preliminary data suggest efficacy, favourable side-effect profile	No PRN experience, only available in tablet form	May have acute use role, more favourable side-effect profile over typical antipsychotics in long-term use

[1] PRN = Pro Re Nata (when required)
[2] EPS = Extra Pyramidal symptoms and signs
[3] NMS = Neuroleptic Malignant Syndrome

potency drugs are more likely to cause sedation, confusion, anticholinergic toxicity and postural hypotension. High potency drugs are more likely to cause acute extrapyramidal side effects (EPS). In some instances, mid-potency agents are preferred because they are more sedative than haloperidol. The typical antipsychotics have retained primacy in the treatment of acute violence because of their efficacy, ease of use/titration (e.g. ability to use PRN dosing; lower liability to induce hypotension) and most particularly, their availability in tablet, liquid and intramuscular forms. Haloperidol is the most commonly used drug in the USA. Loxapine is another choice available in oral and I.M. forms and it has a close homology to clozapine in receptor affinity (likely to be even more pronounced when loxapine is administered intramuscularly) (Singh *et al.*, 1996). Zuclopenthixol acetate has been reported to be more effective than haloperidol, with a more prolonged action (Baastrup *et al.*, 1993). Droperidol is another agent with rapid onset which is used most commonly for acutely agitated patients in psychiatric emergency rooms in the USA. Overall, it is presently unclear whether one drug is superior to another (Royal College of Psychiatrists, 1998). Familiarity and experience in the emergency use of one or another drug is probably the most compelling determinant of choice. While some patients may require high doses of typical antipsychotic medications, clinical observations and objective studies confirm that many schizophrenic patients receive typical antipsychotics at high doses which have limited effect and which may even (by way of inducing akathisia) aggravate violence (Krakowski *et al.*, 1993). Dosing regimens should be critically reviewed over time. The long-term use of oral typical antipsychotics in the face of persistent violence should be discouraged due to inadequate response and the risk of tardive dyskinesia (TD). However, these agents have a specific role in augmentation when an atypical antipsychotic has failed to control aggressive symptoms adequately (Mowerman and Siris, 1996). In addition, the long-acting depot intramuscular form of a typical antipsychotic should be considered when violence persists due to chronic medication non-compliance (Glazer and Kane, 1992). Depot neuroleptics are much less frequently used in the USA than in Europe. They have, however, a clear indication where violence is a risk due to uncontrolled psychosis from non-compliance. In this circumstance, an atypical drug may be added to facilitate a dose reduction of the depot neuroleptic and, thereby, to minimize the long-term risk of TD, although further research is needed on such combinations.

Atypical antipsychotics

There is accruing evidence that novel antipsychotics may be of benefit in managing violence (Buckley, 1998). Moreover, since these agents are generally better tolerated by patients and as these drugs have low or negligible rates of akathisia, violent patients may be more likely to comply with this therapy. Any transition from typical to atypical antipsychotic should be undertaken judiciously and in a gradual manner, with a long period of cross-tapering to minimize the risk of relapse (Weiden *et al.*, 1997).

Most of the available data thus far is on the efficacy of clozapine for violence in schizophrenia (for a thorough review see Glazer and Dickson, 1998). Indeed, recently published Schizophrenic Patient Outcomes Research

Team (PORT) treatment guidelines recommend clozapine therapy for schizophrenic patients with persistent violence (Lehman *et al.*, 1998). With the availability of clozapine in state facilities in the USA, patients who had been hospitalized for years because of persistent violence improved and discharge became possible. A similar pattern has been described in English high security hospitals (the Special Hospitals Treatment Resistant Schizophrenia Research Group, 1996; Dalal *et al.*, 1999). Response rates observed in several studies are highlighted in Table 23.4. The response to clozapine in seriously violent offender patients with schizophrenia who continue on clozapine is comparable to results from the general literature (Dalal *et al.*, 1999). Several studies have also suggested that clozapine possesses a specific antiaggressive effect (Volavka *et al.*, 1993; Buckley *et al.*, 1995; Rabinowitz *et al.*, 1996).

It is important to be creative and persistent when offering clozapine therapy to a patient with persistent violence. Staff may be sceptical about the value of trying clozapine in these patients because of their perceptions of efficacy (Mishara *et al.*, 1995) or of the patients' supposed likelihood of noncompliance (Swinton and Ahmed, in press). These patients are most often distrustful and they have a highly ambivalent therapeutic relationship. Patients may dismiss clozapine out of hand because of the associated blood count monitoring. Persistence, the use of videotapes, the involvement of family members in the decision making, and even enlisting the support of a patient who is doing well on clozapine are all useful approaches to gaining informed consent and patient compliance with this treatment. For violent patients, clozapine therapy should be started by overlapping with the patient's current antipsychotic medication, and the dose of clozapine treated slowly upwards. Typical maintenance doses for clozapine for these patients differ between Europe and the USA, with European doses in the range of 200–400 mg and with USA doses at a higher range of 400–600 mg.

Table 23.4 Efficacy of Clozapine for Violence in Schizophrenia

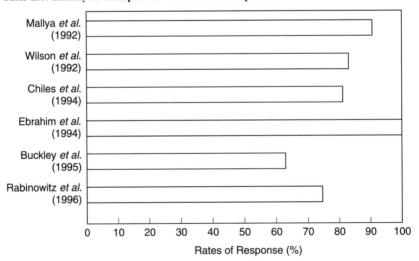

Rates of Response (%)

It is important not to undermedicate with clozapine (or any other drug), but over 600 mg the risk of induced epilepsy rises. Clozapine plasma levels can be a useful adjunct in optimizing therapy (Buckley and Schulz, 1996).

There is emerging evidence that risperidone may be another choice for treating violence in schizophrenia (the Special Hospitals Treatment Resistant Schizophrenia Research Group, 1996; Buckley, 1998). However, the effect does not appear to be as pronounced as with clozapine. Risperidone's efficacy in this regard may be best demonstrated in other conditions such as behavioural disturbance in dementia or in controlling agitation in autistic patients (Katz et al., 1999; McDougle et al., 1998). In a state hospital population, Buckley and colleagues noted that risperidone was of equal efficacy to conventional neuroleptics in ameliorating violence in patients with schizophrenia (Buckley et al., 1997). The availability of risperidone in liquid form is an advantage in the acute management of violence in schizophrenia. More experience (and clinical studies) are required on the emergency/PRN use of risperidone.

There are as yet no published data on the use of olanzapine in schizophrenic patients with persistent violence. In the USA multicentre trial, olanzapine was of similar efficacy to haloperidol in treating aggression (Beasley et al., 1998). The ease of use of olanzapine and single dosing schedule is an advantage. Like risperidone, there is insufficient experience yet with the emergency (PRN) use of this drug.

There are also no published data on the efficacy of quetiapine in patients with persistent violence. In the multicentre trials of quetiapine, a selective effect of quetiapine upon hostility (not observed with haloperidol) was reported (Hellewell et al., 1998). It is presently too early in clinical experience to determine its role in managing violence.

Zotepine, not available in the USA, has been noted to be more efficacious than either haloperidol or thiothixene in BPRS-derived measures of hostility and activation during clinical trials (Prakash and Lamb, 1998). However, more clinical experience is required with this drug in patients prone to violence in order to determine its efficacy accurately. Ziprasidone is another novel antipsychotic (see Chapter 6) which, importantly, has an intramuscular form for the management of acute agitation.

Combinations of drugs

Lithium, carbamazepine, valproate, and beta-blockers have all been proposed for augmentation strategies in patients with schizophrenia and persistent violence (Christison et al., 1991; Ratey et al., 1992; Volavka, 1995; Fava, 1997). A combination of an antipsychotic medication plus any of these drugs may be helpful for some patients with recalcitrant illness and persistent violence, with the following caveats. First, polypharmacy should be used judiciously and should not supplant the optimum use of neuroleptic monotherapy. Secondly, previous medication response and records should be reviewed thoroughly since the patient may have already failed the proposed combination therapy years ago. Third, drug–drug interactions and toxicity must be carefully monitored since additive adverse effects such as sedation can really complicate the management of violence. The practice of combined use of typical and atypical antipsychotic medications has already been noted. Gradual transitions in the medication regimen are important to avoid psychotic relapse with the emergent risk of violent behaviour. Maintenance therapy with a depot low dose antipsychotic may be required to minimize the risk of violence because of a psychotic relapse.

Concluding remarks

Research on violence and schizophrenia has moved well beyond an epidemiologically based debate as to whether this association is present or not; violence is still too broad a concept as a unitary phenomenon. Several contributory factors must be considered to explain the heightened risk of violence by people with schizophrenia; among them, the psychosis itself, the complication of substance abuse, qualities of interpersonal relationships, or lack of them. When considering medication for violence in the context of psychosis, atypical antipsychotics, especially clozapine, offer promise for more effective management of this patient group.

References

Baastrup, P.C., Albfors, U.G. and Bjerkenstedt, L. (1993). A controlled Nordil multicenter study of zuclopenthixol acetate in oil solution, haloperidol, and zuclopenthixon in the treatment of acute psychosis. *Acta Psych. Scand.*, **87**, 48–58.

Ball, G. (1994). Modifying the behavior of the violent patient. *Psych Q.*, **64**, 359–369.

Bartels, S.J., Drake, M.A. and Freeman, D.H. (1991). Characteristic hostility in schizophrenic outpatients. *Schizophrenia Bull.*, **17**, 163–171.

Beasley, C.M., Sayler, M.E., Kiesler, G.M., *et al.* (1998). The influence of pharmacotherapy on self-directed and externally-directed aggression in schizophrenia. *Schizophr. Res.*, **29**, 28.

Buchanan, A., Reed, A., Wessely, S., *et al.* (1993). Acting on delusions 2: the phenomenological correlates of acting on delusions. *Br. J. Psychiatry*, **163**, 77–82.

Buckley, P.F. (1998). The management of aggression in schizophrenia. *Schizophrenia Monitor.*, **8**, 19–22.

Buckley, P.F., Bartell, J., Donenwirth, K., *et al.* (1995). Violence and schizophrenia: clozapine as a specific antiaggressive agent. *Bull. Amer. Acad. Psychiatry Law*, **23**, 607–611.

Buckley, P.F., Ibrahim, Z.Y., Singer, B., *et al.* (1997). Aggression and schizophrenia: efficacy of risperidone. *J. Am. Acad. Psychiatry Law*, **25**, 173–181.

Buckley, P.F. and Schulz, S.C. (1996). Clozapine and risperidone: refining and extending their use. *Harvard Rev. Psychiatry*, **4**, 184–199.

Buckley, P.F., Thompson, P., Way, L., *et al.* (1994). Substance abuse among patients with treatment resistant schizophrenia: characteristics and implications for clozapine therapy. *Am. J. Psychiatry*, **151**, 385–389.

Chaiken, J., Chaiken, M. and Rhodes, W. (1994). Predicting violent behaviour and classifying violent offenders. In: *Understanding and Preventing Violence Vol. 4. Consequences and Control* (A.J. Reiss and J.A. Roth, eds), Washington, DC, National Academy Press.

Chiles, J., Davidson, P. and McBride, D. (1994). Effects of clozapine on use of seclusion and restraint in a state hospital. *Hosp. Comm. Psychiatry*, **45**, 269–271.

Christison, G.W., Kirch, D.G. and Wyatt, R.J. (1991). When symptoms persist: choosing among alternative somatic treatments for schizophrenia. *Schizophrenia Bull.*, **17**, 217–245.

Coid, B., Lewis, S.W. and Reveley, A.M. (1993). A twin study of psychosis and criminality. *Br. J. Psychiatry*, **163**, 77–83.

Corrigan, P., Youdofsky, S. and Silver, J. (1993). Pharmacologic and behavioral treatments for aggressive psychiatric inpatients. *Hosp. Comm. Psychiatry*, **44**, 125–133.

Craig, T. (1982). An epidemiologic study of problems associated with violence among psychiatric in-patients. *Am. J. Psychiatry*, **139**, 1262–1266.

Dalal, B., Larkin, E., Leese, M., *et al.* (1999). Clozapine treatment of long-standing schizophrenia and serious violence. *Crim. Behour. Men. Hlth.*, **9**, 168–178.

Depp, F.C. (1983). Assaults in a public mental hospital. In: *Assaults within Psychiatric Facilities* (J.R. Lion and W.H. Reid, eds), New York, Grune and Stratton.

Ebrahim, G.M., Gibler, B., Gacono, C.B., *et al.* 1994). Patient response to clozapine in a forensic psychiatric hospital. *Hosp. Comm. Psychiatry*, **45**, 271–273.

Fava, M. (ed.) (1997) Psychopharmacologic treatment of pathologic aggression. In: *Psychiatric Clinics of North America*. Philadelphia, W.B. Saunders, pp. 427–452.

Gardner, W., Lidz, C.W., Mulvey, E.P., *et al.* (1986a). Clinical versus actuarial predictions of violence by patients with mental illnesses. *J. Consulting Clin. Psychol.*, **64**, 602–609.

Gardner, W., Lidz, C.W., Mulvey, E.P., *et al.* (1986b). A comparison of actuarial methods for identifying repetitively violent patients with mental illnesses. *Law Hum. Behav.*, **20**, 35–48.

Glazer, W.M. and Dickson, R.A. (1998). Clozapine reduces violence and persistent aggression in schizophrenia. *J. Clin. Psychiatry*, **59**, 8–14.

Glazer, W.M. and Kane, J.M. (1992). Depot neuroleptics therapy: an underutilized treatment option. *J. Clin. Psychiatry*, **53**, 426–430.

Gunn, J. (1997). Maintaining a balanced perspective on risk. *Int. Rev. Psychiatry*, **9**, 163–165.

Gunn, J., Maden, A. and Swinton, M. (1991). Treatment needs of prisoners with psychiatric disorders. *Br. Med. J.*, **303**, pp. 338–340.

Häfner, H. and Böker, W. (1973). (translated by H. Marshall, 1992) *Crimes of Violence by Mentally Abnormal Offenders*, Cambridge, Cambridge University Press.

Hakola, H.P.A. and Laulumaa, V.A. (1982). Carbamazepine in treatment of violent schizophrenics. *Lancet*, **1**, 1358 (letter).

Heads, T.C., Leese, M., Taylor, P.J., *et al.* Schizophrenia and serious violence: an exploration of interaction between social context, symptoms and violence. Available from authors.

Hellerstein, D., Frosch, W. and Koeningsberg, H.W. (1987). The clinical significance of command hallucinations. *Am. J. Psychiatry*, **44**, 219–21.

Hellewell, J.S.E., Cameron-Hands, D. and Cantillon, M. (1998). Seroquel: evidence for efficacy in the treatment of hostility and aggression. *Schizoph. Res.*, **29**, 154–155.

Hirsch, S.R. and Barnes, T.R.E. (1996). High-dose neuroleptic therapy. *Br. J. Psychiatry*, **164**, 81–86.

Hodgins, S. (1992). Mental disorder, intellectual deficiency and crime. *Arch. Gen. Psychiatry*, **49**, 476–483.

Janofsky, J.S., Spears, S. and Newbauer, D.N. (1988). Psychiatrists' accuracy in predicting violent behavior on an inpatient unit. *Hosp. Comm. Psychiatry*, **39**, 1090–1094.

Juninger, J. (1990). Predicting compliance with command hallucinations. *Am. J. Psychiatry*, **147**, 245–247.

Katz, I.R., Jeste, D.V., Mintzer, J.E. (1999). For the Risperidone Study Group. Comparison of Risperidone and placebo for psychosis and behavioural disturbances associated with dementia: a randomized, double-blind study trial. *J. Clin. Psychiatry*, **60**, 107–115.

Krakowski, M.I., Kunz, M., Czolor, P., *et al.* (1993). Long-term high-dose neuroleptic treatment: who gets it and why? *Hosp. Comm. Psychiatry*, **44**, 640–644.

Lehman, A.F., Steinwachs, D.M. and the PORT Co-Investigators (1998). Translating research into practice: the schizophrenia PORT treatment recommendations. *Schizophr. Bull.*, **24**, 1–10.

Lidz, G.W., Mulvey, E.P. and Gardener, W. (1993). The accuracy of predictions of violence to others. *J. Am. Med. Assoc.*, **269**, 1007–1011.

Lindqvist, P. and Alleback, P. (1990) Schizophrenia and crime. A longitudinal follow-up of 644 schizophrenics in Stockholm. *Br. J. Psychiatry*, **157**, 345–350.

Link, B.G. and Stueve, A. (1994). Psychotic symptoms and the violent/illegal behavior of mental patients compared to community controls. In: *Violence and Mental Disorder. Developments in*

Risk Assessment (J. Monahan and H.J. Steadman, eds), Chicago, University of Chicago Press, pp. 137–155.

Link, B.G., Stueve, A. and Phelan, W. (1998). Psychotic symptoms and violent behaviours: probing the components of 'threat/control-override' symptoms. *Soc. Psychiatry Psychiat. Epidemid.*, **33**, S55–60.

Lion, J.R. and Saloff, P.H. (1984). Implementation of seclusion and restraint. In: *The Psychiatric Uses of Seclusion and Restraint*. (K. Tardiff, ed.), Washington DC: American Psychiatric Press.

Luchins, D.J. (1984). Carbamazepine in violent nonepileptic schizophrenics. *Psychopharmacol. Bull.*, **20**, 569–571.

Maden, T., Taylor, C.J.A., Brooke, D. *et al.* (1995). *Mental Disorder in Remand Prisoners*. London, Home Office.

Mallya, A.R., Roos, P.D. and Colgan, K.R. (1992). Restraint, seclusion and clozapine. *J. Clin. Psychiatry*, **53**, 395–397.

McDougle, C.J., Holmes, J.P., Carlson, D.C., *et al.* (1998). A double-blind placebo controlled study of risperidone in adults with autistic disorder and other pervasive developmental disorders. *Arch. Gen. Psychiatry*, **55**, 633–641.

McGauley, G. (1997). The actor, the act and the environment: forensic psychotherapy and risk. *Int. Rev. Psychiatry*, **9**, 257–264.

McNeil, D.E. and Binder, R.L. (1995). Correlates of accuracy in the assessment of psychiatric inpatients: risk of violence. *Am. J. Psychiatry*, **152**, 901–906.

Mishara, A., Orr, B. and Buckley, P.F. (1995). Staff attitudes to clozapine therapy: initial observations. *J. Psychosocial Nursing*, **33**, 44–47.

Mowerman, S. and Siris, S.G. (1996). Adjunctive loxapine in a clozapine-resistant cohort of schizophrenic patients. *Ann. Clin. Psychiatry*, **8**, 193–197.

Monahan, J. (1993). Limiting therapist exposure to *Tarasoff* liability. *Am. Psychol.*, **48**, 242–250.

Morand, C., Young, S.N. and Evin, F.R. (1983). Clinical response of aggressive schizophrenia to oral tryptophan. *Biol. Psychiatry*, **18**, 575–577.

Mullen, P.E., Burgess, P., Wallace, C., *et al.* (1999). Criminal offending in schizophrenics: the influence of community care and substance misuse. Presentation to International Forensic Mental Health Conference, Melbourne, Australia.

Mulvey, E.P., Shaw, E. and Lidz, C. (1994). Why use multiple resources in research on patient violence in the community? *Crim. Behav. Men. Hlth.*, **4**, 253–258.

Neppe, V. (1983). Carbamazepine as adjunctive treatment in non-epileptic chronic inpatients with EEG temporal lobe abnormalities. *J. Clin. Psychiatry*, **44**, 326–331.

Nilsson, K., Palmstierna, T. and Wistedt, B. (1988). Aggressive behaviour in hospitalised psychogeriatric patients. *Acta Psychiatrica Scandin.*, **78**, 172–175.

Podolsky, E. (1964). The manic murderer. *Corrective Psychiatry, J. Soc. Ther.*, **10**, 213–217.

Prakash, A. and Lamb, H.M. (1998). Zotapine: a review of its pharmacodynamic and pharmacokinetic properties and therapeutic efficacy in the management of schizophrenia. *CNS Drugs*, **9**, 153–175.

Rabinowitz, J., Avon, M. and Rosenberg, V. (1996). Effect of clozapine on physical and verbal aggression. *Schizophr. Res.*, **22**, 249–255.

Ratey, J.J., Sorgi, P., O'Driscoll, G.A., *et al.* (1992). Nadolol to treat aggression and psychiatric symptomatology in chronic psychiatric inpatients: a double-blind, placebo-controlled study. *J. Clin. Psychiatry*, **53**, 41–46.

Rogers, R., Nussbaum, D. and Gillis, R. (1988). Command hallucinations and criminality: a clinical quandary. *Bull. Am. Acad. Psychiatry Law*, **16**, 251–258.

Royal College of Psychiatrists (1990). The seclusion of psychiatric patients. *Psychiatric Bull.*, **14**, 754–756.

Royal College of Psychiatrists Special Working Party on Clinical Assessment and Management of Risk (1996). *Assessment and Clinical Management of Risk of Harm to Other People*. London, Royal College of Psychiatrists Council Report CR53.

Royal College of Psychiatrists (1998). *Management of Imminent Violence*. London, Royal College of Psychiatrists, OP41.

Schipkowensky, N. (1968). Affective disorders: cyclophrenia and murder. In: *The Mentally Abnormal Offender* (A.V.S. de Reuck and R. Porter, eds), London, CIBA, Churchill.

Singh, A.N., Barlas, C., Singh, C., *et al.* (1996). A neurochemical basis for the antipsychotic activity of Loxapine: interactions with dopamine D1, D2, D4 and serotonin 5-HT2 receptor subtypes. *J. Psychiatry Neurosci.*, **21**, 29–35.

The Special Hospitals' Treatment Resistant Schizophrenia Research Group (1996). Schizophrenia, violence, clozapine and risperidone: a review. *Br. J. Psychiatry*, **69** (Suppl. 31), 21–30.

Stanko, E.A. (1993). Everyday violence and experience of crime. In: *Violence in Society* (P.J. Taylor, ed.), London, Royal College of Physicians, pp. 169–180.

Steadman, H.J., Monahan, J., Robbins, P.C., *et al.* (1993). From dangerousness to risk assessment: implications for appropriate research strategies. In: *Mental Disorder and Crime* (S. Hodgins, ed.), Newbury Park, CA, Sage: pp. 39–62.

Steadman, H.J., Mulvey, E.P., Monahan, J., *et al.*, (1998). Violence by people discharged from acute psychiatric inpatient facilities and by others in the same neighbourhoods. *Arch. Gen. Psychiatry*, **55**, 393–401.

Swanson, J.W., Holzer, C.E., Ganju, V.K., *et al.* (1990). Violence and psychiatric disorder in the community: evidence from the Epidemilogic Catchment Area surveys. *Hosp. Comm. Psychiatry*, **41**, 761–770.

Swanson, J., Borum, R., Swartz, M., *et al.* (1996). Psychotic symptoms and disorders and the risk of violent behavior in the community. *Crim. Behav. Men. Hlth.*, **6**, 309–329.

Swinton, M. and Ahmed, A.G. (in press) Reasons for non-prescription of clozapine in treatment resistant schizophrenia. *Crim. Behav. Men. Hlth.*

Taylor, P.J. (1985). Motives for offending among violent and psychotic men. *Br. J. Psychiatry*, **147**, 491–498.

Taylor, P.J. (1993). Schizophrenia and crime: distinctive patterns in association. In: *Crime and Mental Disorder* (S. Hodgins, ed.), Newbury Park, CA, Sage Publications, pp. 63–85.

Taylor, P.J., Garety, P., Buchanan, A., *et al.* (1994). Delusions and violence. In: *Violence and Mental Disorder* (J. Monahan and H.J. Steadman, eds), Chicago, Chicago University Press, pp. 161–182.

Taylor, P.J. and Gunn, J. (1999). Homicides by people with mental illness: myth and reality. *Br. J. Psychiatry*, **174**, 9–14.

Taylor, P.J. and Gunn, J.C. (1984). Violence and psychosis. *Br. Med. J.*, **288**, 1945–1949, and **289**, 9–12.

Taylor, P.J. and Hodgins, S. (1994). Violence and psychosis: critical timings. *Crim. Behav. Men. Hlth*, **4**, 267–289.

Taylor, P.J., Leese, M., Williams, D., *et al.* (1998). Mental disorder and violence: a special (high security) hospital study. *Br. J. Psychiatry*, **172**, 218–226.

Taylor, P.J., Mahendra, B. and Gunn, J. (1983). Erotomania in males. *Psychol. Med.*, **13**, 645–650.

Tiihonen, J., Isohanni, M. Räsänen, P., *et al.* (1997). Specific major mental disorders and criminality: A 26 year prospective study of the 1996 Northern Finland Birth Cohort. *Am. J. Psychiatry*, **154**, 840–845.

Tiihonen, J. and Swartz, M.S. (in press). Pharmacological intervention for preventing violence among the mentally ill with secondary alcohol and drug use disorders.

Volavka, J. (1995). *The Neurobiology of Violence.*, Washington, DC, American Psychiatric Press.

Volavka, J., Zito, J., Vitral, J., *et al.* (1993). Clozapine effects on hostility and aggression in schizophrenia, *J. Clin. Psychopharmacol.*, **13**, 287–289.

Walker, N. and McCabe, S. (1973). *Crime and Insanity in England Vol. 2 New Solutions and New Problems*, Edinburgh, Edinburgh University Press.

Wallace, C., Mullen, P.E., Burgess, P., *et al.* (1998). Serious criminal offending and mental disorder: a case linkage study. *Br. J. Psychiatry*, **172**, 477–484.

Weiden, P., Aquila, R., Dalheim, L., *et al.* (1997). Switching antipsychotic medications. *J. Clin. Psychiatry*, **58** (Suppl. 10), 68–72.

Werner, P.D., Rose, T.L., Yesavage, J.A., *et al.* (1984). Psychiatrists' judgements of dangerousness in patients on an acute care unit. *Am. J. Psychiatry*, **141**, 263–266.

Wessely, S., Buchanan, A., Reed, A., *et al.* (1993). Acting on delusions 1: prevalence. *Br. J. Psychiatry*, **163**, 69–76.

Wessely, S., Castle, D., Douglas, A.J., *et al.* (1994). The criminal careers of incident cases of schizophrenia. *Psychol. Med.*, **24**, 483–502.

West, D.J. (1965). *Murder Followed by Suicide*. London, Heinemann.

Wilson, W.H. (1992). Clinical review of clozapine treatment in state hospital. *Hosp. Comm. Psychiatry*, **43**, 700–703.

24

Poor compliance with treatment in people with schizophrenia: causes and management

Thomas Barnes, Daniel Andrews and A. George Awad

Key points

- Redress paternalistic assumptions by placing decisions about treatment within a doctor–patient collaboration in which there is mutual respect of opinions and views.
- Use of depot preparations does not guarantee good compliance although it avoids the problem of covert non-compliance.
- Akathisia may be more of an influence on compliance when treating acute psychotic episodes than during maintenance treatment; not all dysphoria associated with antipsychotic medication can be attributed to akathisia.
- While new antipsychotics have a reduced liability for acute extrapyramidal side effects, they share many other side effects with conventional antipsychotics; hence improved EPS tolerability cannot be assumed to translate directly into substantially improved compliance in the long term.
- Necessity of continuing collaboration with attention to factors unique to each patient in terms of their experience of illness and side effects of medication, health beliefs, broader expectations and the wider impact of illness within a social context.

Introduction

Parsons (1951) described the expectation within society that the ill should comply with prescribed treatment as part of a medically sanctioned 'sick role'. Both the social recognition and privileges afforded by the sick role require the individual passively to accept treatment as prescribed by the doctor. Furthermore, to do otherwise may result in sanctions or disapproval. The values that underpin this process may have become less acceptable, and are undergoing a process of revision. This is reflected in the use of various euphemisms for compliance such as adherence or resistance to treatment, and self-care. The recently advocated model of concordance seeks to redress the paternalistic assumptions implicit in terms such as compliance by placing decisions about treatment within a doctor–patient partnership in which there is mutual respect of opinions and views (Britten, 1998). In that compliance refers to following the doctor's advice, the term may be rather narrow for psychiatric practice, which often depends upon a multidisciplinary approach and advice to the patient from different professional perspectives. Although concordance may be the more appropriate term within psychiatric practice, compliance is used in this chapter to reflect the terminology and emphasis of much of the previous literature, but without prejudice to emerging concepts.

In schizophrenia, the prevalence of non-compliance with maintenance neuroleptics has been reported in the range of 30–50% for oral and 10–15% for depot preparations (Kane and Borstein, 1985; Johnson, 1993). It is often stated that compliance in psychiatric populations is no better or worse than in other medical settings. However, following a review of previous studies of treatment compliance, Cramer and Rosenheck (1998) concluded that a mean of 58% of patients receiving antipsychotics were compliant with medication compared to 76% of patients prescribed medication for physical disorders, although in both groups the inter-individual variation in compliance behaviour was considerable. It seems plausible that clinical factors specific to schizophrenia including lack of insight, delusional beliefs, cognitive and motivational deficits, disorganization and deficits in socio-adaptive functioning would account for any greater liability towards non-compliance in this population.

Pragmatic interventions

There is evidence that compliance is adversely affected when multiple medications are prescribed or administered in frequent, divided doses (Porter, 1969). Furthermore, studies have shown that up to 60% of psychiatric patients may have difficulty in understanding simple drug labelling instructions (Boyd et al., 1974). The simplification of drug regimens, attention to patients' understanding of instructions, and the use of calendar packs and dosset boxes can all be valuable interventions. In settings where supervision is available, the use of liquid or syrup preparations, or crushed tablets in a suspension, may assist in the management of covert non-compliance.

The use of depot antipsychotic preparations has been reported to improve compliance (Crawford and Forrest, 1974). However, their main advantage is that the problem of covert non-compliance is overcome. Non-compliance is inevitably signalled by failure to attend for, or refusal to accept the injection, so appropriate action may be taken by the clinical team who will be aware that stopping medication will increase the risk of relapse and also that non-compliance can be a symptom of deterioration in the mental state. Nevertheless, the use of depot preparations in themselves does not guarantee good compliance; Curson et al. (1985) found that up to 40% of patients well established on depot showed compliance problems at some point during a follow-up period of 7 years.

The context of compliance

The system of care

It has been recognized that structural and administrative problems relating to mental health services can impact upon compliance (Dencker and Dencker, 1995), though there is little systematic research in this area.

Factors such as geographical distance to the clinic, clinic atmosphere, waiting times, opening hours, prescription costs and frequency of change in health care workers are both relevant and amenable to change. There is a need for the provisions of the system to match the needs and expectations of the patient.

Therapeutic relationships

The quality of therapeutic relationships and the attitudes and behaviour of clinicians and other professionals to whom an individual patient relates have gained increasing acceptance as determinants of compliance-related behaviour. As argued by Blackwell (1976), a clinician's own reluctance to recognize this may jeopardize effective clinical management.

Frank and Gunderson (1990) demonstrated the relevance of the quality of the therapeutic relationship in influencing compliance and showed specifically that continuity of involvement improves a therapist's capacity to effect and reinforce change. Irwin et al. (1971) identified the significant positive effects on compliance in schizophrenia when treatment was undertaken by a doctor who regarded medication as an essential part of therapy. However, there may be a negative effect on compliance if doctors fail to empathize with reasons for non-compliance or regard the patient's illness as irremediable (Weiden et al., 1991). Key factors in the doctor–patient relationship within psychiatric practice were identified by Rogers and Pilgrim (1993), and included belief in treatment, the maintenance of hope, willingness to share information, avoidance of confrontation and punishment, mutual involvement in decision making and accessibility to the patient on the patient's terms.

Corrigan et al. (1990) emphasized that working towards compliance should be a collaborative venture. The positive effect of encouraging patients to adopt the role of 'participant consumer' (Kelly et al., 1990) is reflected by the tendency of patients and their advocates to employ non-medical terms such as 'user' or 'client' to affirm self-efficacy and choice and try to establish less asymmetrical relationships with physicians and mental health services. One advantage of multidisciplinary working is that non-medical mental health professionals may be perceived as being less linked to the process of sanctioning the sick role than the doctor and therefore be in a better position to foster more equitable therapeutic relationships with patients (Bebbington, 1995).

Family interventions

Families and carers of people with schizophrenia find problems with treatment compliance among the most difficult to manage. Various studies have confirmed that compliance is positively influenced when a patient has a relative, carer or friend prepared to supervise medication (Young et al., 1986), and negatively influenced by social isolation, living alone, social deprivation and lack of employment. Although it is reasonable to presume that the health beliefs held both within and between families would impact upon compliance, systematic research in this area has not been undertaken. Mantonakis et al. (1985) have demonstrated a range of positive and negative attitudes towards medication in the families of individuals with schizophrenia. Out of several potentially relevant factors only poor general education was found to correlate significantly with negative attitudes.

Bebbington and Kuipers (1994) carried out a systematic review of studies of Expressed Emotion (EE) in the families of individual with schizophrenia and found that the proportion of patients complying with medication was similar between high and low EE families. This suggests that modification of EE alone may have little impact upon compliance and that such interventions should tackle any compliance issues directly.

The value of family involvement and psychoeducation in promoting compliance, either as a general principle or as a formal intervention, has become increasingly evident. There have been consistent reports of a strong association between good discharge planning and improvement in subsequent compliance and outcome (Bebbington, 1995) to which family involvement may well have contributed as part of a collaborative approach. Regarding more structured interventions, Falloon et al. (1985) compared the efficacy of a family based, problem solving behavioural approach with an individual, patient-oriented approach of similar intensity. Over a 2-year follow-up period, only 'family managed' patients were found to show improvements in a range of measures including treatment compliance and overall medication requirement. Similarly, Kelly et al. (1990) found that an active home-based, family psychoeducational and problem solving approach resulted in significantly improved patient compliance, more positive attitudes towards care services and lower rates of rehospitalization. An indirect effect was suggested, in that an improvement in patient attitudes towards medication was not shown.

Legal powers to enforce compliance

In England and Wales, the Mental Health Act (1983) allows for compulsory treatment, but restricted to within an inpatient setting. A similar situation exists in Canada, with the exception of the province of Saskatchewan which recently introduced provisions for compulsory community treatment. There is a continuing debate regarding the desirability and utility of such measures. In England and Wales, The Mental Health (Patients in the Community) Act 1995 makes provision for the conveyance of a patient to attend for treatment by a designated supervisor (usually a community psychiatric nurse) but not the enforcement of treatment itself. The clinical appropriateness and limitations of such a power, itself unlikely to promote compliance strategies within the community, is cogently reviewed by Eastman (1998). Bebbington (1995) points out that while patients may tolerate compulsory measures within an already established long-term therapeutic relationship, in other cases they may serve only as a temporary expedient which may alienate patients and deter future voluntary compliance.

The contribution of substance misuse

Comorbid substance misuse in patients with schizophrenia is recognized to be common, although it seems likely that the true prevalence in this population may be higher than self report by patients might indicate (McPhillips et *al.*, 1997). Consistent associations have been found between substance misuse, poor prognosis and compliance difficulties (Pristach and Smith, 1990). The 'self-medication' hypothesis may be relevant to these associations; patients may titrate their medication and illicit drugs against positive or negative symptoms, side effects or a subjective experience of dysphoria (Liddle and Barnes, 1988, Duke *et al.*, 1994; Voruganti *et al.*, 1997). Alternatively, patients who use illicit substances may be those who reject convention, or are more disorganized generally, or seek to combat the stigma of mental illness by adopting the label of 'substance abuser' (Weiden *et al.*, 1994).

Side-effects of antipsychotic medication

The adverse effects of antipsychotic drugs have been consistently reported to be associated with non-compliance (Young *et al.*, 1986), although there are exceptions (Middelboe, 1995). While the extrapyramidal syndromes such as parkinsonism, akathisia and dystonia are implicated most often as causes of non-compliance (Young *et al.*, 1986; Buchanan, 1992), non-neurological side effects such as sedation, lassitude and weight gain may occur as commonly and be responsible for a greater subjective burden in some patients (Goff and Shader, 1995; Bhavnani and Levin, 1996). The impact and tolerability of particular side effects will vary dramatically from patient to patient, depending on their nature and severity. For example, some patients find drug-related hypersalivation to be ignominious and embarrassing to a degree that is intolerable, even in cases where it might be objectively rated as mild.

Extrapyramidal side effects

Experience of the motor and mental aspects of acute extrapyramidal syndromes is generally considered to be a common reason for patients' reluctance to take antipsychotic medication. A prevailing view is that the early experience of extrapyramidal symptoms, such as bradykinesia, dystonia and the dysphoria associated with akathisia, can sensitize patients and contribute to future non-compliance (Van Putten *et al.*, 1976; Weiden *et al.*, 1986; Buchanan, 1996). For example, Van Putten (1974) showed that refusal of antipsychotic medication was associated with bradykinesia, tremor, dystonia and akathisia, with akathisia being the strongest predictor. Further, Marder *et al.* (1983) found akathisia to be a common reason for patients dropping out of high-dose antipsychotic treatment studies. Nevertheless, Awad (1993) noted that while akathisia has been linked with non-compliance in acute inpatients, Weiden *et al.* (1991) failed to find any association between compliance and akathisia in a study of schizophrenic patients followed up after discharge from hospital. Similarly, in a 2-year prospective study, Buchanan (1992) found that adverse effects, including akathisia, at the time of discharge from hospital, showed no significant relationship with compliance. These findings prompt speculation that akathisia may be more of an influence on compliance when treating acute psychotic episodes than during maintenance treatment.

The contribution of parkinsonism to poor compliance also seems equivocal (Hummer and Fleischhacker, 1996). Buchanan (1992) found a negative correlation between bradykinesia at the time of discharge from hospital and compliance with medication over the following 2 years. Further, Fleischhacker et al., (1994) failed to find any association between the development of parkinsonism during the first 4 weeks of antipsychotic treatment and subsequent compliance. The uncertain findings in this area may partly reflect that measures of parkinsonism tend to reflect rigidity and tremor rather than the subjective effects (particularly the apathy, listlessness, and possibly depressive feelings associated with the bradykinesia component of the condition) which may be more relevant to compliance in the longer term (see below). For example, Weiden et al. (1991) noted that distress relating to bradykinesia at the time of discharge from hospital was a weak correlate of contemporaneous non-compliance but a strong predictor of subsequent non-compliance.

Subjective response

Van Putten (1974) reported a subjective sensation of dysphoria occurring in some patients within 24 hours of taking oral antipsychotics. This and other early work by Van Putten and colleagues led to the idea that the subjective experience of medication might be a determinant of compliance (Van Putten et al., 1984; Awad, 1993) and prompted further work on the nature and clinical correlates of the subjective, psychological aspects of the extrapyramidal syndromes (Halstead et al., 1994; Awad and Hogan, 1994; Casey, 1995). For example, it emerged that not all dysphoria associated with antipsychotic medication can be attributed to akathisia (Goff and Shader, 1995; King et al., 1995). Further, it can be difficult to discriminate between the subjective aspects of extrapyramidal side effects and the overlapping phenomena of the 'neuroleptic-induced deficit syndrome', negative symptoms of schizophrenia and depressive features (Barnes and McPhillips, 1995). Nevertheless, a series of rating scales have been developed to measure the subjective response to antipsychotic medication: the Neuroleptic Dysphoria Scale (Van Putten and May, 1978), the Drug Attitude Inventory (DAI; Hogan and Awad, 1992; Awad et al., 1995), The Subjective Well-being on Neuroleptics (Naber et al., 1994) and the Rating of Medication Influences (Weiden et al., 1994). Studies using such scales have demonstrated a relationship between negative subjective response to antipsychotic treatment and non-compliance (Van Putten and May, 1978; Van Putten, et al., 1981; Hogan et al., 1983; Naber et al., 1994). For example, using the DAI in a sample of 150 patients with schizophrenia, Hogan et al. (1983) were able to classify patients, with 89% accuracy, as either compliant or non-compliant with medication.

The impact of the new antipsychotic drugs

A feature of all the new, so-called atypical antipsychotic drugs, is a reduced liability for acute extrapyramidal side effects. While the individual drugs available (such as amisulpride, clozapine, olanzapine, quetiapine, risperidone, sertindole, ziprasidone and zotepine) show differences in their side-effect profiles, as a group they share many other side effects seen with the conventional antipsychotic drugs, including sedation, dysphoria, sexual dysfunction, weight gain, adverse endocrine effects, autonomic and cardiovascular effects, and seizures. These side effects can contribute to the subjective side-effect burden and thus, a patient's decision whether or not to take medication. Therefore, while the lower risk of extrapyramidal symptoms with these new drugs may improve their tolerability, it cannot be assumed to translate directly into substantially improved compliance in the long term. How the conventional and new antipsychotic drugs compare on subjective response and treatment compliance is starting to be investigated (Rammsayer and Gallhofer, 1995; Franz *et al.*, 1997; Awad and Voruganti, 1999), and prospective, long-term investigations are required, in which patients are randomly allocated to optimal treatment with either a conventional or new antipsychotic.

Attitudes, beliefs and behaviour

There is increasing awareness of the contribution of lack of insight, specific delusional beliefs and individual health belief constructs in determining compliance behaviour in schizophrenia. The individual's health beliefs may represent preserved premorbid attitudes that themselves reflect social and cultural values as fashioned by that individual's experience and not necessarily attitudes distorted by psychopathology or experience of treatment. As proposed by Baldessarini (1994), the acceptance of prolonged medical treatment may, indeed, be fundamentally inconsistent with human nature.

It may be erroneous to consider insight as a unitary concept. As proposed by David (1990), insight rests on a tripartite relationship between acknowledgement of illness, appropriate attribution of abnormal mental phenomena and acceptance of the need for treatment. These components of insight as reflected in health beliefs, rather than global insight, may be significant in determining compliance. Budd *et al.* (1996) confirmed this view in a comparison of insight and health beliefs in compliant and non-compliant patients receiving depot medication. Overall assessments of insight were similar between the two groups; however, good compliers expressed stronger beliefs in the likelihood of relapse, envisaged more serious consequences of relapse and perceived greater benefits from medication. In a study of first-episode schizophrenia patients, Barnes *et al.* (1997) reported similar findings; only the 'need for treatment' variable of the Birchwood Insight Scale (Birchwood *et al.*, 1994) was significantly associated with compliance.

The Health Belief Model (Rosenstock, 1974) predicts that individuals are more likely to comply with treatment if certain conditions are met. These include the individual's perception that they are susceptible to illness, that their illness is severe, that treatment is effective and that the costs of compliance are low. It is also proposed that health behaviour is influenced by motivational cues to action. Many of the interventions to promote compliance using psychoeducation, behavioural interventions or cognitive approaches would seem to accord with this model in that they have sought to modify health beliefs or cues to action rather than effect change in global insight.

Psychoeducation

Soskis (1978) found that although inpatients with schizophrenia were considerably more knowledgeable about their medication in comparison to medical inpatients, their intention to comply with medication was significantly less. Whilst psychoeducational interventions have been shown to increase knowledge, their effect on compliance has tended to be modest and not sustained over time (Streicker *et al.*, 1986; Goldman and Quinn, 1988; Lowe *et al.*, 1995). Hornung *et al.* (1993) found improved compliance and attitudes in patients regularly attending for psychoeducational training for medication management, but the effect was not significant; patients became more cautious about medication but not more satisfied with their knowledge.

There would seem to be limitations to adopting a purely didactic approach to psychoeducation. Clary *et al.* (1992) found that over half of discharged patients who had received 'medication instruction' neither knew the name of nor the reason for their prescription. Munetz and Roth (1985) found that information regarding antipsychotics was more likely to be retained if given in the context of an informal discussion with the patient rather than in written form. Neither approach, however, was found to promote patients' retention of information deemed most relevant to decisions about treatment. The authors thus advocated the repeated presentation of relevant information within the context of an ongoing therapeutic relationship.

Given these limitations, psychoeducational interventions may need to be embraced within wider management strategies if they are to be effective (Goldstein, 1992), and perhaps draw upon patients' own concepts of illness (Tuchett, 1982).

Behavioural interventions

Strategies including environmental cues, positive reinforcement and prompting strategies to promote compliance can take various forms and there is scope for their implementation by a variety of mental health professionals and carers. Carrion *et al.* (1993) demonstrated the efficacy of prompting by clinical staff in improving compliance. Common interventions include reminders in the form of letters or telephone calls to patients (Thomas *et al.*, 1992). In the USA the efficacy of financial incentives to reward compliance in medical settings has been reported (Giuffrida and Torgerson, 1998), although the applicability of such an approach in psychiatric settings and in other cultures remains to be established.

The effective use of integrated behavioural techniques to promote compliance was described by Falloon (1984). These incorporate a behavioural analysis of non-compliance episodes and interventions tailored to the individual patient, including self-monitoring of medication, environmental cues such as diaries and calendar packs and positive reinforcement of compliance with praise. An assertive approach to non-compliance was supported in addition to the use of psychoeducation and cognitive structuring through repeated rehearsal of the rationale for medication. Boczkowski *et al.* (1985) described the implementation and efficacy of 'behavioural tailoring', an approach involving fitting the drug regimen within the daily routine and the use of a calendar as a prompt and to allow self-monitoring of compliance. At 3 months, following this approach, compliance as derived from pill counts was reported as significantly greater in comparison to that measured in controls.

Cognitive-behavioural approaches

Kemp *et al.* (Kemp and David, 1996; Kemp *et al.*, 1998) have reported the development and efficacy of 'compliance therapy' which draws on 'motivational interviewing' techniques (Miller and Rollnick, 1991). The approach involves four to six sessions of 20–60 minutes each during which the therapist focuses on the patient's conceptualization of their illness, experience of side effects, ambivalence about treatment, the role of stigma, and the benefits and drawbacks of treatment. Emphasis is placed on the value of staying well through the use of medication, which is re-framed as a freely chosen strategy to promote quality of life. The approach both depends on and fosters a high degree of collaboration and is highly compatible with the principles of concordance. In comparison to supportive counselling, patients receiving compliance therapy with intermittent 'booster' sessions were found to show significantly greater improvements in attitude to medication, insight and compliance. These benefits were maintained over a follow-up period of 18 months (Kemp *et al.*, 1998). However, 30% of those considered eligible refused to participate in the study and a further 35% became lost to follow-up. Those who dropped out of the study were found to have lower baseline levels of insight and more severe extrapyramidal side effects.

Conclusions

The published literature suggests that the behaviours, attitudes and motivations that underpin compliance with treatment are multifaceted and liable to vary over time both within and independently of illness episodes. No single factor or explanatory model is likely to account fully for compliance behaviour and, therefore, interventions fashioned according to a careful, multidimensional appraisal of the individual patient, may have a better chance of success.

Much of this chapter has focused on formal interventions that would have implications in clinical practice regarding both the availability of appropriate expertise and manpower. However, particularly in regard to the quality and nature of the therapeutic relationship, there are general principles applicable to all clinicians. These include the need for a process of continuing collaboration with attention to factors unique to each patient in terms of their experience of illness and the side effects of medication, their health beliefs, broader expectations and the wider impact of their illness within a social context. This may allow for the development of interventions responsive to the individual and a style of working with patients that reflects true concordance.

Notwithstanding the potential benefits of such an approach, the effect of most interventions appears to depend, in part, upon a baseline level of compliance or compliance promoting factors sufficient to allow engagement and change. Patients who have proved to be persistently non-compliant therefore represent a particular challenge, in that they may be less amenable to such strategies. Indeed, a central limitation of clinical studies testing interventions to improve compliance is that such patients are unlikely to have consented to participate (Bowen and Barnes, 1994), and therefore there may be limits to the generalizability of the findings to wider clinical practice.

References

Awad, A.G. (1993). Subjective response to neuroleptics in schizophrenia. *Schizophrenia Bull.*, **19**, 609–618.

Awad, A.G. and Hogan, T.P. (1994). Subjective response to neuroleptics and the quality of life: implications for treatment outcome. *Acta Psychiatrica Scand.*, **89** (Suppl. 380), 27–32.

Awad, A.G. and Voruganti, L.N.P. (1999). Neuroleptics and quality of life in Schizophrenia. In: *Quality of Life and Mental Health Care* (S. Priebe *et al.*, ed.), London, Wrightson Biomedical Publishing, pp. 19–24.

Awad, A.G., Hogan, T.P., Vorungati, L.N.P., *et al.* (1995). Patients' subjective experiences on antipsychotic medications: implications for outcome and quality of life. *Int. Clin. Psychopharmacol.*, **10** (Suppl. 3), 123–132.

Baldessarini, R. (1994). Enhancing treatment with psychotropic medicines. *Bull Menninger Clin.*, **58**, 224–241.

Barnes, T.R.E. and McPhillips, M.A. (1995). How to distinguish between the neuroleptic-induced deficit syndrome, depression and disease-related negative symptoms in schizophrenia. *Int. Clin. Psychopharmacol.*, **10** (Suppl. 3), 115–121.

Barnes, T.R.E., McPhillips, M.A., Hillier, R. *et al.* (1997). Compliance with medication in first-episode schizophrenia (abstract). *Schizophrenia Res.*, **24**, 205.

Bebbington, P.E. (1995). The content and context of compliance. *Int. J. Psychopharmacol.*, **9** (Suppl. 5), 41–50.

Bebbington, P.E. and Kuipers, L. (1994). The predictive utility of Expressed Emotion in schizophrenia: an aggregate analysis. *Psychol. Med.*, **24**, 707–718.

Bhavnani, S.M. and Levin, G.M. (1996). Antipsychotic agents: a survey of the prevalence, severity and burden of side effects. *Int. Clin. Psychopharmacol.*, **11**, 1–12.

Birchwood, M., Smith, J., Drury, V., *et al.* (1994). A self report insight scale for psychosis: reliability, validity and sensitivity to change. *Acta Psychiatrica Scand.*, **89**, 62–67.

Blackwell, B. (1976). Treatment adherence. *Br. J. Psychiatry*, **129**, 513–531.

Boczkowski, J., Zeichner, A. and DeSanto, N. (1985). Neuroleptic compliance among chronic schizophrenic out-patients: an intervention outcome report. *Consulting Clin. Psychol.*, **53**, 666–671.

Bowen, J. and Barnes, T.R.E. (1994). The clinical characteristics of schizophrenic patients consenting and not consenting to a placebo-controlled trial. *Hum. Psychopharmacol.*, **9**, 423–433.

Boyd, J.R., Covington, T.R., Stanaszek, W., *et al.* (1974). Drug defaulting II. Analysis of non-compliance patterns. *Am. J. Hosp. Pharm.*, **31**, 485–491.

Britten, N. (1998). Psychiatry, stigma and resistance. *Br. Med. J.*, **317**, 763–764.

Buchanan, A. (1992). A two-year prospective study of treatment compliance in patients with schizophrenia. *Psychol. Med.*, **22**, 787–797.

Buchanan, A. (1996). *Compliance with Treatment in Schizophrenia*, Hove, Sussex, Psychology Press.

Budd, R.J., Hughes, I.T.C. and Smith, J.A. (1996). Health beliefs and compliance with antipsychotic medication. *Br. J. Clin. Psychol.*, **35**, 393–397.

Carrion, P.G., Swann, A., Kellert-Cecil, H., *et al.* (1993). Compliance with clinic attendance by outpatients with schizophrenia. *Hosp. Comm. Psychiatry*, **44**, 764–767.

Casey, D.E. (1995). Motor and mental aspects of extrapyramidal syndromes. *Int. Clin. Psychopharmacol.*, **10** (Suppl. 3), 105–114.

Clary, C., Dever, A. and Schweizer, E. (1992). Psychiatric inpatients' knowledge about medication at hospital discharge. *Hosp. Comm. Psychiatry*, **43**, 140–144.

Corrigan, P.W., Liberman, R.P. and Engel, J.D. (1990). From non-compliance to collaboration in the treatment of schizophrenia. *Hosp. Comm. Psychiatry*, **41**, 1203–1211.

Cramer, J.A. and Rosenheck, R. (1998). Compliance with medication regimes for mental and physical disorders. *Psychiatric Serv.*, **49** (2) 196–201.

Crawford, R. and Forrest, A. (1974). Controlled trial of depot fluphenazine in out-patient schizophrenics. *Br. J. Psychiatry*, **124**, 385–391.

Curson, D.A., Barnes, T.R.E., Bamber, R.W., *et al.* (1985). Seven year follow-up study of the MRC 'Modecate' trial. *Br. J. Psychiatry*, **146**, 446–480.

David, A. (1990). Insight and psychosis. *Br. J. Psychiatry*, **156**, 798–908.

Dencker, S.J. and Dencker, K. (1995). The need for quality assurance for a better compliance and increased quality of life in chronic schizophrenic patients. *Clin. Psychopharmacol.*, **9** (Suppl. 5), 5–40.

Duke, P.J., Pantelis, C. and Barnes, T.R.E. (1994). South Westminster Schizophrenia Survey II. Alcohol use in schizophrenia: symptomatology, relationship with tardive dyskinesia, akathisia and age of onset. *Br. J. Psychiatry*, **164**, 630–636.

Eastman, N. (1998). The Mental Health (Patients in the Community) Act. A clinical analysis. *Br. J. Psychiatry*, **170**, 492–496.

Falloon, I.R.H. (1984). Developing and maintaining adherence to long term drug taking regimes. *Schizophrenia Bull.*, **10**, 412–417.

Falloon, I.R.H., Boyd, J.L., McGill, C.W., *et al.* (1985). Family management in the prevention of schizophrenia. *Arch. Gen. Psychiatry*, **42**, 887–896.

Fleischhacker, W.W., Meise, U., Gunther, V., *et al.* (1994). Compliance with antipsychotic drug treatment: influence of side effects. *Acta Psychiatrica Scand.*, **89** (Suppl. 382), 11–15.

Frank, A.F. and Gunderson, J.G. (1990). The role of the therapeutic alliance in the treatment of schizophrenia. Relationship to course and outcome. *Arch. Gen. Psychiatry*, **47**, 228–236.

Franz, M., Lis, S., Pluddemann, K., *et al.* (1997). Conventional versus atypical antipsychotics: subjective quality of life in schizophrenic patients. *Br. J. Psychiatry*, **170**, 422–425.

Giuffrida, A. and Torgerson, D.J. (1998). Should we pay the patient? Review of financial incentives to enhance patient compliance. *Br. Med. J.*, **315**, 703–707.

Goff, D.C. and Shader, R.J. (1995). Non-neurological side effects of antipsychotic agents. In: *Schizophrenia* (S.R. Hirsch and D.R. Weinberger, eds), Oxford, Blackwell Science, pp. 566–584.

Goldman, C.R. and Quinn, F.L. (1998). Effects of a patient education programme in the treatment of schizophrenia. *Hosp. Comm. Psychiatry*, **39**, 282–286.

Goldstein, M.J. (1992). Psychosocial strategies for maximising the effects of psychotropic medications for schizophrenia and mood disorder. *Psychopharmacol. Bull.*, **28**, 237–240.

Halstead, S.M., Barnes, T.R.E. and Speller, J.C. (1994). Akathisia: prevalence and associated dysphoria in an inpatient population with chronic schizophrenia. *Br. J. Psychiatry*, **164**, 177–183.

Hogan, T.P. and Awad, A.G. (1992). Subjective response to the neuroleptics and outcome in schizophrenia: a re-examination comparing two measures. *Psychol. Med.*, **22**, 347–352.

Hogan, T.P., Awad, A.G. and Eastwood, M.R. (1983). A self-report scale predictive of drug compliance in schizophrenics: reliability and discriminative ability. *Psychol. Med.*, **13**, 177–183.

Hornung, W.P., Buchkremer, G., Redbrake, M., *et al.* (1993). Patientmodifizierte medikation: wie gehen schizophrene patienten mit ihren neuroleptika um? *Nervenarzt*, **64**, 434–439.

Hummer, M. and Fleischhacker, W.W. (1996). Compliance and outcome in patients treated with antipsychotics. *CNS Drugs*, **5** (Suppl. 1), 13–20.

Irwin, D.S., Witzel, W.D. and Morgan, D.W. (1971). Phenothiazine intake and staff attitudes. *Am. J. Psychiatry*, **127**, 1631–1635.

Johnson, D.A.W. (1993). Depot neuroleptics. In: *Antipsychotic Drugs and their Side Effects* (T.R.E. Barnes, ed.), London, Academic Press, pp. 205–212.

Kane, J.M. and Borstein, M. (1985). Compliance in the long-term treatment of schizophrenia. *Psychopharmacol. Bull.*, **21**, 23–27.

Kelly, G.R., Scott, J.E. and Mamon, J. (1990). Medication compliance and health education among outpatients with chronic mental disorders. *Med. Care.*, **28**, 1181–1197.

Kemp, R. and David, A. (1996). Compliance therapy, an intervention targeting insight and treatment adherence in psychotic patients. *Behav. Cognitive Psychother.*, **24**, 331–350.

Kemp, R., Kirov, G., Everitt, B., *et al.* (1998) Randomised controlled trial of compliance therapy. *Br. J. Psychiatry*, **172**, 413–419.

King, D.J., Burke, M. and Lucas, R.A. (1995). Antipsychotic drug-induced dysphoria. *Br. J. Psychiatry*, **167**, 480–482.

Liddle, P.F. and Barnes, T.R.E. (1998). The subjective experience of deficits in schizophrenia. *Comprehensive Psychiatry*, **29**, 157–164.

Lowe, C.J., Raynor, D.K., Courtney, E.A., *et al.* (1995). Effects of self medication programme on knowledge of drugs and compliance with treatment in elderly patients. *Br. Med. J.*, **310**, 1129–1231.

Mantonakis, J., Markidis, M., Kontaxakis, V., *et al.* (1985). A scale for detection of negative attitudes towards medication among relatives of schizophrenic patients. *Acta Psychiatrica Scand.*, **71**, 186–189.

Marder, S.R., Mebane, A., Chie, C.P., *et al.* (1983). A comparison of patients who refuse and consent to neuroleptic treatment. *Am. J. Psychiatry*, **140**, 470–472.

McPhillips, M.A., Kelly, F., Barnes, T.R.E., *et al.* (1997). Detecting co-morbid substance misuse among people with schizophrenia living in the community: a study comparing the results of questionnaires with analysis of hair and urine. *Schizophrenia Res.*, **25**, 141–148.

Middelboe, T. (1995). Predictors of treatment compliance in long-term mentally ill. *Eur. Neuropsychopharmacol.*, **5**, 318.

Miller, W.R. and Rollnick, S. (1991). *Motivational Interviewing: Preparing People to Change.* New York, Guildford Press.

Munetz, M.R. and Roth, L.H. (1985). Informing patients about tardive dyskinesia. *Arch. Gen. Psychiatry*, **42**, 866–871.

Naber, D., Walther, A., Kircher, T., *et al.* (1994). Subjective effects of neuroleptics predict complianace. In: *Prediction of Neuroleptic Treatment Outcome in Schizophrenia: Concepts and Methods* (W. Gaebel and G.R. Awad, eds), Heidelberg, Springer-Verlag, pp. 111–122.

Parsons, T. (1951). Illness and the role of the physician: a sociological perspective. *Orthopsychiatry*, **21**, 452.

Porter, A.M.W. (1969). Drug defaulting in a general practice. *Br. Med. J.*, **1**, 218–222.

Pristach, C.A. and Smith, C.M. (1990). Medication compliance and substance abuse among schizophrenic patients. *Hosp. Comm. Psychiatry*, **41**, 1345–1348.

Rammsayer, T. and Gallhofer, B. (1995). Remoxipride versus haloperidol in healthy volunteers: psychometric performance and subjective tolerance profiles. *Int. Clin. Psychopharmacol.*, **10**, 31–37.

Rogers, A. and Pilgrim, D. (1993). Service users' views of psychiatric treatments. *Sociol. Hlth Illness*, **15**, 612–631.

Rosenstock, I.M. (1974). Historical origins of the health belief model. *Hlth Educ. Monogr.*, **2**, 328.

Soskis, D.A. (1978). Schizophrenic and medical in-patients as informed drug consumers. *Arch. Gen. Psychiatry*, **35**, 645–649.

Streicker, S.K., Amdur, M. and Dincin, J. (1986). Educating patients about psychiatric medications: failure to enhance compliance. *Psychosoc. Rehab. J.*, **4**, 15–28.

Tuchett, D. (1982). *Final report on the Patient Project*. London, Health Education Council.

Thomas, B.H., Ernst, C. and Ernst, K. (1992). How can one achieve compliance? On the aftercare of psychiatric patients after clinic discharge. *Nervenartz*, **63**, 442–443.

Van Putten, T. (1974). Why do schizophrenic patients refuse to take their drugs? *Arch. Gen. Psychiatry*, **31**, 67–72.

Van Putten, T. and May, P.R.A. (1978). Subjective response as a predictor of outcome in pharmacotherapy. *Arch. Gen. Psychiatry*, **35**, 477–480.

Van Putten, T., Crumpton, E. and Yale, C. (1976). Drug refusal in schizophrenia and the wish to be crazy. *Arch. Gen. Psychiatry*, **31**, 1443–1445.

Van Putten, T., May, P.R.A., Marder, S.R., *et al.* (1981). Subjective response to antipsychotic drugs. *Arch. Gen. Psychiatry*, **38**, 187–190.

Van Putten, T., May, P.R.A., Marder, S.R., *et al.* (1984). Akathisia with haloperidol and thiothixene. *Arch. Gen. Psychiatry*, **41**, 1036–1039.

Voruganti, L.P., Heslegrave, R.J. and Awad, A.G. (1997). Neuroleptic dysphoria may be the missing link between schizophrenia and substance misuse. *J. Nerv. Ment. Dis.*, **185**, 463–465.

Weiden, P.J., Shaw, E. and Mann, J.J. (1986). Causes of neuroleptic non-compliance. *Psychiatric Ann.*, **16**, 571–575.

Weiden, P.J., Dixon, L., Frances, A., *et al.* (1991). Neuroleptic non-compliance in schizophrenia. In: *Advances in Neuropsychiatry and Psychopharmacology* (C. Tamminga and S.C. Schulz, eds), New York, Raven Press, vol. 1, pp. 285–295.

Weiden, P.J., Rapkin, B., Mott, T., *et al.* (1994). Rating of Medication Influences (ROMI) scale in schizophrenia. *Schizophrenia Bull.*, **20**, 297–310.

Young, J.L., Zonana, H.V. and Shepler, L. (1986). Medication non-compliance in schizophrenia: codification and update. *Bull. Am. Acad. Psychiatric Law.*, **14**, 105–122.

25

Pharmacoeconomics and resource allocation: lessons from North America

William Glazer and Ruth Dickson

Key points

- While acquisition costs for atypical antipsychotics are clearly much higher than for typical drugs, all indications are that they pay for themselves by reducing utilization of expensive services.
- There is an uncoupling of pharmacoeconomic data and payment systems in North America which results in disjointed pharmacotherapy with atypical antipsychotics.
- There is a misalignment of incentives for single service points to use atypical antipsychotics, in spite of demonstrated savings for the system as a whole.
- An emerging risk sharing strategy may provide a more parsimonious approach to delivering high acquisition cost, high quality effective care within complex mental health systems.

Introduction

American and Canadian mental health delivery systems have experienced increases in antipsychotic drug (unit) costs since clozapine and the first line atypical antipsychotic medications were introduced to practice. This chapter will examine the responses of the care systems to these increases – both rational and irrational.

A US government contracted study (Medstat group, 1998) of the growth of mental health, alcohol and other drug abuse (MHAOD) treatment expenditures between 1986 and 1996 (Chapter 5) found that:

'Psychotropic medication use has been increasing over time, due in part to the increasing availability and application of new and older psychotropic medications. Estimates from the National Ambulatory Medical Care Survey (NAMCS) (a large nationally representative survey of ambulatory care services) indicate that the number of visits during which a psychotropic medication was prescribed increased from 32.7 million to 45.6 million from 1985 to 1994. Consistent with this growth in utilization, expenditures for retail psychotropic medications grew by 9.6 percent annually between 1986 and 1996 (from $2.4 billion in 1986).'

This measured increase of 9.6% exceeds the average increase in total expenditures of 7.2%, which is actually a decline as a share of total health spending over the last decade. While the interpretation of studies such as these is complex, it is tempting to associate the increased drug costs at least in part with the trend for a decrease in total spending for mental health care over the 10-year period, i.e. the newer, and more expensive medications have reduced spending in other areas, resulting in part in lower overall expenditures.

The magnitude of the increase in costs of the newer atypical antipsychotic agents is abundantly clear. A recent publication (*Medical Letter*, 1997) displayed a striking difference in monthly acquisition costs to the pharmacist for a 30-day supply of atypical and typical antipsychotic medications based on the average wholesale price or Health Care Financing Administration's listings in the Drug Topics Red Book 1996 and March 1997. Among the antipsychotic agents described, the generic version of the 'typical' drug haloperidol (Haldol) cost one hundredth that of the first-line 'atypical' agents olanzapine (Zyprexa) and risperidone (Risperdal).

The administrators and managers of delivery systems in both Canada and the USA are acutely aware of this increase in acquisition costs. It is common to see efforts by these delivery systems to contain or restrict access to the atypical antipsychotic medications *because* of this cost increase. Yet, at the same time, reviews of pharmacoeconomic studies of the atypical antipsychotic medications (Buckley, 1998; Fichtner *et al.*, 1998; Zito, 1998) as well as a strong letter of endorsement for use by the Director of the National Institute of Mental Health to the Director of the Federal Medicaid Program (Hyman, 1998), are indications that they pay for themselves by reducing utilization of expensive services. There is good reason to believe that the use of these medications, at least in subgroups of or possibly all schizophrenia patients and other psychotic disorders, will result in economic efficiencies when looking at the total direct costs for the illness. Nevertheless, more states and provinces are looking for means to reduce expenditures on budget lines, and it is anticipated that much more attention will be placed on the costs of the new antipsychotic medications. Why the discrepancy between the pharmacoeconomic data and the day-to-day operations of mental health care delivery systems? Why does administrative and clinical policy not reflect the science? This chapter will illustrate some of the obstacles and possible solutions to reducing and eliminating this 'disconnect'.

Why do delivery systems ignore pharmacoeconomic data?

The reasons for this uncoupling of pharmacoeconomic data and payment systems are quite complex. On a macro level, it is abundantly clear that funding patterns in US and Canadian mental health delivery systems are disorganized, fragmented and suffer from lack of a shared vision. In the USA, funding flows for serious mental illnesses vary by state, but there are patterns that can be identified. Figure 25.1 illustrates how a patient's care is typically funded within a given state.

Requisite treatments for psychotic illnesses are comprehensive and extend beyond medical services such as hospitalization, doctor visits and medication. They include housing, transportation and rehabilitation. As illustrated in the diagram, at the state level such services are covered via multiple administrative channels. For example, the Department of Corrections and the Department of Mental Health, Substance Abuse and Developmental Disability (which may be separated into three separate departments in

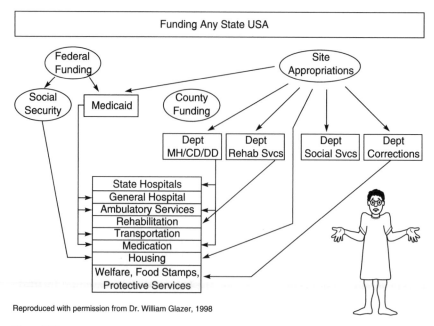

Reproduced with permission from Dr. William Glazer, 1998

Figure 25.1
Funding for the treatment of schizophrenia in 'Any State', USA

some states) fund the patient's treatment plan separately. In addition to State level funding, there is Federal level funding through Medicaid, Medicare and the Veterans' Administration. To make matters even more complicated, some states utilize county funding channels as well. In this effort, American administrators and clinicians alike operate out of the *silo mentality*, i.e. the funding of care for the seriously mentally ill is distributed in bundles or units that do not relate to each other, resulting in uncoordinated services. There are experiments with the delivery of Medicaid funded services in a number of states in the USA. These experiments are called 'managed care' and involve efforts to organize and coordinate services more efficiently, although in some cases, critics feel that the intent is simply to cut costs or, even more cynically stated, to increase profits. As of this writing, it is unclear how successful or dominant these experiments will be.

The Canadian system is less complex than the USA as each person has health insurance coverage through a national health care plan administered provincially and is therefore eligible for medical care, both inpatient and outpatient. However, the silo mentality exists as well. The federal government 'transfers' health, welfare and education funds to each province and the provinces set up services for the seriously mentally ill populations using federal, provincial and local monies. A disability plan exists for each eligible individual to cover medical, dental, and medication requirements. The funding flow for medical care has been fragmented where funding to institutions (both psychiatric and general medical) is separated from that of the community agencies. There is no national policy for medications, and the patients with schizophrenia have their medications paid as a disability benefit funded by the provincial drug plan (assuming they are eligible), separate from funds that go for hospital care or physician visits. Thus, care providers in the provinces do not see an integrated budget that reflects how a prescribed medication impacts on the population's utilization of inpatient or community services.

Here are examples to illustrate the fragmentation of service delivery and its impact on medication use in both countries.

Example 1: institutional vs community based care

In many states and in the Veterans' Administration (VA) system (until recently), the institutional budget is often separated from the community budget, and there occurs, as one prominent pharmacist in a state system put it 'a patchwork quilt effect – a tower of babble' in which it is impossible to integrate the data. For example, in institutionalized patient populations, states often have adequate data systems to track utilization and service indicators such as days hospitalized, time in restraints, use of medications, etc. But once that patient is transferred to the community, they lose this tracking capacity. Community data are fragmented. For example, the patient's physician may not be a part of the mental health centre that provides psychiatric care, and his or her vocational rehabilitation may come from yet another system of care with no links to a common data base. In the USA, medications are usually covered by Medicaid, assuming that the patient is eligible, but they may be dispensed from private pharmacies that are usually separate from any central data collection system. Under Health Care Financing Administration guidelines, if an individual is aged between 20–65 and institutionalized for 26 days or more, there is a loss of Medicaid eligibility and it takes 45–60 days to reinstate cover after the patient is discharged. The inpatient staff will discharge the patient with 2 weeks of medication, and after that, there is no resource to cover the costs until Medicaid is reinstated. Thus, fragmentation in coverage for inpatient and outpatient care is a deterrent to coordinated use of medications. There is proposed legislation to change this situation in some states where they are attempting to get 'emergent medical approval' in place to cover the break in continuity. Fortunately, in the Canadian system that is less of a problem, but gaps in medication coverage still do occur as social services determine eligibility for medication and there may be bureaucratic delays in reinstating benefits as the person moves from the hospital to the community.

It should go without saying that in such fragmented 'systems', savings from medications' impact on reduced hospitalization costs do not flow between the institution and community budgets. In fact, no party is given credit for financial savings related to reduced hospital use. While pharmacoeconomic studies demonstrate that the atypical antipsychotic medications reduce hospital days, and in so doing pay for their high costs, the management of an institution does not see this cost saving, and therefore has no financial incentive to reduce hospital days in order to fund expensive medications. The manager of the institutional budget is not rewarded or informed about the contribution his or her services makes to the total budget for the population. While there may be administrative edicts to reduce the use of expensive inpatient services, there is rarely a *financial* incentive for an institution to reduce utilization rates. In facts, in most settings, the incentives are perverse.

For example, in Canada, the service providers in general hospitals and institutions providing acute psychiatric care in areas with very limited number of acute inpatient beds that operate at full capacity may actually be penalized with increased work load. A 6-year mirror study in a Day Program in the Calgary system (Dickson, 1998) showed that hospital days decreased with clozapine treatment but the programme did not directly benefit from these savings, although time was saved with the resultant reduction in admissions. At the same time, patients discharged earlier because of more rapid improvement on the new medications, may mean that more admissions are possible, thus increasing the acuity on the wards and the amount of necessary paper work with new admissions and discharges. If the hospital uses atypical antipsychotic medication and reduces length of stay and rehospitalization rates, it is rarely in a position to reduce the number of beds in its facility and generate funds for community services for the 'discharged' patients. It is a socioeconomic and political reality that state and provincial hospitals constitute important sources of jobs and services in their communities. Elimination of these revenues hurt the economies of local communities and, additionally, the institutions often have unions that prohibit changes in jobs that would be required to enhance community services at the expense of inpatient services. It is our observation that whether in the USA or in Canada, obscuring the amount of savings realized from reduced use of inpatient services allows the state or province to apply such savings to non-health care related purposes such as building bridges, schools and roads. By keeping the exact amount of savings in one system unclear, it is easy to shift those monies to other areas of government.

In the midst of the chaos lie examples of emerging solutions. For example, the Province of Saskatchewan has been able to merge data from both the institutional, community and medication budgets for defined patient groups. This arrangement allowed researchers to conduct a mirror design study of the impact of risperidone on the direct costs for treating persons with schizophrenia (Albright *et al.*, 1996). The results suggested a savings in hospital costs when patients were treated with risperidone relative to when they had been treated previously with typical antipsychotic agents. In Illinois, the Director of the Department of Human Services (DHS) Pharmacy Services, Mr Randy Malan RPh, has worked on the integration of his Department's clinical data base. The Department of Human Services is capable of tracking patients in state run institutions, while the Department of Public Aid which, in Illinois, is managed separately from DHS, tracks charges for all medical services in the community. The result is that under usual circumstances, both groups have not been able to track patients discharged from inpatient to community-based care. To solve the problem, the two departments have begun to collaborate on tracking their shared patients. They identify patients by merging identification numbers into a shared data system, and then extracting data by time frame – a very primitive methodology. Having accomplished this step, they meet to identify issues of mutual interest, e.g. the percentage of kept first appointments in community clinics by patients discharged from state institutions. The two agencies require shared service agreements and approved changes in confidentiality procedures to allow this work to proceed. According to Mr Malan, 'If the hardware and software for patient tracking exist in the Medicaid and Mental Health systems, any state can integrate their data as long as a common desire for understanding of clinical outcomes exist in both departments'. With such obstacles to coordinating data, it is commendable that the State of Illinois is able to track outcomes of patients who move from inpatient to community-based care. Their experience demonstrates the need for substantial flexibility in clinical and administrative procedures if such goals are to be reached.

Example 2: Managed care and the atypical antipsychotic medications

Over the last 5 years, states have been experimenting with managed care options for seriously mentally ill (SMI) patients through creative programming allowed by flexible federal policy in the Medicaid programme. The approaches vary from state to state, and change rapidly as they are implemented. One popular approach is exemplified by the State of Michigan where Medicaid funds are administered by Qualified Health Plans (QHPs), which are capitated entities responsible for the physical health care of all eligible recipients, including SMI individuals. The QHPs 'carve out' capitated payments for specialty mental health services to county-sponsored community mental health services programmes (CMHSPs) that have been the traditional caretakers for this population (Figure 25.2).

Commensurate with these managed care initiatives for the SMI, states are attempting to reorganize their services to create 'smarter government' that is more responsive to the needs of the persons covered. Model programmes, such as the one that was studied in Monroe Livingston County in Upstate New York, have shown that under a 'single-source' funding model (Reed *et al.*, 1992) with centralized control of dollars, it is easier to coordinate the services that are required by the treated population. The State of Michigan is ahead of the curve in its organizational strategy for the SMI population. Planners and administrators at the state level understand that the silo mentality is ineffective in caring for persons with serious illnesses. The silo mentality sees multiple governmental entities focused on the same patient,

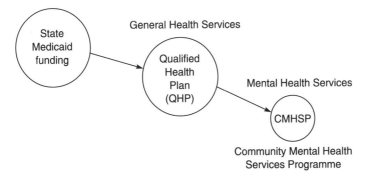

Figure 25.2
Michigan's Medicaid carve-out for psychiatric services

but in an antagonistic not synergistic fashion. In Michigan, to reduce the silo effect, they organized under one agency – the Department of Community Health – agencies that had had independent responsibility to oversee public finances reaching persons with physical, mental and specialized disability groups. The Department of Community Health oversees the Federal Medicaid Programme, the former Departments of Mental Health, Substance Abuse and Developmental Disabilities, Public Health, and the Office of Aging. In the past, a substance abusing person with schizophrenia received his mental health services from an agency that was controlled by the Department of Mental Health, his substance abuse services from an agency that was controlled by the Department of Substance Abuse, and his physical health care via an agency funded by the Department of Public Health, and the chances of coordination of his care were low. Under the reorganization plan, all of these agencies exist under one administrative roof, thus maximizing the chances that the patient will receive appropriate services in a timely fashion.

In spite of Michigan's cutting edge macro-level administrative programming, and a publically stated interest in getting atypical antipsychotic medications to the appropriate persons (Haveman, 1998), Michigan still has problems with access to these agents. In the carve-out arrangement described above, the QHPs take the financial risk for the medications prescribed by the CMHSPs. The CMHSPs are at risk for the costs of inpatient and other intensive subacute services, but not the cost of the medications. If the CMHSPs spend too much on medications, then this will disrupt the QHPs' budget and jeopardize their financial viability. A closer look at the budgetary arrangement between the QHPs and the CMHSPs illuminates this *misalignment of incentives* in more detail.

The CMHSPs, but not the QHPs, realize the savings from reducing state hospital days because this cost is in the former's budget. Similarly, under the Medicaid capitation, the CMHSPs keep up to 5% of all savings from service utilization (including community inpatient care) from their aggregate capitation payment – the QHP realizes nothing of this savings. Neither the CMHSP nor the QHP realize savings in physical health care utilization that may occur from the use of the atypical antipsychotic medications. In other words, there is no tracking of total health care costs (both medical and psychiatric) for SMI individuals, nor is there any estimation of total savings that are related to the use of the atypical antipsychotic agents. The payers for the medication (the QHP) are 'blind' to the impact of these agents on total costs for SMI illnesses and 'short-sighted' in their vision of funding services for SMI persons over time. As a result, the QHPs do not absorb or integrate the pharmacoeconomic knowledge that is emerging from studies of the atypical antipsychotic medications. A top administrator in the Michigan Department of Community Health recently commented that he was 'shocked' to see such a lack of knowledge about atypical antipsychotic medications by administrators in these QHPS who are responsible for their payment. He noted that they seemed to have a 'disdain' for these agents in a 'keep 'em on Haldol' mentality that he felt reflected the stigma of mental illness. These payers become fixated on the 'front end costs' – they become focused on the increase in acquisition costs for these agents and they are unable (or unwilling) to trace their potential offsets. A medical director for one of the CMHSPs told us that they were trying to work with the QHPS to solve this dilemma from a utilization review perspective.

In short, states lack a reimbursement system that promotes payers or providers to share financially from the efficiencies that should be realized from the atypical antipsychotic medications.

Example 3: the clinical level

Unfortunately, the dynamics described in case examples 1 and 2 are often translated to the level of the clinician-prescriber. While clinicians want to see their patients treated effectively, they are often forced to adapt to administrative realities, and in so doing, rationalize the use of cheaper antipsychotic medications as 'standard' care. Of course, rationalization breeds distorted perceptions. The first author has heard US clinicians, in informal discussions, admit that they fear prescribing the expensive antipsychotic agents because they will 'break the bank', and thus threaten the financial viability of their organization and even their own jobs. Others fear that if they reduce hospital days with these medications, they will reduce the need for the hospital and will be prescribing themselves out of a job! One psychiatrist working in a VA setting said, 'I feel that I will be fired if I write too many prescriptions for brand medications'. It is common to see a misperception between institutional and community practitioners. An institutional doctor may initiate treatment with an atypical antipsychotic agent, which is switched to a typical agent as soon as the patient reaches the outpatient clinic!

In both the Canadian and US systems, where accessibility to the new antipsychotic medications varies between provinces or agencies, attempts to restrict access to the atypicals operates in subtle ways. Canadian physicians are for the most part paid to see patients on a fee for service basis through provincial Medicare insurance plans. In provinces where some but not all of the atypical antipsychotics are considered to be second line drugs, the physician must complete burdensome forms or obtain telephone authorization through the provincial drug plan for the patient to receive the medication; this is all unbillable time for the physician and, therefore, represents a reduction in his or her income and also resented by the physicians as a 'waste of time' better spent on actually seeing patients as they are trained to do.

Recently, one of the authors (WMG) consulted to a large American HMO that was treating a large population of SMI persons. The HMO had decided to choose one of the three available atypical antipsychotic medications for its formulary. While the two excluded medications were available, the clinicians had to fill out time-consuming 'pre-certification' forms to use them. The decision to include only one of the three first-line atypicals on the formulary was not based on knowledge about the impact of these medications on total costs for the HMO. Rather, it was based on acquisition costs over the last 6 months. The decision makers had no scientific or clinical rationale to justify the exclusion of the other two agents. They had little interest in a comparative study (Tran *et al.*, 1997), which would have argued, from the most conservative interpretation, that there are important differences in the safety and efficacy profiles of these agents.

Another example at the clinical level comes from one of the author's (RAD) experience several years ago in a large hospital-based day hospital clinic specialized in treating individuals with schizophrenia. In the past, payment for patients' depot antipsychotic medications were covered by the hospital budget. This was convenient for the patients and for the nursing staff, as depot medications would be directly ordered by the programmes as medication ward stock. However, when the hospital administrators were pressed to reduce costs, this service was eliminated and all patients were required to have their prescriptions for depot medications filled at private pharmacies who then charged dispensing fees and variable but often increased dollar amounts for these medications. Thus, budgetary restraints led administrators to set a policy to help shift medication costs away from the hospital to the disability plan drug coverage, both ultimately funded by the provincial government. This change left no way to calculate the costs of private vs hospital dispensing and therefore calculating the most efficient cost effective way to deliver these drugs to the patients. While no follow-up study of this procedural change was performed, it is also possible that non-compliance increased by virtue of this change. The extra step of having to go to the pharmacy may have acted as a deterrent to some patients. While it made good budgetary sense to shift the costs for medications away from the agency's budget, it may not have made clinical sense to ask patients to undergo the necessary changes. Nursing time previously utilized for direct patient care was also wasted on ensuring the medication was obtained from the private pharmacies. It made neither clinical nor global financial sense for this change to occur, yet the hospital produced 'cost savings' on a budget line item and appeared to be saving money.

Risk sharing: an emerging solution

All three examples of coordination failures described above can be improved or solved by the application of *risk-sharing arrangements*. Risk sharing encourages a joint effort or an alignment of incentives between or among involved parties to attain health in a designated population. Risk-sharing arrangements have expanded in the general medical sector as a result of the managed care movement in the USA, but they have thus far not affected mental healthcare systems appreciably. There may be capitated reimbursement structures in place for mental health providers, but this format is limited to per member per month revenues that are usually distributed on a fee-for-service basis, e.g. the agencies or institutions are paid on a *per diem* basis, while the providers are reimbursed by salary or a negotiated fee-for-service basis. It is rare to see a provision for risk sharing based on the outcomes of care where surpluses and deficits are shared among the stakeholders. Take the three examples above. There is no risk sharing between the institution and the community agencies (example 1), the payer and the provider (example 2) or the facility and the provider (example 3). Risk sharing can promote efficient alignment of incentives among these parties.

Recently, Melek (1996) discussed methods to promote risk sharing between behavioural and medical healthcare providers to achieve medical cost offset effects. The methodology is applicable to other relationships as well, including ones that aim to achieve pharmacoeconomic efficiencies. Melek describes methods of structuring such risk-sharing programmes between mental health and medical providers:

a major task is to obtain agreement between the medical and behavioral groups on the amount of 'risk overlap' between the groups. That is, how much medical cost influence do the groups agree is attributable to the behavioral healthcare providers. For example, if the expected medical costs are projected to be $100 PM/PM and the groups agree that $10 of these costs are highly correlated with behavioral healthcare delivery, then 10% can be established as the risk overlap rate. The higher degree of behavioral healthcare delivery influence that is established, the higher the amount of risk overlap and risk sharing (both for excess funds and fund shortfalls) are structured into the arrangement.

Is it possible to apply this type of risk-sharing agreement to achieve pharmacoeconomic efficiencies? Take a drug like clozapine, the first of the atypical antipsychotic medications. Clozapine is unique in that it has an indication for a specific population of patients, i.e. the refractory or treatment-resistant schizophrenia group. While clozapine is the treatment of choice for non-responder patients as outlined by both the American and Canadian practice guidelines, there is reason to believe that in both systems it is not used as widely as it might be for this population. There are approximately 65 000 patients receiving clozapine in the USA today. If there are 2.5 million patients with psychotic illness (a very conservative estimate), then the prevalence of clozapine use is 2.6%. Most experts agree that at least 20% (another conservative estimate) of the universe of schizophrenic patients is treatment refractory. This crude estimate would suggest that only one-eighth of eligible patients are receiving the drug!

The refractory patient population is easily identified through claims that reflect service utilization/costs, or clinically via records. The patient population is of great interest to payers because they are at 'high risk' for the utilization of expensive resources such as inpatient care. In addition, clozapine carries a clinical tracking mandate. All patients receiving clozapine must get weekly/bi-monthly blood tests for signs of agranulocytosis[1]. Novartis tracks these blood tests through it's 'Clozaril National Registry' or CNR, which alerts the clinical facility when abnormal tests are found. The CNR will not allow dispensing of the drug if the patients fails to get blood tests as prescribed by the standards set by the FDA.

---

[1]One reason for the apparent underutilization of clozapine is the requirement for weekly blood samples – an inconvenience to patients, families and providers alike. A second explanation is that physicians are not comfortable prescribing the drug because of the side effects and the need for blood monitoring. Yet another explanation is the cost. Clozapine has cost considerably more than other antipsychotic medication of the typical and atypical classes. In spite of reasonable pharmacoeconomic evidence that clozapine *at least* pays for itself by reducing inpatient days, payers and delivery systems have been limited in their ability to meet the acquisition cost requirement for clozapine. In short, clozapine is a relatively expensive drug that is tracked closely and used in a defined population of patients that interests payers because they are potential higher utilizers of clinical services. These characteristics make clozapine a likely candidate for risk sharing.

In Canada there are examples of risk sharing in several areas. Novartis offers a reimbursement programme if the patients do not stay on clozapine for 6 months. However, with the absence of any alignments in incentives among the prescribing physician, the hospital pharmacies and the provincial drug payment system for persons with disabilities, this had had little impact on physician's willingness to initiate clozapine treatment. This manufacturer has also funded nursing positions to facilitate the start ups of clozapine clinics. Unfortunately there is no mechanism in place to pass cost savings accrued secondary to reduced inpatient hospitalizations to these outpatient clinics.

In both the USA and Canada, 'sampling' medication is a form of risk sharing traditionally/historically offered by the pharmaceutical companies. For example, companies such as Janssen, Lilly and Zeneca will give free medications to bridge the gap between the hospital and community care when Medicaid benefits for the patient are restored. They will also provide samples for 'indigent' patients who, presumably, will obtain benefits once stabilized. In Canada, quetiapine was approved by the Health Protection Branch in January, 1998 but not approved by the Alberta provincial formulary until October, 1998. During that interlude, Zeneca took the risk of providing drug for patients until approval so that when payment became available, there were already patients on the drug.

One of the authors (WMG) is consulting with Novartis and state systems that are interested in developing a risk-sharing contract for Clozaril (brand form of clozapine). Novartis is interested in developing such a model in the USA because it is facing generic competition and is interested in maintaining its current book of business. The creation of a risk-sharing model would insure long-term contracts with its customers. To develop the risk-sharing model[2], the pharmacoeconomic studies of clozapine need to be considered. Two of the most useful studies are prospective and randomized comparisons of clozapine to standard 'typical' antipsychotic medications.

The first study, by Essock et al. (1996a) from the State of Connecticut, screened some 1300 long-term inpatients from the state hospitals for clozapine eligibility on a given day. They found that 60% of the population met criteria for treatment resistance, and they conducted a trial of clozapine vs. usual care, i.e. typical antipsychotics, in 227 of these patients who volunteered to be randomized (Essock et al., 1996b). The authors found that discharge rates did not differ, but once discharged, patients on clozapine were less likely to be readmitted. More recently, the authors have reported in meetings that overall direct costs for the two groups were relatively equal, i.e. clozapine's expensive cost was offset by its ability to reduce inpatient utilization. However, the authors point out a reality that all states must face: to make clozapine available to all eligible patients, the State of Connecticut must invest approximately $140 million in order to give patients hospitalized on a single day a year's access to clozapine.

The second study by Rosenheck et al. (1997) from 15 Veterans Administration Medical Centers, compared clozapine to haloperidol in a

[2]This model was developed with Mr Dennis Dionne, CNS Marketing Director, Novartis Pharmaceuticals and Mr Michael Kenyon, Principle, Phildius, Kenyon & Scott.

random assignment, double-blind design over a 1-year period. The study found that clozapine-treated patients had higher treatment retention rates, greater symptomatic improvement, fewer extrapyramidal side effects, comparable quality of life ratings and $2441 per patient per year lower total health care costs (not statistically significant). Presumably, this lack of statistical significance resulted because of the small number of patients studied in the fact of tremendous variability of costs that were found across the medical centres participating in the study. A study of a larger patient sample would probably yield statistically significant results. But in the absence of such an investigation, it is most prudent to conclude that this study demonstrates that clozapine's high acquisition cost is offset by its ability to reduce expensive service utilization.

A model for risk sharing

How might these data apply to a risk-sharing agreement between the manufacturer of clozapine and a State? The key issue is the degree to which the two parties share responsibility for the cost of the drug. They must agree on the amount of *risk overlap* – the degree to which total direct costs are influenced by the medication. To determine the risk overlap, the seller and buyer must define the population that will be treated. For example, since the cost savings related to clozapine appear to occur in the high-risk, high utilizer population, which uses hospital level care frequently, an approach would be to define a costly patient population, perhaps those patients who have cost over $20 000 or more in inpatient days over the last year. Now assume further that clozapine would reduce these costs in this population on average by 15%[3]. The manufacturer of clozapine agrees to take a risk by selling the drug to the State for less, e.g. a negotiated amount well below the usual cost. Both parties agree that if the drug 'does its job' and achieves some, all or more than the 15% cost savings in a defined time period, e.g. a year, then the State will share the savings by paying up to (or more than) the full cost of the drug, consistent with the degree of savings measured.

In order for a risk-sharing agreement such as this to occur, the State must be able to track the cost and utilization outcomes in the defined population. Ideally, tracking can occur though the use of claims data *and* the findings from the Clozaril National Registry (see above). It is possible to merge data from the state and the CNR provided patient confidentiality is protected. Such a merger would allow the state to track compliance more accurately, since the attainment of blood tests regularly is a reasonable proxy for medication compliance. Another important consideration in outcome measurement is the time frame. The time frame for this risk-sharing agreement should extend beyond a year, because outcome research on schizophrenia has found that once a high utilizer patient is stabilized in the first year of

[3]In the VA collaborative study (Rosenheck *et al.*, 1997), the clozapine-treated patients experienced 24.3 fewer psychiatric inpatient days than the haloperidol-treated patients. This reduction constituted a 14% reduction in utilization, which translated to a 15.8% reduction in costs. Of course, the actual percentage of savings attributable to the use of clozapine would have to be estimated carefully, depending on the population and the total number of clinical and economic parameters under consideration.

treatment, even greater savings may be appreciated in the second year. Unfortunately, there are no data available to help estimate how much these savings would be in the risk-sharing agreement under discussion.

Assuming that a risk-sharing agreement can be reached, the state will need to educate the clinicians about the opportunity in order to align them with the overall goals. A risk-sharing agreement at the department level cannot and should not dictate prescribing decisions at the clinical level. On the other hand, many clinicians might change their attitudes about prescribing clozapine if they understood that: (1) their leadership had solved the acquisition cost problem that had been related to this medication; and (2) savings resulting from the use of clozapine would be directed back to clinical programmes. If clinical programmes are in a position to apply savings from the use of a drug like clozapine to improving patient services, then there is an incentive in place that would probably encourage greater use of the drug. The problem is that most States do not yet have the luxury of applying their savings to their own services (see the discussion about the silo mentality above).

In the absence of administrative clarity, a strategy would be to operationalize the definition of treatment refractoriness for the clinicians. For example, a patient with a psychotic diagnosis who has been chronically hospitalized for a defined number of days or who has exhibited a revolving door pattern of admissions, e.g. three admissions in one year, and who has been treated with adequate doses of two antipsychotic agents should be a candidate for clozapine. This definition could be taught across the State and implemented in drug utilization reviews. Another strategy would be to provide physicians with consulting pharmacists or psychiatrists to educate clinicians who have not had experience prescribing the drug. In the future, clinicians will be motivated to prescribe medications that save money and do not jeopardize quality of care, if these savings can be used to strengthen programming to treat patients more effectively.

It is probable that this risk-sharing model is too complex for many state systems. While a State is able to identify eligible patients for a risk-sharing agreement, it may be unequipped to track what happens to them clinically or financially because the data collection systems are fragmented. There are many ways to tailor a risk-sharing agreement to work with existing administrative and clinical procedures in a given setting.

Other examples of risk sharing

Consider the State of Michigan described above in example 2. An immediate strategy for the problem of access to atypical antipsychotic medications in Michigan is to make these health issues community issues and require the same collaboration at the local level that is occurring at the state level. Incentives need to be extended to the QHP and the CMHSPs to identify their 'risk overlap' related to these medications, track their use and identify total cost savings that will benefit both parties. In the case of Michigan, the risk overlap is how much the atypicals use influences the psychiatric-related costs for SMI individuals within the CMHSPs and the physical health care costs for SMI clients in the QHPs. In the case of clozapine, the studies cited above suggest that at a minimum, clozapine pays for itself by reducing expensive service utilization. If this is true, then the CMHSPs could share the savings from reduced service utilization with the QHP by reimbursing them for the cost of the clozapine. Of course, such arrangements could be developed for all atypical antipsychotic medications, not just clozapine. Pharmaceutical companies could join such a risk-sharing agreement in a manner similar to the example cited above from Illinois.

Conclusions

Risk-sharing models will be the rule rather than the exception within the next decade. Mental health care delivery systems are only beginning to understand how treatments such as the atypical antipsychotic medications impact on the total costs of care for psychotic disorders like schizophrenia. As these systems improve in their ability to track longitudinally clinical and cost outcomes within defined patient populations, they will become naturally motivated to achieve efficiencies, without jeopardizing quality of care, via the alignment of both financial and clinical incentives among the various stakeholders.

References

Albright, P.S., Livingstone, S., Keegan, D.L., et al. (1996). Reduction of healthcare resource utilization and costs following the use of risperidone for patients with schizophrenia previously treated with antipsychotic therapy: a retrospective analysis using the Saskatchewan Health linkable databases. Clin. Drug. Invest., 11, 289–299.

Buckley, P.F. (1998). Treatment of schizophrenia: let's talk dollars and sense. Am. J. Managed Care, 4, 369–383.

Dickson, R.A. (1998). Hospital days in clozapine-treated patients. Can. J. Psychiatry, 43, 945–948.

Essock, S.M., Hargreaves, W.A., Dohm, F.A., et al. (1996a). Clozapine eligibility among State Hospital Patients. Schizophrenia Bull., 22, 15–25.

Essock, S.M., Hargreaves, W.A., Vovell, N.H., et al. (1996b). Clozapine's effectiveness for patients in state hospitals: results from a randomized trial. Psychopharmacol. Bull., 32, 683–697.

Fichtner, C.G., Hanrahan, P. and Luchins, D.J. (1998). Pharmacoeconomic studies of atypical antipsychotics: review and perspective. Psychiatric Ann., 28, 381–396.

Haveman, J.K. (1998). Access to atypical antipsychotics: a public payor's perspective. Behav. Hlth Care Tomorrow, 7, 45–48.

Hyman, S.E. (1998). Letter to Ms Sally K. Richardson, Director, Center for Medicaid and State Operations, January 16.

Medical Letter (1997). 39, 38.

Medstat Group for Substance Abuse and Mental Health Services Administration (SAMSHA) (1998). DHS Contract no. 270-96-007, Joan Dilonardo, Project Officer.

Melek, S.P. (1996). Behavioral healthcare risk-sharing and medical cost offsets, Milliman & Robertson, Inc. Research Reports.

Reed, S., Hennesy, K., Brown, S.W., et al., (1992). Capitation from a provider's perspective. Hosp. & Comm. Psych., 43, (12), 1173–1175.

Rosenheck, R., Thomas, J., Henderson, W., et al. (1997). A comparison of clozapine and haloperidol in hospitalized patients with refractory schizophrenia. N. Engl. J. Med., 337, 809–815.

Tran, P.V., Hamilton, S.H., Kuntz, A.J., *et al.* (1997). Double-blind comparison of olanzapine versus risperidone in the treatment of schizophrenia and other psychotic disorders. *J. Clin. Psychopharmacol.*, **17**, 407–418.

Zito, J.M. (1998). Pharmacoeconomics of the new antipsychotics for the treatment of schizophrenia. *Psychiatric Clin. N. Am.*, **21**, 181–202.

Index